Nutrition, Diet and Healthy Aging

Nutrition, Diet and Healthy Aging

Editors

Emiliana Giacomello
Luana Toniolo

MDPI • Basel • Beijing • Wuhan • Barcelona • Belgrade • Manchester • Tokyo • Cluj • Tianjin

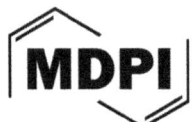

Editors
Emiliana Giacomello
University of Trieste
Italy

Luana Toniolo
University of Padova
Italy

Editorial Office
MDPI
St. Alban-Anlage 66
4052 Basel, Switzerland

This is a reprint of articles from the Special Issue published online in the open access journal *Nutrients* (ISSN 2072-6643) (available at: https://www.mdpi.com/journal/nutrients/special_issues/nutrition_diet_and_healthy_aging).

For citation purposes, cite each article independently as indicated on the article page online and as indicated below:

LastName, A.A.; LastName, B.B.; LastName, C.C. Article Title. *Journal Name* **Year**, *Volume Number*, Page Range.

ISBN 978-3-0365-4841-8 (Hbk)
ISBN 978-3-0365-4842-5 (PDF)

© 2022 by the authors. Articles in this book are Open Access and distributed under the Creative Commons Attribution (CC BY) license, which allows users to download, copy and build upon published articles, as long as the author and publisher are properly credited, which ensures maximum dissemination and a wider impact of our publications.

The book as a whole is distributed by MDPI under the terms and conditions of the Creative Commons license CC BY-NC-ND.

Contents

About the Editors vii

Emiliana Giacomello and Luana Toniolo
Nutrition, Diet and Healthy Aging
Reprinted from: *Nutrients* **2021**, *14*, 190, doi:10.3390/nu14010190 1

Nurul Izzati Mohd Suffian, Siti Nur 'Asyura Adznam, Hazizi Abu Saad, Yoke Mun Chan, Zuriati Ibrahim, Noraida Omar and Muhammad Faizal Murat
Frailty Intervention through Nutrition Education and Exercise (FINE). A Health Promotion Intervention to Prevent Frailty and Improve Frailty Status among Pre-Frail Elderly—A Study Protocol of a Cluster Randomized Controlled Trial
Reprinted from: *Nutrients* **2020**, *12*, 2758, doi:10.3390/nu12092758 5

Arnold Markovics, Attila Biró, Andrea Kun-Nemes, Mónika Éva Fazekas, Anna Anita Rácz, Melinda Paholcsek, János Lukács, László Stündl and Judit Remenyik
Effect of Anthocyanin-Rich Extract of Sour Cherry for Hyperglycemia-Induced Inflammatory Response and Impaired Endothelium-Dependent Vasodilation
Reprinted from: *Nutrients* **2020**, *12*, 3373, doi:10.3390/nu12113373 17

Qinran Liu, Jianjun Guo, Liang Hu, Nicola Veronese, Lee Smith, Lin Yang and Chao Cao
Association between Intake of Energy and Macronutrients and Memory Impairment Severity in US Older Adults, National Health and Nutrition Examination Survey 2011–2014
Reprinted from: *Nutrients* **2020**, *12*, 3559, doi:10.3390/nu12113559 31

Maha Hussain Alhussain, Shaea Alkahtani, Osama Aljuhani and Syed Shahid Habib
Effects of Nutrient Intake on Diagnostic Measures of Sarcopenia among Arab Men: A Cross-Sectional Study
Reprinted from: *Nutrients* **2020**, *13*, 114, doi:10.3390/nu13010114 45

Jinhee Kim, Yunhwan Lee, Chang Won Won, Mi Kyung Kim, Seunghee Kye, Jee-Seon Shim, Seungkook Ki and Ji-hye Yun
Dietary Patterns and Frailty in Older Korean Adults: Results from the Korean Frailty and Aging Cohort Study
Reprinted from: *Nutrients* **2021**, *13*, 601, doi:10.3390/nu13020601 59

Toshiko Tanaka, Sameera A. Talegawkar, Yichen Jin, Stephania Bandinelli and Luigi Ferrucci
Association of Adherence to the Mediterranean-Style Diet with Lower Frailty Index in Older Adults
Reprinted from: *Nutrients* **2021**, *13*, 1129, doi:10.3390/nu13041129 69

Ana Moradell, Ángel Iván Fernández-García, David Navarrete-Villanueva, Lucía Sagarra-Romero, Eva Gesteiro, Jorge Pérez-Gómez, Irene Rodríguez-Gómez, Ignacio Ara, Jose A. Casajús, Germán Vicente-Rodríguez and Alba Gómez-Cabello
Functional Frailty, Dietary Intake, and Risk of Malnutrition. Are Nutrients Involved in Muscle Synthesis the Key for Frailty Prevention?
Reprinted from: *Nutrients* **2021**, *13*, 1231, doi:10.3390/nu13041231 79

Chwan-Li Shen, Sivapriya Ramamoorthy, Gurvinder Kaur, Jannette M. Dufour, Rui Wang, Huanbiao Mo and Bruce A. Watkins
Dietary Annatto-Extracted Tocotrienol Reduces Inflammation and Oxidative Stress, and Improves Macronutrient Metabolism in Obese Mice: A Metabolic Profiling Study
Reprinted from: *Nutrients* **2021**, *13*, 1267, doi:10.3390/nu13041267 93

Qiumin Huang, Xiaofang Jia, Jiguo Zhang, Feifei Huang, Huijun Wang, Bing Zhang,
Liusen Wang, Hongru Jiang and Zhihong Wang
Diet–Cognition Associations Differ in Mild Cognitive Impairment Subtypes
Reprinted from: *Nutrients* **2021**, *13*, 1341, doi:10.3390/nu13041341 113

Larry A. Tucker
Fruit and Vegetable Intake and Telomere Length in a Random Sample of 5448 U.S. Adults
Reprinted from: *Nutrients* **2021**, *13*, 1415, doi:10.3390/nu13051415 129

Dominika Jamioł-Milc, Jowita Biernawska, Magdalena Liput, Laura Stachowska
and Zdzisław Domiszewski
Seafood Intake as a Method of Non-Communicable Diseases (NCD) Prevention in Adults
Reprinted from: *Nutrients* **2021**, *13*, 1422, doi:10.3390/nu13051422 147

Jaqueline C. Avila, Rafael Samper-Ternent and Rebeca Wong
Malnutrition Risk among Older Mexican Adults in the Mexican Health and Aging Study
Reprinted from: *Nutrients* **2021**, *13*, 1615, doi:10.3390/nu13051615 165

Jian Zhang and Ai Zhao
Dietary Diversity and Healthy Aging: A Prospective Study
Reprinted from: *Nutrients* **2021**, *13*, 1787, doi:10.3390/nu13061787 175

Marina Martín, Amaia Rodríguez, Javier Gómez-Ambrosi, Beatriz Ramírez, Sara Becerril,
Victoria Catalán, Miguel López, Carlos Diéguez, Gema Frühbeck and María A. Burrell
Caloric Restriction Prevents Metabolic Dysfunction and the Changes in Hypothalamic
Neuropeptides Associated with Obesity Independently of Dietary Fat Content in Rats
Reprinted from: *Nutrients* **2021**, *13*, 2128, doi:10.3390/nu13072128 191

Emiliana Giacomello and Luana Toniolo
The Potential of Calorie Restriction and Calorie Restriction Mimetics in Delaying Aging: Focus
on Experimental Models
Reprinted from: *Nutrients* **2021**, *13*, 2346, doi:10.3390/nu13072346 205

Nikolina Jukic Peladic, Giuseppina Dell'Aquila, Barbara Carrieri, Marcello Maggio,
Antonio Cherubini and Paolo Orlandoni
Potential Role of Probiotics for Inflammaging: A Narrative Review
Reprinted from: *Nutrients* **2021**, *13*, 2919, doi:10.3390/nu13092919 221

Won Jang, Yoonjin Shin and Yangha Kim
Dietary Pattern Accompanied with a High Food Variety Score Is Negatively Associated with
Frailty in Older Adults
Reprinted from: *Nutrients* **2021**, *13*, 3164, doi:10.3390/nu13093164 231

Katherine Marie Ottolini, Elizabeth Vinson Schulz, Catherine Limperopoulos
and Nickie Andescavage
Using Nature to Nurture: Breast Milk Analysis and Fortification t o I mprove G rowth and
Neurodevelopmental Outcomes in Preterm Infants
Reprinted from: *Nutrients* **2021**, *13*, 4307, doi:10.3390/nu13124307 243

About the Editors

Emiliana Giacomello

Emiliana Giacomello works as an Assistant Professor at the Department of Medicine, Surgery and Health at the University of Trieste. Her main interests are focused on the study of skeletal muscle plasticity in the differentiation and development of different physiological conditions, such as ageing. In this context, her most recent research centered on the study of the diet and calorie restriction mimetics in ageing animal models. Her research encompasses in vitro and vivo studies, which include cell culture, animal models and human tissues. She specializes in the characterization of the skeletal muscle cells using histomorphology methodologies. She has expertise in the application of conventional and confocal fluorescence microscopy, which allows for collaboration with multiple groups to share and implement the obtained knowledge. In parallel to her research activity, she fulfills her didactic commitments in the courses of Medicine and Surgery and Technical Health Professions.

Luana Toniolo

Luana Toniolo is a university researcher and works as an Assistant Professor in the muscle physiology and biophysics laboratory of the Department of Biomedical Sciences as a member of the "Muscle Contractility and Plasticity" research group. The research activity is centered on muscle physiology, particularly the cellular and molecular aspects of the diversity between skeletal muscle fibers. She specializes in the preparation and manipulation of single-skinned cells and ex vivo muscle preparations for the study of the physiological characteristics of mammalian skeletal muscle. She is interested in various problems related to muscle tissue, particularly the physiological responses of skeletal muscle and its adaptations to stimuli such as training, immobilization, denervation or physiological changes such as aging. Alongside her research activity, she has various didactic commitments. Her teaching activities were mainly carried out in the context of her degree in Medicine and Surgery. Since 2011 she has been a member of the Italian Society of Physiology.

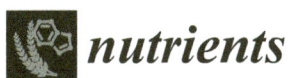

Editorial

Nutrition, Diet and Healthy Aging

Emiliana Giacomello [1,*] and Luana Toniolo [2,*]

[1] Department of Medicine, Surgery and Health Sciences, University of Trieste, 34149 Trieste, Italy
[2] Laboratory of Muscle Biophysics, Department of Biomedical Sciences, University of Padova, 35131 Padova, Italy
* Correspondence: egiacomello@units.it (E.G.); luana.toniolo@unipd.it (L.T.)

Citation: Giacomello, E.; Toniolo, L. Nutrition, Diet and Healthy Aging. *Nutrients* **2022**, *14*, 190. https://doi.org/10.3390/nu14010190

Received: 22 December 2021
Accepted: 29 December 2021
Published: 31 December 2021

Publisher's Note: MDPI stays neutral with regard to jurisdictional claims in published maps and institutional affiliations.

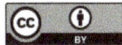

Copyright: © 2021 by the authors. Licensee MDPI, Basel, Switzerland. This article is an open access article distributed under the terms and conditions of the Creative Commons Attribution (CC BY) license (https://creativecommons.org/licenses/by/4.0/).

The current increase in life expectancy is confirmed by data from different sources (i.e., The World Population Prospects 2019 issued by the United Nations; https://population.un.org/wpp/ (accessed on 20 December 2021)), which predict that, in the near future, individuals who are over 65 and over 80 will be the fastest-growing portion of the population.

Although the increase in lifespan is a positive effect of the world's improved sanitary, nutritional, and socioeconomic conditions, it is not free of complications. Actually, this improved lifespan is associated with an intensification of chronic diseases, such as cardiovascular disease, diabetes, cancer, sarcopenia, and degenerative disorders, which are grouped into what are called non-communicable diseases.

Aging is determined by the functional alteration of cell- and organ-related mechanisms that contribute to the functional decline of the individual. These alterations converge to a complex condition called frailty, where the individual experiences a loss of physical and psychological abilities, leading to a state of increased risk for adverse health outcomes in several pathologies.

At present, the frailty index is a clinically evaluated method that can be used to assess the quality of aging, which depends on the individual's exposition to different physical activities, nutritional regimens, and other socioeconomic characteristics. Therefore, frailty results in a modifiable condition that can be improved with affordable adjustments in lifestyle, such as following a nutritional regimen that meets the needs of aged people.

The aim of this Special Issue titled "Nutrition and Healthy Ageing" is to provide an overview on the connection between nutrition and aging, update knowledge on the mechanisms that are responsible for aging, and report on nutritional strategies that can be implemented to overcome age-related diseases.

This Special Issue collects 14 research articles and 4 reviews that span from studies in the population to basic research on experimental models. Overall, the collection touches themes such as dietary diversity, calorie restriction regimens, physical exercise, antiaging agents, social issues, and strategies to promote healthy aging. Attesting to the widespread interest in the correlation between nutrition and healthy aging, the current issue reports data on the correlation between diet and healthy aging from China, Italy, Korea, Malaysia, Mexico, Saudi Arabia, Spain, and the United States of America.

The most marked message that emerges from this collection is the correlation between the frailty index and dietary diversity. Studies from different countries with very diverse nutritional habits show that aged individuals with a good diet variety score present a better frailty index [1–10]. Evidently, due to the diverse geographical origin of the data, it is difficult to infer what the best diet to avoid or to postpone the occurrence of frailty is. Moreover, as determined by the study of Avila and collaborators [11], other socioeconomic factors can increase the risk of malnutrition and can negatively influence the health status of aging people.

The maintenance of mental capacities is one important factor that characterizes healthy aging. As raised by work from Liu and collaborators [7] from and Zhang [2] and collaborators, the psychological conditions of aged people could also be correlated with dietary variety, and a high intake of carbohydrates and fat could be associated with memory impairment.

Although we are far from identifying an ideal diet for a healthy aging, it can be summarized that adherence to Mediterranean diet for Europeans [5], the use of a balanced diet rich in vegetables in U.S. [3], and the general balanced equilibrium of vegetables, oil, fish, and meat in the diet seems to have a major role in maintaining a lower frailty index and in the prevention of the non-communicable diseases.

The fact that aging is a multifaceted phenomenon that results from one or more failures at the molecular, cellular, physiologic, and functional levels, makes age-related diseases challenging therapeutic targets. Moreover, studies on aging and antiaging agents in humans can be difficult and can provide heterogeneous results due to the above-mentioned sanitary, geographical, and socioeconomic characteristics. In this issue, an example is provided by the review of Peladic and collaborators [12], which analyzes the literature on the role of probiotics on the modulation of inflammaging. The authors report heterogeneous evidence and come to the conclusion that probiotics have a limited effect on the modulation of low-grade inflammatory conditions in old individuals.

Although research based on the use of experimental models has several hurdles [13], it represents an important resource to study the molecular mechanisms underlying aging, therefore helping in the search for potential targets. The use of these experimental models provides the opportunity to understand the mechanisms of action of micronutrients and to search for dietary regimens or molecules that can ameliorate the signs of aging or that can postpone aging. This Special Issue also provides a contribution to the broad field of antiaging strategies that have been tested in experimental models. Shen and collaborators show that attano-extracted tocotrienols improve the inflammatory and oxidative condition and the metabolism of macronutrients in obese mice [14]. Markovics and collaborators report that the anthocyanin-rich extract of sour cherry can improve the hyperglycemia-induced dysfunction of the endothelium in cultured human umbilical cord vein endothelial cells [15]. Martin and collaborators show that calorie restriction prevents the changes in the hypothalamic neuropeptides that are associated with obesity and metabolic dysregulation in rats [16].

In line with the sentence reported on the Pan American Health organization website, "Healthy aging is a continuous process of optimizing opportunities to maintain and improve physical and mental health, independence, and quality of life throughout the life course" (https://www.paho.org/en/healthy-aging (accessed on 20 December 2021)), prevention will have a central role in limiting age-related consequences. In this regard, Ottolini and collaborators [17] stress the influence of milk quality for feeding premature neonates on neurodevelopment. Additionally, as reported in the study protocol by Mohd Suffian and collaborators [18], there is an increasing interest in interventions aimed at promoting the prevention of frailty.

Being that the field of healthy aging is the subject of continuous modifications, future studies that are aimed at elucidating the processes that are involved in aging and their correlation with nutrition would be helpful to improve the diet quality in the population to prevent or reduce age-related complications.

Author Contributions: E.G. and L.T. conceptualized and wrote the paper. All authors have read and agreed to the published version of the manuscript.

Funding: This research received no external funding.

Institutional Review Board Statement: Not applicable.

Informed Consent Statement: Not applicable.

Data Availability Statement: Not applicable.

Conflicts of Interest: The authors declare no conflict of interest.

References

1. Jang, W.; Shin, Y.; Kim, Y. Dietary Pattern Accompanied with a High Food Variety Score Is Negatively Associated with Frailty in Older Adults. *Nutrients* **2021**, *13*, 3164. [CrossRef] [PubMed]
2. Zhang, J.; Zhao, A. Dietary Diversity and Healthy Aging: A Prospective Study. *Nutrients* **2021**, *13*, 1787. [CrossRef] [PubMed]
3. Tucker, L.A. Fruit and Vegetable Intake and Telomere Length in a Random Sample of 5448 U.S. Adults. *Nutrients* **2021**, *13*, 1415. [CrossRef] [PubMed]
4. Huang, Q.; Jia, X.; Zhang, J.; Huang, F.; Wang, H.; Zhang, B.; Wang, L.; Jiang, H.; Wang, Z. Diet–Cognition Associations Differ in Mild Cognitive Impairment Subtypes. *Nutrients* **2021**, *13*, 1341. [CrossRef] [PubMed]
5. Tanaka, T.; Talegawkar, S.A.; Jin, Y.; Bandinelli, S.; Ferrucci, L. Association of Adherence to the Mediterranean-Style Diet with Lower Frailty Index in Older Adults. *Nutrients* **2021**, *13*, 1129. [CrossRef] [PubMed]
6. Kim, J.; Lee, Y.; Won, C.W.; Kim, M.K.; Kye, S.; Shim, J.-S.; Ki, S.; Yun, J. Dietary Patterns and Frailty in Older Korean Adults: Results from the Korean Frailty and Aging Cohort Study. *Nutrients* **2021**, *13*, 601. [CrossRef] [PubMed]
7. Liu, Q.; Guo, J.; Hu, L.; Veronese, N.; Smith, L.; Yang, L.; Cao, C. Association between Intake of Energy and Macronutrients and Memory Impairment Severity in US Older Adults, National Health and Nutrition Examination Survey 2011–2014. *Nutrients* **2020**, *12*, 3559. [CrossRef] [PubMed]
8. Jamioł-Milc, D.; Biernawska, J.; Liput, M.; Stachowska, L.; Domiszewski, Z. Seafood Intake as a Method of Non-Communicable Diseases (NCD) Prevention in Adults. *Nutrients* **2021**, *13*, 1422. [CrossRef] [PubMed]
9. Moradell, A.; Fernández-García, Á.I.; Navarrete-Villanueva, D.; Sagarra-Romero, L.; Gesteiro, E.; Pérez-Gómez, J.; Rodríguez-Gómez, I.; Ara, I.; Casajús, J.A.; Vicente-Rodríguez, G.; et al. Functional Frailty, Dietary Intake, and Risk of Malnutrition. Are Nutrients Involved in Muscle Synthesis the Key for Frailty Prevention? *Nutrients* **2021**, *13*, 1231. [CrossRef] [PubMed]
10. Alhussain, M.H.; Alkahtani, S.; Aljuhani, O.; Habib, S.S. Effects of Nutrient Intake on Diagnostic Measures of Sarcopenia among Arab Men: A Cross-Sectional Study. *Nutrients* **2021**, *13*, 114. [CrossRef] [PubMed]
11. Avila, J.C.; Samper-Ternent, R.; Wong, R. Malnutrition Risk among Older Mexican Adults in the Mexican Health and Aging Study. *Nutrients* **2021**, *13*, 1615. [CrossRef] [PubMed]
12. Jukic Peladic, N.; Dell'Aquila, G.; Carrieri, B.; Maggio, M.; Cherubini, A.; Orlandoni, P. Potential Role of Probiotics for Inflammaging: A Narrative Review. *Nutrients* **2021**, *13*, 2919. [CrossRef] [PubMed]
13. Giacomello, E.; Toniolo, L. The Potential of Calorie Restriction and Calorie Restriction Mimetics in Delaying Aging: Focus on Experimental Models. *Nutrients* **2021**, *13*, 2346. [CrossRef] [PubMed]
14. Shen, C.-L.; Ramamoorthy, S.; Kaur, G.; Dufour, J.M.; Wang, R.; Mo, H.; Watkins, B.A. Dietary Annatto-Extracted Tocotrienol Reduces Inflammation and Oxidative Stress, and Improves Macronutrient Metabolism in Obese Mice: A Metabolic Profiling Study. *Nutrients* **2021**, *13*, 1267. [CrossRef] [PubMed]
15. Markovics, A.; Biró, A.; Kun-Nemes, A.; Fazekas, M.É.; Rácz, A.A.; Paholcsek, M.; Lukács, J.; Stündl, L.; Remenyik, J. Effect of Anthocyanin-Rich Extract of Sour Cherry for Hyperglycemia-Induced Inflammatory Response and Impaired Endothelium-Dependent Vasodilation. *Nutrients* **2020**, *12*, 3373. [CrossRef] [PubMed]
16. Martín, M.; Rodríguez, A.; Gómez-Ambrosi, J.; Ramírez, B.; Becerril, S.; Catalán, V.; López, M.; Diéguez, C.; Frühbeck, G.; Burrell, M.A. Caloric Restriction Prevents Metabolic Dysfunction and the Changes in Hypothalamic Neuropeptides Associated with Obesity Independently of Dietary Fat Content in Rats. *Nutrients* **2021**, *13*, 2128. [CrossRef] [PubMed]
17. Ottolini, K.M.; Schulz, E.V.; Limperopoulos, C.; Andescavage, N. Using Nature to Nurture: Breast Milk Analysis and Fortification to Improve Growth and Neurodevelopmental Outcomes in Preterm Infants. *Nutrients* **2021**, *13*, 4307. [CrossRef] [PubMed]
18. Mohd Suffian, N.I.; Adznam, S.N.; Abu Saad, H.; Chan, Y.M.; Ibrahim, Z.; Omar, N.; Murat, M.F. Frailty Intervention through Nutrition Education and Exercise (FINE). A Health Promotion Intervention to Prevent Frailty and Improve Frailty Status among Pre-Frail Elderly—A Study Protocol of a Cluster Randomized Controlled Trial. *Nutrients* **2020**, *12*, 2758. [CrossRef] [PubMed]

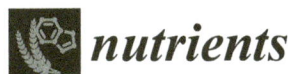

Article

Frailty Intervention through Nutrition Education and Exercise (FINE). A Health Promotion Intervention to Prevent Frailty and Improve Frailty Status among Pre-Frail Elderly—A Study Protocol of a Cluster Randomized Controlled Trial

Nurul Izzati Mohd Suffian [1], Siti Nur 'Asyura Adznam [1,2,*], Hazizi Abu Saad [1,3], Yoke Mun Chan [1,2], Zuriati Ibrahim [1], Noraida Omar [1,2] and Muhammad Faizal Murat [1]

1. Department of Nutrition and Dietetics, Faculty of Medicine and Health Sciences, Universiti Putra Malaysia, Serdang, Selangor 43400, Malaysia; nurulizzatisuffian@gmail.com (N.I.M.S.); hazizi@upm.edu.my (H.A.S.); cym@upm.edu.my (Y.M.C.); zuriatiib@upm.edu.my (Z.I.); noraidaomar@upm.edu.my (N.O.); muhammadfaizalmurat@gmail.com (M.F.M.)
2. Malaysian Research Institute of Ageing, (My Ageing) Universiti Putra Malaysia, Serdang, Selangor 43400, Malaysia
3. Sports Academy, Universiti Putra Malaysia, Serdang, Selangor 43400, Malaysia
* Correspondence: asyura@upm.edu.my; Tel.: +60-(39)-7692481

Received: 19 June 2020; Accepted: 17 August 2020; Published: 10 September 2020

Abstract: The ageing process has been associated with various geriatric issues including frailty. Without early prevention, frailty may cause multiple adverse outcomes. However, it potentially may be reversed with appropriate interventions. The aim of the study is to assess the effectiveness of nutritional education and exercise intervention to prevent frailty among the elderly. A 3-month, single-blind, two-armed, cluster randomized controlled trial of the frailty intervention program among Malaysian pre-frail elderly will be conducted. A minimum of total 60 eligible respondents from 8 clusters (flats) of Program Perumahan Rakyat (PPR) flats will be recruited and randomized to the intervention and control arm. The intervention group will receive a nutritional education and a low to moderate multi-component exercise program. To date, this is the first intervention study that specifically targets both the degree of frailty and an improvement in the outcomes of frailty using both nutritional education and exercise interventions among Malaysian pre-frail elderly. If the study is shown to be effective, there are major potential benefits to older population in terms of preventing transition to frailty. The findings from this trial will potentially provide valuable evidence and serve as a model for similar future interventions designed for elderly Malaysians in the community.

Keywords: community-dwelling; elderly; exercise; frailty; intervention; multi-component; nutrition education; randomized controlled trial

1. Introduction

A developing country such as Malaysia is not exempt from the fast changing demographic patterns in society and is expected to achieve the status of an ageing country by 2035 [1,2]. In line with this, the ageing process has been associated with various geriatric issues including frailty [3]. Frailty is a term commonly used by health care professionals to describe the condition of an older person who has chronic health problems, has lost functional abilities, and is likely to deteriorate further [4]. Frailty is a continuum process, and researchers commonly classify frailty into three categories (normal, pre-frail, and frail) according to the degree of deterioration [5]. Interestingly, it is not unidirectional but a dynamic and reversible process [6].

Several risk factors lead to frailty including socio-demographic status (advanced age, female, low educational, and socio-economic status), chronic disease, malnutrition, physical inactivity, cognitive impairment, poor functional status, and history of falls [2,7–9]. A clear relationship is also shown with adverse outcomes, such as disability/dependency, hospitalization, institutionalization, falls, poor mobility, depression, and death in community-dwelling older adults [5,10,11]. While those in an intermediate stage of frailty (pre-frail) present an increased risk of becoming frail within just three years [5].

The recent review on the global prevalence of pre-frail and frail elderly in the community ranged from 34.6% to 50.9% and 4.9% to 27.3%, respectively [12]. Asian countries recorded a higher prevalence range of pre-frailty (40% to 72%) and frailty (5% to 28%) than the global range [13,14]. Consistent with the worldwide trend, the frailty problem among Malaysian elderly has also emerged as a cause for concern [2]. In a large scale study conducted among community-dwelling elderly in an urban area in Malaysia, it was found that pre-frailty and frailty affected 61.7% and 8.9% of the older adults, respectively [15]. In addition, on the east coast of the peninsula, there are about 18.3% frail elders [16], and in Perak and Kelantan, the frailty affected 23.0% of the older adults [17].

Although the prevalence of the pre-frail elderly population is already at an alarming state, only a few interventions have focused on the pre-frail elderly population [18–20]. Pre-frail individuals have more than twice the risk of becoming frail compared to non-frail people [5]. However, because frailty appears to be a dynamic process and potentially reversible, implementing interventions for pre-frail elderly may prevent the development of frailty. Evidence shows that pre-frail elderly may respond better to interventions than elderly who have already moved to a frail state [21], probably due to less disability than that of the frail elderly [5]. Thus, there is potential for more intensive interventions among pre-frail elderly.

Unfortunately, research to improve frailty outcomes for frail elderly is still in its infancy, especially in Asian countries. Despite several nutritional interventions that were applied in a previous study, few convincing effects in improving frailty outcomes were apparent. Moreover, most of the studies involved supplementation and meal support, which are obviously costly [22–25] and hence run the risk of poor sustainability [3]. Even though there are limited interventions on nutrition education that have been conducted among frail elders but few studies able to report positive outcomes [26,27]. It includes the education on healthy food choices and dietary habit change [27,28].

In contrast, the evidence concerning the effectiveness of exercise intervention on the frailty outcome was undoubtedly more convincing [29–32]. In fact, exercise seems to play an essential role in any combination interventions, whereby additional intervention (e.g., nutritional intervention) can only lead to further improvement [33]. A recent systematic review suggests the importance of a combination intervention as these tend to be more effective than a single intervention [33], especially when diet and exercise are both included [33,34]. It has been shown that the characteristics of exercise programs that seem to result in better outcomes should include multicomponent training that is performed 3 days per week, with a duration of 3 months or longer and less than 60 min per session [35,36]. However, uncertainty still exists with regard to which exercise characteristics (type, frequency, and duration) are the most effective.

Evidence shows that elderly people living in rural areas have an economic disadvantage [37], which may put them at risk of being malnourished [38] and thus at high risk of being frail [39]. However, less is known about the poor elderly population living in urban areas such as the Program Perumahan Rakyat (PPR) flats in Kuala Lumpur area. In the 2000 census, Kuala Lumpur reached the status of 100 percent urban population [40]. Meanwhile, the PPR flats are low-cost public subsidized high-rise flats (5 to 18 floors) built for the resettlement of squatters and to provide housing to the economically disadvantaged individuals. According to Loh et al. [1], the PPR flats are places where the urban poor and a growing aging population reside. Thus, probably, the elderly who are living in the PPR flats are also at risk of being frail.

To the best of knowledge, there is no published frailty intervention that specifically targets both the degree of frailty and an improvement in the outcome using a combination of nutrition education and exercise interventions among Malaysian pre-frail elderly. Although a recent trial was conducted among the pre-frail elderly in Malaysia [20], the study only included single intervention and the focus was on the supplementation. Even though the supplementation given has the potential to reverse frailty and its outcomes, the efficacy remains doubtful. To address this gap, this study aims to develop, implement, and evaluate the effectiveness of a Frailty Intervention through Nutrition Education and Exercise (FINE) intervention program targeted at both improving the degree of frailty and the outcomes by using a combination of nutrition education and exercise interventions, and compare it with the general health education among Malaysian pre-frail elderly in a poor urban setting.

2. Materials and Methods

This study is designed and will be conducted and reported in keeping with the Consolidation Standards of Reporting (CONSORT) 2010 statement and its extension to cluster randomized trials [41].

2.1. Trial Design

The "FINE" project is a 3-month (12 weeks) intervention program, single-blind, two-armed cluster randomized controlled trial (cluster RCT), conducted among pre-frail elderly with a pre- and post-intervention and 3-month follow-up assessments to assess the effectiveness of the program. The trial mainly comprises nutritional education and exercise intervention among older people aged 60 years and above in the PPR flats in Kuala Lumpur. The trial is registered prospectively at ClinicalTrial.gov with registration number NCT04327544 on 30 March 2020.

2.2. Participants

2.2.1. Ethics Approval

The clinical trial is conducted in accord with the guidelines of the Declaration of Helsinki and the guidelines of Good Clinical Practice (GCP). Written informed consent will be sought from all the study participants prior to the commencement of the study. The study already has been approved by the Ethics Committee for Research involving Human Subjects Universiti Putra Malaysia (JKEUPM) (JKEUPM-2019-335). Permission for field data collection in the PPR flats has already been attained from the Dewan Bandaraya Kuala Lumpur (DBKL), as well as the Head Officer of the PPR flats in Kuala Lumpur.

2.2.2. Screening of Frailty Status

In total, there are 32 PPR flats listed under Kuala Lumpur area (DBKL, 2019). One of the PPR flats is excluded for the purpose of acceptability study as part of the development process of education materials, while the remaining 31 flats are divided into four different zones. Two zones with the highest prevalence of pre-frail elderly will be selected for the intervention study. However, due to no previous data having been recorded regarding the frailty status of the elderly, a cross-sectional study will be conducted to assess the current frailty status of the elderly. Using the one proportion formula by Daniel [42] with estimated prevalence of pre-frailty, 72.4% [14] and additional 20% subjects, the number of samples included in the screening study is 368.

Meanwhile, the minimum required cluster recruited from each zone is based on the calculation in the actual intervention study which is 4. Since there are 4 zones, in total 16 flats (cluster) will be included and randomly selected. Note that a cluster refers to one PPR building that has at least 50 residents aged 60 years and above. A proportionate sampling technique will be used for the recruitment of the respondents from each PPR to ensure that the total number of respondents will fairly represent each PPR flats. Frailty status will be assessed using Malay language standardized phenotype of frailty questionnaire [5]. The frailty phenotype evaluates five components of the frailty syndrome and allocates one point for each criterion met; respondents meeting zero criteria are defined as non-frail, whereas those meeting one or two criteria are defined as pre-frail, and those meeting three, four, or five criteria are defined as frail.

2.2.3. Eligibility and Recruitment

Based on the result from the screening, two zones with the highest number of pre-frail elderly will be selected. Pre-frail people 60 years and older from the selected PPR flats will be invited to participate in this FINE program. After the invitation process, the information sheets will be distributed and explained. Those individuals that agree to participate will be requested to provide written informed consent, and subsequently, they will be further screened to identify their eligibility to participate. The inclusion and exclusion criteria are as in Table 1. Once individuals have been screened as being eligible to participate, they will be invited to attend a pre-intervention data collection (baseline assessment). The overview of the frailty intervention study flow is shown in Figure 1.

Table 1. The summary of the inclusion and exclusion criteria for the Frailty Intervention through Nutrition Education and Exercise (FINE) program.

Inclusion Criteria	Exclusion Criteria
• Men or women aged 60 years and above	• Self-reported chronic diseases and mental illnesses (heart-related disease, chronic obstructive pulmonary disease (COPD), stroke, cancer, asthma, renal dysfunction, terminally ill, major depression, bipolar, disorder, obsessive compulsive disorder and post-traumatic disorder)
• Meet one or two frailty phenotype score (pre-frail)	• Physical Activity Readiness-Questionnaire (PAR-Q & YOU) (Yes $\geq$ 1) [43]
• Able to ambulate without personal assistance	• Bedridden
• Residing in the PPR flats in Kuala Lumpur	• Cognitive impairment (ECAQ < 6) [44]
• Willing to participate in the intervention program with informed consent	• Sensory impairment (visual & hearing) that will interfere with communication
	• Unable to read and write
	• Already involved or still participating in any health interventional study
	• Any sustained fracture (hip, vertebrae) in past six months
	• Any surgery (hip, abdominal area) in past six months

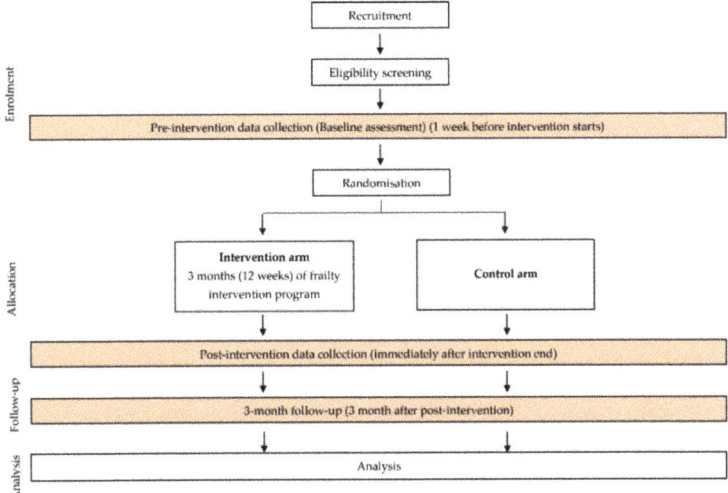

Figure 1. The overview of the frailty intervention study flow. Adapted from the CONSORT 2010 flow diagram (extension to cluster randomized trails) [41].

2.2.4. Sample Size Calculation

The sample size for each arm was calculated by using two group mean comparison formula [25]. Both the mean and standard deviation from the study conducted by Tarazona-Santabalbina et al. [29] in Spain was used as the reference, and based on the calculation using the result for the variable of the Short Physical Performance Battery (SPPB), the sample size required for each intervention and control arm is 15 respondents.

With a hypothesized intra-cluster correlation coefficient (ICC) 0.02 [1], fixed cluster size of 4 [45], and a minimum of 15 respondents required under individual randomization, the calculated minimum required cluster size and sample size is 4 and 16 per arm, respectively. After an adjustment for the estimated response rate, a sample size of 30 respondents per arm is required to provide of 80%, with $\alpha = 0.05$. In total, the respondents for both arms are 60 elderlies with approximately 8 respondents from each cluster (4 clusters for each arm).

2.2.5. Randomization and Allocation

Randomization will be conducted after the baseline assessment is completed. Randomization takes place at the zone level to reduce the risk of exposure of the control arm to the intervention effect. PPR flats with the highest prevalence of pre-frail elderly in two zones resulting from the screening will be randomized into the intervention arm and the control. Using a computer-generated random number sequence, the study statistician will allocate the PPR flats into the intervention and control group based on their zones.

2.3. Intervention

Prior to the commencement of the FINE program, a process of development of the frailty intervention module and education materials will be conducted. The educational materials will be developed based on the frailty intervention module to serve as a reference or reading materials for the respondents throughout the program. It includes flipchart, PowerPoint slides, booklet, and posters. During a 12-week (3-month) intervention period, in overall, participants attend one session of frailty, exercise, and healthy eating talk; 20 sessions of a low to moderate intensity multi-component exercise course; and 5 sessions of nutrition education intervention. Additionally, there is one session during the following 3 months after the intervention ends. It should be noted that each session will be held in the facility area or hall of the PPR flats for around 60 min.

As an introduction, a few talk sessions and an exercise demonstration will be conducted for few days of the first week regarding frailty, exercise, and nutrition with the aims of introducing, refreshing, and improving the knowledge regarding the topic. Each topic will be delivered by the research team based on the frailty intervention module. In the following week, the exercise activities will be conducted two days per week [19] concurrently with the nutrition session, which is only once per week. The multicomponent exercise program is an adaptation with a slight modification of the frailty intervention study conducted by Tarazona-Santabalbina, which involves a progressive combination of activities including proprioception and balance exercises, aerobic training, resistance training, and stretching [29]. All exercise sessions will be delivered in group as it is effective in reducing or postponing frailty [46] and will be supervised by qualified physiotherapists [29]. For nutrition education intervention, five sessions of group discussion are conducted among participants; the main idea being to educate the elderly to improve their intake of calories, protein [47,48], calcium, and vitamin D [49]. Thus, every week they will receive an explanation about the importance of each nutrient, its sources, and the recommendation for daily intake. The session will also be interspersed with a few quizzes and hands-on activities, such as cooking practice [18] and games [50], to reinforce the learning objectives. In the following 12 weeks after the intervention ends, one session is added with the purpose of doing revision regarding the previous education session and to supervise the exercise routine practice by the elderly. The session will be conducted at week 6 after the intervention ends and will be delivered by a dietitian and a physiotherapist from the research team, lasting for one hour. The respondents in the control group will not receive any intervention program. A summary of the FINE program is shown in Table 2.

Table 2. Summary of the frailty FINE program.

	Intervention Group				Control Group
	Week	Day 1	Day 2	Day 3	
12 weeks intervention program	1	Talk on frailty	Talk on exercise	Talk on healthy eating	* No intervention
	2	Multicomponent exercise *			
	3	Multicomponent exercise *		Nutrition education class	
	4	Multicomponent exercise *			
	5	Multicomponent exercise *		Nutrition education class	
	6	Multicomponent exercise *			
	7	Multicomponent exercise *		Nutrition education class	
	8	Multicomponent exercise *			
	9	Multicomponent exercise *		Nutrition education class	
	10	Multicomponent exercise *			
	11	Multicomponent exercise *		Nutrition education class	
	12	INTERVENTION END			

* exercise intervention.

2.4. Outcome Measures

In this research study, the primary and secondary outcomes will focus on three key domains, which are physical changes, cognitive performance, and functional improvement. This includes the changes in frailty status and score, knowledge, attitude, and practice (KAP) towards frailty, nutrition and exercise, dietary intake, anthropometric measurements, cognitive status, functional ability status, mobility status, and risk of falls. Apart from that, demographic data (e.g., gender, race, age, monthly income, education level, and marital status) will be assessed as well.

2.4.1. Primary Outcome

Frailty Score/Status

The frailty status will be assessed using the well-established Malay language standardized phenotype of the frailty questionnaire; as proposed by Fried et al. [5]. The questionnaire evaluates five components of the frailty syndrome (weight loss, exhaustion, weakness, slowness, and low activity) and allocates one point for each criterion met; respondents meeting zero criteria are defined as non-frail, whereas those meeting one or two criteria are defined as pre-frail, and those meeting three, four, or five criteria are defined as frail.

2.4.2. Secondary Outcomes

Knowledge, Attitude, and Practice (KAP) towards Frailty, Nutrition, and Exercise

The KAP questions will be developed prior to data collection to measure the construct of knowledge, attitude, and practice in relation to frailty, nutrition, and exercise among the elderly. The questions will consist of items based on the content of the developed educational materials. A validation and reliability study will be conducted after it is developed.

Dietary Intake

The amount of food items consumed by the respondents in the past week will be recorded by the validated Malay language of Diet History Questionnaire (DHQ) via the interview method. The data will be analyzed using the Nutritionist Pro™ Diet Analysis Software and then compared to the Malaysian Recommended Nutrient intake [51].

Anthropometric Measurements

- Body weight will be measured using an electronic flat scale (SECA 803, Hamburg, Germany).
- Height of the participant will be measured using stadiometer (SECA 213, Hamburg, Germany).
- When no valid measurement can be obtained due to particularities (e.g., kyphosis, scoliosis), an alternative method will be used to measure the height using a demi-span measurement. The height will be measured using equations developed for the Malaysian elderly [52].
- Body Mass Index (BMI) will be derived using the calculation: weight in kilograms divided by the height in meters squared [weight (kg)/height^2 (m^2)] [53]
- Body part circumference including mid-upper arm circumference (MUAC) and calf circumference (CC) will be measured using a flexible non-stretchable measuring tape (SECA 201, Hamburg, Germany) [52].
- Body composition including body fat percentage and muscle percentage will be assessed using a portable body composition analyzer (OMRON HBF-375, Japan).

Cognitive Status

This study will use the validated Malay language version of the Mini-Mental State Examination (M-MMSE) questionnaire to assess the cognitive functioning of the respondents [54].

Functional Ability

The well-established Malay language version of the Lawton Instrumental Activities of Daily Living (IADL) questionnaire will be used to assess the respondents' ability to perform eight daily activities (i.e., ability to use telephone, shopping, preparing meals, housekeeping, doing laundry, using public transport, taking medications, and handling finances) [1,15].

Mobility Status

A well-established Malay language version of the Short Physical Performance Battery (SPPB) will be used for this study to test the respondents' mobility status [55] to evaluate lower limb extremity functioning in three components (balance test, gait speed test, and repeated chair stand test).

Risk of Falls

The Malay language version of the Berg Balance Scale (BBS) will be used to assess the risk of falls among the respondents [56]. A process of back translation and monolingual testing will be conducted for the questionnaire prior to the evaluation process [57].

2.5. Statistical Analysis

The description of the respondents' characteristics will be reported by group (control and intervention). Depending on the distribution of the variable of interest, the descriptive statistics of continuous data will be presented by using the mean and standard deviation and the median and the inter-quartile range. Categorical data will be presented as frequencies and percentages. For primary analysis, since there are small number of cluster, as recommended by Hayes and Moulton (2017), analysis will be conducted at cluster level instead of individual level [58]. Thus, the primary and secondary outcomes will be compared within and between groups using 2-way repeated ANOVA by general linear model. Any covariate data at baseline value will be adjusted and further test will be conducted using a repeated measure analysis of covariance (ANCOVA). If the data is not distributed normally, Kruskall–Wallis test will be used to analyze the data. Statistical significance is set at $p < 0.05$. Data will be entered and analyzed using SPSS 25.0 software.

Intention-to-treat (ITT) will be applied in the data management and analysis. All data will be processed according to their arm even if the participant did not manage to come to all the intervention sessions. It is assumed that majority of the participant in the intervention arm will receive adequate number of the intervention sessions. Action will be taken in order to prevent lower attendance from the participants such as conducting extra exercise classes for participants who could not come to a certain session. For every nutrition session, class will start with the revision on the topic that had been discussed in previous session. This can help participants who could not come to the previous nutrition session to learn the topic they missed.

3. Discussion

The FINE intervention program presents a unique approach, delivering a multi-domain intervention for pre-frail elderly men and women who live in the urban community. Often, research had been made among poor rural elderly, showing their high risk of getting malnutrition and becoming frail, but less is known among poor elderly population that live in urban areas such as the elderly community in PPR, Kuala Lumpur. Considering the high prevalence of the pre-frail elderly in urban areas [15], this target group should not be neglected. Aligned with the main objectives to improve the frailty status of the elderly, the program will have a highly positive impact in many ways, i.e., physically, mentally, and in social life.

The major strength of the proposed study design is the implementation of a multi-domain intervention that was considered to be more effective that a single intervention, especially through nutrition and exercise [33,34]. In addition, the designated nutritional education intervention was made based on the study that had demonstrated positive outcomes among frail elderly [18,26,59]. A few elderly-related local nutrition-education programs were also reviewed during the design process [1,60], considering the cultural values of local elderly population.

The strength of the nutrition education in this study mainly highlights the strategy to tackle the unintentional weight loss problem, which is also one of the main problems among frail elderly people [61]. Targeting one of the risk factors of frailty is also one of the key strategies for frailty prevention, as highlighted in the report of Asia Pacific CPGs for the management of frailty. The multicomponent exercises were applied in this study because of the strong evidence that performing different types of exercise assists in frailty prevention and improves the outcomes [35,36], and it is strongly recommended by Asia Pacific CPGs. The multi-component exercises were adapted from the exercise programs that were feasibly delivered to frail older people [29,32] with slight modifications to ensure better adherence to the exercise program by the local elderly.

An additional advantage of this community-based intervention is that it will be conducted in a natural setting, allowing respondents to integrate changes into their daily lives in a real-life context. This implies that the intervention delivered can be potentially transferable to other community settings. Moreover, it is also readily transferable to routine clinical practice in a health service setting, and the interdisciplinary approach is relevant to several professional groups in health care such as nutritionists, dietitians, and physiotherapists.

4. Conclusions

In overall, this FINE intervention program has been designed to be interactive, enjoyable, and manageable to encourage adherence among the respondents. Based on the evidence, we are convinced that this intervention program will be able to prevent frailty and the adverse effects associated with pre-frail elderly people. If the intervention produces significant positive effects, the findings will potentially provide valuable evidence and serve as a model of locally acceptable strategies to prevent frailty and reduce adverse health outcomes among older Malaysians.

Author Contributions: N.I.M.S., M.F.M., S.N.A.A., H.A.S., Y.M.C., Z.I., and N.O. conceived the study design and secured the necessary funding. S.N.A.A. led and was responsible for the overall project. N.I.M.S. is a doctoral student involved in the overall project and was responsible for the writing of the manuscript. H.A.S., Y.M.C., Z.I., and N.O. acted as co-supervisors of the doctoral student and provided critical input. All authors have read and agreed to the published version of the manuscript.

Funding: This research was funded by Universiti Putra Malaysia IPS grant, grant number GP-IPS/2017/9547700. The APC was funded by Research Management Centre, Universiti Putra Malaysia.

Acknowledgments: The authors sincerely thank all the study respondents and their families for their cooperation and confidence in our research team. We are also extremely thankful for the assistance and cooperation received from the DBKL and PPR flat leaders.

Conflicts of Interest: The authors declare no conflict of interest. The funders had no role in the design of the study; in the collection, analyses, or interpretation of data; in the writing of the manuscript, or in the decision to publish the results.

References

1. Loh, D.A.; Hairi, N.N.; Choo, W.Y.; Mohd Hairi, F.; Peramalah, D.; Kandiben, S.; Lee, P.L.; Gani, N.; Madzlan, M.F.; Abd Hamid, M.A.I.; et al. MultiCfomponent Exercise and theRApeutic lifeStyle (CERgAS) intervention to improve physical performance and maintain independent living among urban poor older people—A cluster randomised controlled trial. *BMC Geriatr.* **2015**, *15*, 8. [CrossRef] [PubMed]
2. Sathasivam, J.; Bahyah Kamaruzzaman, S.; Hairi, F.; Wan Ng, C.; Chinna, K. Frail elders in an urban district setting in Malaysia: Multidimensional frailty and its correlates. *Asia Pacific J. Public Health* **2015**, *27*, 52–61. [CrossRef] [PubMed]
3. Gallucci, M.; Ongaro, F.; Amici, G.P.; Regini, C. Frailty, disability and survival in the elderly over the age of seventy: Evidence from "The Treviso Longeva (TRELONG) Study". *Arch. Gerontol. Geriatr.* **2009**, *48*, 281–283. [CrossRef] [PubMed]
4. Fairhall, N.; Aggar, C.; Kurrle, S.E.; Sherrington, C.; Lord, S.; Lockwood, K.; Monaghan, N.; Cameron, I.D. Frailty intervention trial (FIT). *BMC Geriatr.* **2008**, *8*, 27. [CrossRef] [PubMed]
5. Fried, L.P.; Tangen, C.M.; Walston, J.; Newman, A.B.; Hirsch, C.; Gottdiener, J.; Seeman, T.; Tracy, R.; Kop, W.J.; Burke, G.; et al. Frailty in older adults: Evidence for a phenotype. *J. Gerontol. Ser. A Biol. Sci. Med. Sci.* **2001**, *56*, 146–157. [CrossRef]

6. Van Kan, G.A.; Rolland, Y.; Bergman, H.; Morley, J.E.; Kritchevsky, S.B.; Vellas, B. The I.A.N.A. task force on frailty assessment of older people in clinical practice. *J. Nutr. Health Aging* **2008**, *12*, 29–37. [CrossRef]
7. Sánchez-García, S.; Sánchez-Arenas, R.; García-Peña, C.; Rosas-Carrasco, O.; Ávila-Funes, J.A.; Ruiz-Arregui, L.; Juárez-Cedillo, T. Frailty among community-dwelling elderly Mexican people: Prevalence and association with sociodemographic characteristics, health state and the use of health services. *Geriatr. Gerontol. Int.* **2014**, *14*, 395–402. [CrossRef]
8. Robertson, D.A.; Savva, G.M.; Kenny, R.A. Frailty and cognitive impairment—A review of the evidence and causal mechanisms. *Ageing Res. Rev.* **2013**, *12*, 840–851. [CrossRef]
9. Etman, A.; Burdorf, A.; Van der Cammen, T.J.M.; Mackenbach, J.P.; Van Lenthe, F.J. Socio-demographic determinants of worsening in frailty among community-dwelling older people in 11 European countries. *J. Epidemiol. Community Health* **2012**, *66*, 1116–1121. [CrossRef]
10. Soysal, P.; Veronese, N.; Thompson, T.; Kahl, K.G.; Fernandes, B.S.; Prina, A.M.; Solmi, M.; Schofield, P.; Koyanagi, A.; Tseng, P.T.; et al. Relationship between depression and frailty in older adults: A systematic review and meta-analysis. *Ageing Res. Rev.* **2017**, *36*, 78–87. [CrossRef]
11. Ensrud, K.E.; Ewing, S.K.; Taylor, B.C.; Fink, H.A.; Stone, K.L.; Cauley, J.A.; Tracy, J.K.; Hochberg, M.C.; Rodondi, N.; Cawthon, P.M.; et al. Frailty and risk of falls, fracture, and mortality in older women: The study of osteoporotic fractures. *J. Gerontol. A Biol. Sci. Med. Sci.* **2007**, *62*, 744–751. [CrossRef] [PubMed]
12. Choi, J.; Ahn, A.; Kim, S. Global prevalence of physical frailty by fried's criteria in community-dwelling elderly with national population-based surveys. *J. Am. Med. Dir. Assoc.* **2015**, *16*, 548–550. [CrossRef] [PubMed]
13. Liu, L.K.; Lee, W.J.; Chen, L.Y.; Hwang, A.C.; Lin, M.H.; Peng, L.N.; Chen, L.K. Association between frailty, osteoporosis, falls and hip fractures among community-dwelling people aged 50 years and older in Taiwan: Results from I-Lan longitudinal aging study. *PLoS ONE* **2015**, *10*, e0136968. [CrossRef] [PubMed]
14. Ng, T.P.; Feng, L.; Nyunt, M.S.Z.; Feng, L.; Niti, M.; Tan, B.Y.; Chan, G.; Khoo, S.A.; Chan, S.M.; Yap, P.; et al. Nutritional, physical, cognitive, and combination interventions and frailty reversal among older adults: A randomized controlled trial. *Am. J. Med.* **2015**, *128*, 1225–1236. [CrossRef]
15. Badrasawi, M.; Shahar, S.; Singh, D.K.A. Risk factors of frailty among multi-ethnic malaysian older adults. *Int. J. Gerontol.* **2017**, *11*, 154–160. [CrossRef]
16. Mohd Hamidin, F.A.; Adznam, S.N.; Ibrahim, Z.; Chan, Y.M.; Abdul Aziz, N.H. Prevalence of frailty syndrome and its associated factors among community-dwelling elderly in East Coast of Peninsular Malaysia. *SAGE Open Med.* **2018**, *6*. [CrossRef]
17. Nur Farhana, M.; Suzana, S.; Manal, S.; Devinder, K.A. Frailty and nutritional status among older adults in Perak and Kelantan. In Proceedings of the NSM Conference, Renaissance Hotel, Kuala Lumpur, Malaysia, 3–4 June 2014.
18. Kwon, J.; Yoshida, Y.; Yoshida, H.; Kim, H.; Suzuki, T.; Lee, Y. Effects of a combined physical training and nutrition intervention on physical performance and health-related quality of life in prefrail older women living in the community: A randomized controlled trial. *J. Am. Med. Dir. Assoc.* **2015**, *16*, 2631–2638.
19. Drey, M.; Zech, A.; Freiberger, E.; Bertsch, T.; Uter, W.; Sieber, C.C.; Pfeifer, K.; Bauer, J.M. Effects of strength training versus power training on physical performance in prefrail community-dwelling older adults. *Gerontology* **2012**, *58*, 197–204. [CrossRef]
20. Badrasawi, M.; Shahar, S.; Zahara, A.M.; Nor Fadilah, R.; Singh, D.K.A. Efficacy of L-carnitine supplementation on frailty status and its biomarkers, nutritional status, and physical and cognitive function among prefrail older adults: A double-blind, randomized, placebo-controlled clinical trial. *Clin. Interv. Aging* **2016**, *11*, 1675–1686. [CrossRef]
21. Faber, M.J.; Bosscher, R.J.; Chin, A.; Paw, M.J.; Van Wieringen, P.C. Effects of exercise programs on falls and mobility in frail and pre-frail older adults: A multicenter randomized controlled trial. *Arch. Phys. Med. Rehabil.* **2006**, *87*, 885–896. [CrossRef]
22. Hutchins-Wiese, H.L.; Kleppinger, A.; Annis, K.; Liva, E.; Lammi-Keefe, C.J.; Durham, H.A.; Kenny, A.M. The impact of supplemental n-3 long chain polyunsaturated fatty acids and dietary antioxidants on physical performance in postmenopausal women. *J. Nutr. Health Aging.* **2013**, *17*, 76–80. [CrossRef] [PubMed]
23. Kim, C.O.; Lee, K.R. Preventive effect of protein-energy supplementation on the functional decline of frail older adults with low socioeconomic status: A community-based randomized controlled study. *J. Gerontol. A Biol. Sci. Med. Sci.* **2013**, *68*, 309–316. [CrossRef] [PubMed]

24. Tieland, M.; Van de Rest, O.; Dirks, M.L.; Van der Zwaluw, N.; Mensink, M.; Van Loon, L.J.C.; De Groot, L.C.P.G.M. Protein supplementation improves physical performance in frail elderly people: A randomized, double-blind, placebo-controlled trial. *J. Am. Med. Dir. Assoc.* **2012**, *13*, 720–726. [CrossRef]
25. Smoliner, C.; Norman, K.; Scheufele, R.; Hartig, W.; Pirlich, M.; Lochs, H. Effects of food fortification on nutritional and functional status in frail elderly nursing home residents at risk of malnutrition. *Nutrition* **2008**, *24*, 1139–1144. [CrossRef] [PubMed]
26. Chan, D.C.; Tsou, H.H.; Yang, R.S.; Tsauo, J.Y.; Chen, C.Y.; Hsiung, C.A.; Kuo, K.N. A pilot randomized controlled trial to improve geriatric frailty. *BMC Geriatr.* **2012**, *12*, 5. [CrossRef]
27. Nykänen, I.; Rissanen, T.H.; Sulkava, R.; Hartikainen, S. Effects of individual dietary counseling as part of a comprehensive geriatric assessment (CGA) on frailty status: A population-based intervention study. *J. Clin. Gerontol. Geriatr.* **2012**, *3*, 89–93. [CrossRef]
28. Manal, B.; Shahar, S.; Singh, D.K.A. Nutrition and frailty: A review of clinical intervention studies. *J. Frailty Aging* **2015**, *4*, 100–106.
29. Tarazona-Santabalbina, F.J.; Gómez-Cabrera, M.C.; Pérez-Ros, P.; Martínez-Arnau, F.M.; Cabo, H.; Tsaparas, K.; Salvador-Pascual, A.; Rodriguez-Mañas, L.; Viña, J. A multicomponent exercise intervention that reverses frailty and improves cognition, emotion, and social networking in the community-dwelling frail elderly: A randomized clinical trial. *J. Am. Med. Dir. Assoc.* **2016**, *17*, 426–433. [CrossRef]
30. Langlois, F.; Vu, T.T.M.; Chassé, K.; Dupuis, G.; Kergoat, M.-J.; Bherer, L. Benefits of physical exercise training on cognition and quality of life in frail older adults. *J. Gerontol. B Psychol. Sci. Soc. Sci.* **2012**, *68*, 400–404. [CrossRef]
31. Giné-Garriga, M.; Guerra, M.; Unnithan, V.B. The effect of functional circuit training on self-reported fear of falling and health status in a group of physically frail older individuals: A randomized controlled trial. *Aging Clin. Exp. Res.* **2013**, *25*, 329–336. [CrossRef]
32. Brown, M.; Sinacore, D.R.; Ehsani, A.A.; Binder, E.F.; Holloszy, J.O.; Kohrt, W.M. Low-intensity exercise as a modifier of physical frailty in older adults. *Arch. Phys. Med. Rehabil.* **2000**, *81*, 960–965. [CrossRef] [PubMed]
33. Dedeyne, L.; Deschodt, M.; Verschueren, S.; Tournoy, J.; Gielen, E. Effects of multi-domain interventions in (pre) frail elderly on frailty, functional, and cognitive status: A systematic review. *Clin. Interv. Aging* **2017**, *12*, 873–896. [CrossRef] [PubMed]
34. Lee, P.H.; Lee, Y.S.; Chan, D.C. Interventions targeting geriatric frailty: A systemic review. *J. Clin. Gerontol. Geriatr.* **2012**, *3*, 47–52. [CrossRef]
35. Theou, O.; Stathokostas, L.; Roland, K.P.; Jakobi, J.M.; Patterson, C.; Vandervoort, A.A.; Jones, G.R. The effectiveness of exercise interventions for the management of frailty: A systematic review. *J. Aging Res.* **2011**. [CrossRef]
36. Nash, K.C.M. The effects of exercise on strength and physical performance in frail older people: A systematic review. *Rev. Clin. Gerontol.* **2012**, *22*, 274–285. [CrossRef]
37. Çakmur, H. Frailty among elderly adults in a rural area of Turkey. *Med. Sci. Monit.* **2015**, *21*, 1232–1242. [CrossRef]
38. Timpini, A.; Facchi, E.; Cossi, S.; Ghisla, M.K.; Romanelli, G.; Marengoni, A. Self-reported socio-economic status, social, physical and leisure activities and risk for malnutrition in late life: A cross-sectional population-based study. *J. Nutr. Health Aging* **2011**, *15*, 233–238. [CrossRef]
39. Lilamand, M.; Kelaiditi, E.; Cesari, M.; Raynaud-Simon, A.; Ghisolfi, A.; Guyonnet, S.; Vellas, B.; Abellan van Kan, G.; The Toulouse Frailty Platform Team. Validation of the mini nutritional assessment-short form in a population of frail elders without disability. Analysis of the toulouse frailty platform population in 2013. *J. Nutr. Health Aging* **2015**, *19*, 570–574. [CrossRef]
40. Tee, G.A.; Ahmad, Y. Public low-cost housing in malaysia: Case studies on PPR low-cosr flats in Kuala Lumpur. *J. Des. Built Environ.* **2012**, *8*, 1–18.
41. Campbell, M.K.; Piaggio, G.; Elbourne, D.R.; Altman, D.G. Consort 2010 statement: Extension to cluster randomised trials. *BMJ* **2012**, *345*, e5661. [CrossRef]
42. Daniel, W. *Biostatistics: A Foundation for Analysis in the Health Sciences*, 7th ed.; John Wiley & Sons: New York, NY, USA, 1999.
43. Gledhill, N. *Physical Activity Readiness Questionnaire (PAR-Q) and You*; Canadian Society for Exercise Physiology: Ottawa, ON, Canada, 2002.

44. Kua, E. H.; Ko, S.M. A questionnaire to screen for cognitive impairment among elderly people in developing countries. *Acta Psychiatr. Scand.* **1992**, *85*, 119–122. [CrossRef]
45. Tokolahi, E.; Hocking, C.; Kersten, P.; Vandal, A.C. Quality and reporting of cluster randomized controlled trials evaluating occupational therapy interventions: A systematic review. *OTJR Occup. Particip. Health* **2016**, *36*, 14–24. [CrossRef]
46. Apóstolo, J.; Cooke, R.; Bobrowicz-Campos, E.; Santana, S.; Marcucci, M.; Cano, A.; Vollenbroek-Hutten, M.; Germini, F.; D'Avanzo, B.; Gwyther, H.; et al. Effectiveness of interventions to prevent pre-frailty and frailty progression in older adults. *JBI Database Syst. Rev. Implement. Rep.* **2018**, *16*, 140–232. [CrossRef] [PubMed]
47. Dent, E.; Lien, C.; Lim, W.S.; Wong, W.C.; Wong, C.H.; Ng, T.P.; Woo, J.; Dong, B.; De la Vega, S.; Hua Poi, P.J.; et al. The asia-pacific clinical practice guidelines for the management of frailty. *J. Am. Med. Dir. Assoc.* **2017**, *18*, 564–575. [CrossRef] [PubMed]
48. Alibhai, S.M.H.; Greenwood, C.; Payette, H. An approach to the management of unintentional weight loss in elderly people. *Can. Med. Assoc. J.* **2005**, *172*, 773–780. [CrossRef] [PubMed]
49. National Coordinating Committee on Food and Nutrition. *Malaysian Dietary Guidelines*, 1st ed.; Technical Working Group on Nutritional Guidelines: Putrajaya, Malaysia, 2010; p. 27.
50. Dorner, T.E.; Lackinger, C.; Haider, S.; Luger, E.; Kapan, A.; Luger, M.; Schindler, K.E. Nutritional intervention and physical training in malnourished frail community-dwelling elderly persons carried out by trained lay "buddies": Study protocol of a randomized controlled trial. *BMC Public Health* **2013**, *13*, 1232. [CrossRef] [PubMed]
51. Ministry of Health (MOH). Recommended Nutrient Intakes for Malaysia (RNI). In *A Report of the Technical Working Group on Nutritional Guidelines*; National Coordinating Committee on Food and Nutrition (NCCFN): Putrajaya, Malaysia, 2017; pp. 519–523.
52. Ngoh, H.J.; Sakinah, H.; Harsa Amylia, M.S. Development of demi-span equations for predicting height among the Malaysian elderly. *Malays. J. Nutr.* **2012**, *18*, 149–159. [PubMed]
53. Muhamad, A.R.; Hamirudin, A.H.; Zainudin, N.; Sidek, S.; Rahman, N.A.A. Nutritional risk according to mini nutritional assessment-short form amonng community dwelling elderly in Kuantan, Pahang: A pilot study. *Int. J. Allied Health Sci.* **2019**, *3*, 247–667.
54. Ibrahim, N.M.; Shohaimi, S.; Chong, H.T.; Rahman, A.H.A.; Razali, R.; Esther, E.; Basri, H.B. Validation study of the mini-mental state examination in a Malay-speaking elderly population in Malaysia. *Dement. Geriatr. Cogn. Disord.* **2009**, *27*, 247–253. [CrossRef]
55. Singh, D.K.A.; Pillai, S.G.K.; Tan, S.T.; Tai, C.C.; Shahar, S. Association between physiological falls risk and physical performance tests among community-dwelling older adults. *Clin. Interv. Aging* **2015**, *10*, 1319–1326. [CrossRef]
56. Berg, K.; Wood-Dauphinee, S.; Ivan Williams, J.; Maki, B. Measuring balance in the elderly: Development and validation of an instrument. *Can. J. Public Health* **1992**, *83*, 1–130.
57. Maneesriwongul, W.; Dixon, J.K. Instrument translation process: A methods review. *J. Adv. Nurs.* **2004**, *48*, 175–186. [CrossRef] [PubMed]
58. Hayes, R.J.; Moulton, L.H. *Cluster Randomised Trials*, 2nd ed.; CRC Press Taylor & Francis Group: Boca Raton, FL, USA, 2017; pp. 197–199.
59. Haider, S.; Dorner, T.E.; Luger, E.; Kapan, A.; Titze, S.; Lackinger, C.; Schindler, K.E. Impact of a home-based physical and nutritional intervention program conducted by lay-volunteers on handgrip strength in prefrail and frail older adults: A randomized control trial. *PLoS ONE* **2017**, *12*, e0169613. [CrossRef] [PubMed]
60. Shahar, S.; Kamaruddin, N.S.; Badrasawi, M.; Mohamed Sakian, N.I.; Manaf, Z.A.; Yassin, Z.; Joseph, L. Effectiveness of exercise and protein supplementation intervention on body composition, functional fitness, and oxidative stress among elderly Malays with sarcopenia. *Clin. Interv. Aging* **2013**, *8*, 1365–1375. [CrossRef] [PubMed]
61. Fougère, B.; Morley, J.E. Weight loss is a major cause of frailty. *J. Nutr. Health Aging* **2017**, *21*, 933–935. [CrossRef]

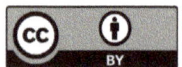

© 2020 by the authors. Licensee MDPI, Basel, Switzerland. This article is an open access article distributed under the terms and conditions of the Creative Commons Attribution (CC BY) license (http://creativecommons.org/licenses/by/4.0/).

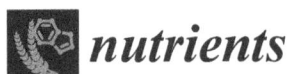

Article

Effect of Anthocyanin-Rich Extract of Sour Cherry for Hyperglycemia-Induced Inflammatory Response and Impaired Endothelium-Dependent Vasodilation

Arnold Markovics [1], Attila Biró [1], Andrea Kun-Nemes [1], Mónika Éva Fazekas [1], Anna Anita Rácz [2], Melinda Paholcsek [2], János Lukács [3], László Stündl [1] and Judit Remenyik [1,*]

1. Institute of Food Technology, University of Debrecen, H-4032 Debrecen, Hungary; arnoldmarkovich@gmail.com (A.M.); biro.attila@agr.unideb.hu (A.B.); andrea.nemes83@gmail.com (A.K.-N.); fazekas.monika@agr.unideb.hu (M.É.F.); stundl@agr.unideb.hu (L.S.)
2. Department of Human Genetics, University of Debrecen, H-4032 Debrecen, Hungary; racz.anna@med.unideb.hu (A.A.R.); paholcsek.melinda@med.unideb.hu (M.P.)
3. Department of Obstetrics and Gynaecology, University of Debrecen, H-4032 Debrecen, Hungary; lukacs.janos@med.unideb.hu
* Correspondence: remenyik@agr.unideb.hu; Tel.: +36-52-51-8600

Received: 11 August 2020; Accepted: 27 October 2020; Published: 2 November 2020

Abstract: Diabetes mellitus (DM)-related morbidity and mortality are steadily rising worldwide, affecting about half a billion people worldwide. A significant proportion of diabetic cases are in the elderly, which is concerning given the increasing aging population. Proper nutrition is an important component in the effective management of diabetes in the elderly. A plethora of active substances of plant origin exhibit potency to target the pathogenesis of diabetes mellitus. The nutraceutical and pharmaceutical effects of anthocyanins have been extensively studied. In this study, the effect of Hungarian sour cherry, which is rich in anthocyanins, on hyperglycemia-induced endothelial dysfunction was tested using human umbilical cord vein endothelial cells (HUVECs). HUVECs were maintained under both normoglycemic (5 mM) and hyperglycemic (30 mM) conditions with or without two concentrations (1.50 ng/µL) of anthocyanin-rich sour cherry extract. Hyperglycemia-induced oxidative stress and inflammatory response and damaged vasorelaxation processes were investigated by evaluating the level of reactive oxygen species (ROS) and gene expression of four proinflammatory cytokines, namely, tumor necrosis factor-alpha (TNF-α), interleukin-6 (IL-6), interleukin-8 (IL-8), and interleukin-1α (IL-1α), as well as the gene expression of nitric oxide synthase (NOS) endothelin-1 (ET-1) and endothelin-converting enzyme-1 (ECE-1). It was found that hyperglycemia-induced oxidative stress was significantly suppressed by anthocyanin-rich sour cherry extract in a concentration-dependent manner. The gene expression of the tested proinflammatory cytokines increased under hyperglycemic conditions but was significantly reduced by both 1 and 50 ng/µL anthocyanin-rich sour cherry extract. Further, although increased ET-1 and ECE-1 expression due to hyperglycemia was reduced by anthocyanin-rich sour cherry extract, NOS expression was increased by the extract. Collectively, these data suggest that anthocyanin-rich sour cherry extract could alleviate hyperglycemia-induced endothelial dysfunction due to its antioxidant, anti-inflammatory, and vasorelaxant effects.

Keywords: hyperglycemia; anthocyanins; endothelial dysfunction; vasodilation

1. Introduction

Life expectancy has increased as a result of novel scientific and technological advances and a decline in poverty, which has facilitated a reduction of communicable diseases [1]. This has shifted the attention of the medical community to treatment of noncommunicable, or chronic, conditions, such as diabetes mellitus (DM). Diabetes mellitus is one of the most common disorders in older adults. In old age (≥60–65 years), DM exhibits higher prevalence than in younger people, posing a serious public health problem in both developed and developing countries [2].

Diabetes mellitus is a condition characterized by persistent hyperglycemia in the blood. Cases of diabetes can be largely classified into two types. In type 1 diabetes (T1D), the cause is an absolute deficiency of insulin secretion due to an autoimmune-mediated response. Type 2 diabetes (T2D), which is much more prevalent in the elderly, is caused by a combination of resistance to insulin action and insufficient compensatory insulin secretory response [3]. Although the progression of diabetes and the emergence of complications have been extensively studied, the molecular mechanisms have not yet been fully elucidated [4]. Nevertheless, there is common agreement that microvascular damage is a key early event in the development of many diabetic complications [5]. The microvascular endothelium is thought to be a major target of hyperglycemic damage as endothelial cells take up glucose passively in an insulin-independent manner and cannot downregulate the glucose transport rate when glucose concentration is elevated, resulting in intracellular hyperglycemia, which significantly affects endothelial cell biology [5].

Hyperglycemia causes tissue damage through four major mechanisms: increased intracellular formation of advanced glycation end products (AGEs), activation of protein kinase C (PKC) isoforms, increased flux of polyol, and via the hexosamine pathway. The collective intensification of these pathways results in a single upstream event: mitochondrial overproduction of reactive oxygen species (ROS) [6]. This consequence of intracellular hyperglycemia contributes to degeneration of microvasculature and leads to progression of diabetic complications [5].

The close relationship between oxidative stress and inflammation has been extensively studied and well documented [7]. Persistent hyperglycemia triggers expression of various proinflammatory cytokines and chemokines, including interleukin-6 (IL-6), interleukin-8 (IL-8), interleukin-1α (IL-1α), and tumor necrosis factor-alpha (TNF-α, which in turn leads to an increase in the inflammatory response. Hyperglycemia-induced inflammation, in synergy with oxidative stress, plays a key role in the pathogenesis of vascular complication of diabetes [8].

The endothelial dysfunction caused by hyperglycemia and consequent inflammation as well as oxidative stress is characterized by impaired endothelium-dependent vasodilation. Several studies have demonstrated that an imbalance of mediators of endothelium-dependent vasodilation is eventuated in hyperglycemic conditions [9]. Amongst the major factors that regulate vasodilation are nitric oxide (NO) and endothelin (ET)-1 [10]. NO is a potent vasodilator produced by nitric oxide synthase (NOS) from the amino acid precursor L-arginine. ET-1 is a locally acting vasoconstrictor produced in endothelial cells by endothelin-converting enzyme (ECE)-1 [11]. Several studies have demonstrated that NO-mediated vasodilation is abnormal in patients with T2D [12]. Increased circulating levels of ET-1 have been found in patients with diabetes [13]. NOS is downregulated while endothelin-1 expression is increased in hyperglycemic conditions [14].

Epidemiological studies have indicated an inverse association between fruit and vegetable intake and the risk of DM. Several dietary patterns consisting of combinations of different foods or food groups are beneficial for diabetes management [15]. Proper nutrition and diet are important factors in the prevention and management of DM. A recent study highlighted the effect of anthocyanin-rich foods or extracts on vascular function in adults [16].

Anthocyanins are nutrients that belong to polyphenols and are mainly found in dark fruits and vegetables [17]. Anthocyanins are polyhydroxy or polymethoxy derivatives of 2-phenylbenzophyryllium in terms of their chemical structure. A phenolic compound consists of two aromatic rings (A and B rings) linked by a three-carbon chain that forms an oxygenated heterocyclic ring (C ring) [18]. Anthocyanins are able to exert, inter alia, antidiabetic effects. In vitro, in vivo, and a few clinical studies have suggested that dietary anthocyanins could ameliorate insulin resistance and offer health benefits in diabetic conditions [19–21].

Interestingly, the molecular mechanisms mentioned above, including excessive ROS production, increased expression of proinflammatory cytokines, and deterioration of vasorelaxant function, can have severe consequences in old age, regardless of diabetes. Vascular aging is a key process affecting the health status of the aged population [22].

In this study, the effect of anthocyanin-rich sour cherry extract was investigated on hyperglycemia-induced inflammatory response, oxidative stress, and impaired endothelium-dependent vasodilation using a culture of human umbilical vein endothelial cells (HUVECs) in order to obtain information on the possible beneficial effect of anthocyanin-rich sour cherry extract. The results may highlight the importance of a diversified diet for healthy aging, especially with regard to cherry consumption.

2. Material and Methods

2.1. Materials

Purified anthocyanin-rich sour cherry extract was prepared by solid-phase extraction procedure following an established protocol [23]. Glucose was purchased from Biosera (Biosera, Nuaille, France).

2.2. Methods

2.2.1. Isolation and Cell Culturing

The HUVECs originated from human umbilical cords that were collected from normal-term placenta and obtained from the Department of Obstetrics and Gynecology, Clinical Centre, University of Debrecen, Debrecen, Hungary. HUVECs were maintained according to the method previously described [24]. Cells were cultured in M199 medium (Biosera, Nuaille, France) supplemented with 10% (v/v) fetal bovine serum (Biosera, Nuaille, France), 10% (v/v) endothelial cell growth (EGM)-2 complex medium (Lonza, Basel, Switzerland), 1.2% (v/v) 2 mM glutamine (1:500; Biosera, Nuaille, France) 1.2% (v/v) 1X penicillin/streptomycin (Biosera, Nuaille, France), 1.2% (v/v) 1X penicillin/streptomycin (Biosera, Nuaille, France), and 1% amphotericin B. Cells were subcultured at 80–100% confluence and incubated at 37 °C with 5% CO_2 level.

2.2.2. Determination of Cellular Viability

MTT Assay

The viability of HUVECs was determined by 3-(4,5-dimethylthiazol-2-yl)-2,5 diphenyltetrazolium bromide (MTT) assay (Duchefa Biochemie, Haarlem, the Netherlands). Cells were plated in 96-well plates (15,000 cells/well) in quadruplicate and treated as indicated. Cells were then incubated with 0.5 mg/mL MTT reagent for 3 h. The formazan crystals were dissolved in 100 µL solubilizing solution (81% (v/v) isopropyl alcohol (Serva, Heidelberg, Germany), 9% (v/v) 1 M HCl (Serva, Heidelberg, Germany), and 10% (v/v) Triton X-100 (Serva, Heidelberg, Germany)) and determined colorimetrically at 465 nm using a Clariostar microplate reader (BMG Labtech, Ortenberg, Germany). The results are expressed as a percentage of vehicle control, regarded as 100%.

Nile Red Assay

For quantitative measurement of polar lipid content of HUVECs, 1 µg/mL Nile Red (Sigma-Aldrich, St. Louis, MO, USA) was used. Cells were cultured in black 96-well plates (15,000 cells/well) in quadruplicate and treated as indicated. The plates were then incubated at 37 °C for 30 min, and fluorescence was measured (485 nm excitation and 565 nm emission wavelengths) using a Clariostar microplate reader (BMG Labtech, Ortenberg, Germany). The results are expressed as a percentage of vehicle control, regarded as 100%.

Determination of Apoptosis

One of the earliest markers of apoptosis is the decrease in mitochondrial membrane potential. The membrane potential of HUVECs was determined using $DilC_1(5)$ fluorescence dye (ENZO, Farmingdale, NY, USA). Cells were seeded into 96-well plates (15,000 cells/well) in quadruplicate and treated as indicated. After removal of the medium, cells were incubated for 30 min with $DilC_1(5)$ solution and then washed with PBS. The fluorescence intensity of $DilC_1(5)$ was measured at 630 nm excitation and 670 nm emission wavelengths using a Clariostar microplate reader (BMG Labtech, Ortenberg, Germany). The results are expressed as a percentage of vehicle control, regarded as 100%.

Determination of Necrosis

Necrotic processes were determined by SYTOX Green staining (Thermo Fisher Scientific, Waltham, MA, USA). Cells were plated into 96-well plates (15,000 cells/well) in quadruplicate and treated as indicated. After the removal of medium, HUVECs were incubated for 30 min with 1 µM SYTOX Green solution. Following incubation, cells were washed with phosphate-buffered saline (PBS), and the fluorescence intensity of SYTOX Green was measured at 490 nm excitation and 520 nm emission wavelengths using a Clariostar microplate reader (BMG Labtech, Ortenberg, Germany). The results are expressed as a percentage of vehicle control, regarded as 100%.

Determination of Level of ROS

Production of ROS by HUVECs was determined by 2′,7′-dichlorofluorescin diacetate (DCFDA) staining (Sigma-Aldrich, St. Louis, MO, USA). Cells were seeded into 24-well plates (100,000 cells/well) in quadruplicate. To label intracellular ROS, cells were incubated with 100 µM DCFDA solution. After 1 h of incubation, cells were washed with PBS and treated as indicated. The fluorescence intensity (excitation = 485 nm; emission = 530 nm) of DCFDA was measured using a Clariostar microplate reader (BMG Labtech, Ortenberg, Germany). The results are expressed as a percentage of vehicle control, regarded as 100%.

Gene Expression Studies by qPCR

qPCR was performed on a Roche LightCycler 480 System (Roche, Basel, Switzerland) using the 5′ nuclease assay. Total RNA was isolated using Extrazole (Blirt, Gdansk, Poland). One microgram of total RNA was reverse transcribed into cDNA using a LunaScript RT SuperMix kit (PCR Biosystems, London, UK). Amplification was performed using the Luna Universal Probe qPCR Master Mix (PCR Biosystems, London, UK). Glyceraldehyde-3-phosphate dehydrogenase (GAPDH) was determined as internal control. The results are expressed relative to 100% for the control group.

Statistical Analysis

Data were analyzed and presented by GraphPad Prism 8.3.1 (GraphPad Software, La Jolla, CA, USA). For multiple comparisons, results were analyzed by ANOVA followed by modified *t*-test for repeated measures according to Bonferroni's method. The data are presented as mean ± SEM (in the case of PCR analysis, results are presented as mean ± SD).

2.3. Ethics

The study was conducted in accordance with the Declaration of Helsinki, and the protocol was approved by the ethics committee of the University of Debrecen (registration number RKEB/IKEB 3712-2012).

3. Results

3.1. Preliminarily Experiments

The main anthocyanin components of sour cherry are cyanidin-3-rutinoside, cyanidin-3-o-glucoside, and cyanidin-3-o-glucosil-rutinoside based on our preliminarily chromatographic analysis [23].

Isolated HUVECs were characterized to positive and negative marker expression using flow cytometry, a method that was routinely used in our recent HUVEC-oriented studies [25].

The optimal concentration of anthocyanin-rich sour cherry extract was decided based on MTT, apoptosis, and necrosis assays [25].

3.2. Effect of Anthocyanin-Rich Sour Cherry Extract on the Viability of HUVECs Maintained in a Hyperglycemic State

Based on the optimal anthocyanin-rich sour cherry extract concentration determined as described above and in a recent study [26] discussing the absorption of anthocyanins and flavanones in humans, we selected anthocyanin-rich sour cherry extract at 1 and 50 ng/µL for further experiments. To investigate the combined effect of the hyperglycemic environment and anthocyanin-rich sour cherry extract, HUVECs were maintained at high glucose levels and treated with anthocyanin-rich sour cherry extract as indicated. Our experiments with MTT assay showed that the combined use of anthocyanin-rich sour cherry extract and high glucose concentration did not significantly reduce cell viability, even after 48 h treatment (Figure 1A). This was also tested using the Nile Red assay, and the same result was observed. While MTT determines cell viability based on mitochondrial dehydrogenase activity, the fluorescent dye Nile Red determines the relative cell number based on the polar lipid content [27]. The results (Figure 1B) of Nile Red assay showed that the combined use of anthocyanin-rich sour cherry extract and high glucose concentration, in line with the MTT data, did not evoke change in cell viability.

Our results required further verification as the onset of early apoptotic and necrotic processes was certainly not detectable in the experiments used above. For this purpose, we examined early apoptotic processes by $DilC_1(5)$ assay (Figure 1C) and early necrotic processes by SYTOX Green labeling (Figure 1D). Although the initiation of a small necrotic process was observed with high glucose treatment, anthocyanin-rich sour cherry extract was able to prevent this and, when used in combination with high glucose, did not cause either necrosis or apoptosis in our delayed conditions on HUVECs.

These results showed that the combined use of anthocyanin-rich sour cherry extract and high glucose concentration had no cytotoxic effect.

3.3. Anthocyanin-Rich Sour Cherry Extract Exerts a Potent Antioxidant Effect

A study has reported the strong antioxidant effect of anthocyanins [28]. We intended to investigate the potential antioxidant effect of anthocyanin-rich sour cherry extract. To assess the antioxidant capacity of anthocyanin-rich sour cherry extract, the level of ROS was measured in hyperglycemic conditions with or without the extract. As expected, high glucose concentrations resulted in elevated ROS levels in our HUVECs model. Anthocyanin-rich sour cherry extract was able to eliminate this increment (Figure 2), indicating the potent antioxidant effect of the extract.

3.4. Anthocyanin-Rich Sour Cherry Extract Reduces Gene Expression of Proinflammatory Cytokines

Numerous studies have shown a strong association between persistent hyperglycemia and inflammation. Increased secretion of proinflammatory cytokines is a manifestation of hyperglycemia-induced inflammatory processes [7]. In order to obtain insight into the inflammatory processes induced by hyperglycemia, we examined the expression levels of four proinflammatory cytokines, namely, TNF-α, IL-6, IL-8, and IL-1α, under hyperglycemic conditions with or without anthocyanin-rich sour cherry extract. First, these genes were examined after 48 h of incubation, when ROS production was the most obvious in our experimental setup. No significant change in the expression of proinflammatory cytokines was observed at this sampling time. Therefore, we assessed whether a differential expression occurred long-term by evaluating the expression after seven days. After seven days, high glucose concentration significantly increased the expression of the previously mentioned proinflammatory cytokines compared to the untreated control maintained at normal glucose levels (Figure 3). Anthocyanin-rich sour cherry extract was able to significantly suppress this effect at both 1 and 50 ng/µL concentrations, except for the case of TNF-α (Figure 3A), which was decreased significantly by 1 ng/µL concentration of anthocyanin-rich sour cherry extract.

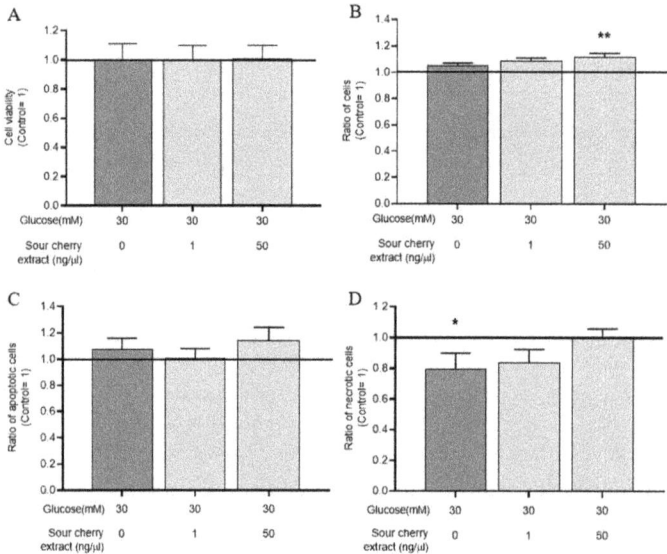

Figure 1. Combined use of anthocyanin-rich sour cherry extract and high glucose does not influence viability of human umbilical cord vein endothelial cells (HUVECs). Viability of HUVECs was monitored following 48 h treatment by 3-(4,5-dimethylthiazol-2-yl)-2,5 diphenyltetrazolium bromide (MTT) (**A**) and Nile Red (**B**) assays. Early necrotic and apoptotic processes of HUVECs were monitored following 48 h treatment by DilC1(5) (**C**) and SYTOX Green (**D**) assays. Results are expressed as percentage of untreated control (100%, solid line), with normoglycemia (5 mM) as mean ± SEM of four independent determinations. * and ** mark significant ($p < 0.05$ and $p < 0.01$, respectively) differences compared to the vehicle control group.

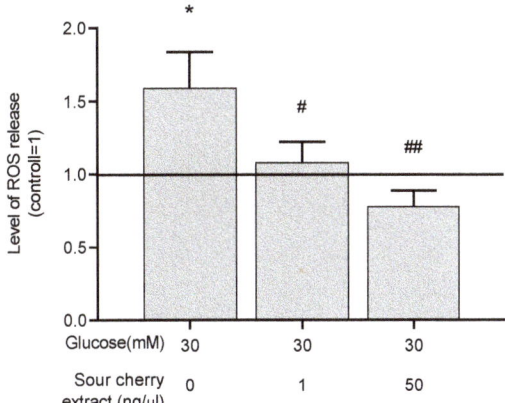

Figure 2. Anthocyanin-rich sour cherry extract decreases production of reactive oxygen species (ROS) under hyperglycemic condition. Production of ROS by HUVECs was monitored following 48 h treatment by 2′,7′-dichlorofluorescin diacetate (DCFDA) staining. Results are expressed as the percentage of untreated control (100%, solid line) with normoglycemia (5 mM) as mean ± SEM of four independent determinations. * marks a statistically significant difference ($p < 0.05$) compared to the vehicle control group. #, ## marks significant ($p < 0.05$, $p < 0.001$) differences as indicated compared to the untreated control with hyperglycemia (30 mM).

3.5. Anthocyanin-Rich Sour Cherry Extract Enhances Expression of NOS and Decreases Expression of ET-1 and ECE-1

As a result of prolonged and direct contact with the hyperglycemic milieu, the vasorelaxation process is impaired [29]. Deficiency in bioavailable NO is one of the major features of hyperglycemia-induced endothelial dysfunction [30]. Moreover, the biosynthesis of certain vasoconstrictors, such as ET-1, is increased. Given the increase in the inflammatory response of cells exposed to persistent hyperglycemia (seven days), we investigated the expression levels of proteins that play a key role in endothelial cell vasorelaxation processes. Because a substantial inflammatory effect could only be elicited following seven days of treatment, the effect of high glucose levels on vasorelaxation was examined at this time. HUVECs treated at a concentration of 30 mM glucose significantly increased the gene expression of ET-1 (Figure 4A) as well as the expression of ECE-1 (Figure 4B), which produces its active form. Anthocyanin-rich sour cherry extract was able to significantly reduce the hyperglycemia-induced enhanced gene expression of ET-1 (Figure 4A) and ECE-1 (Figure 4B).

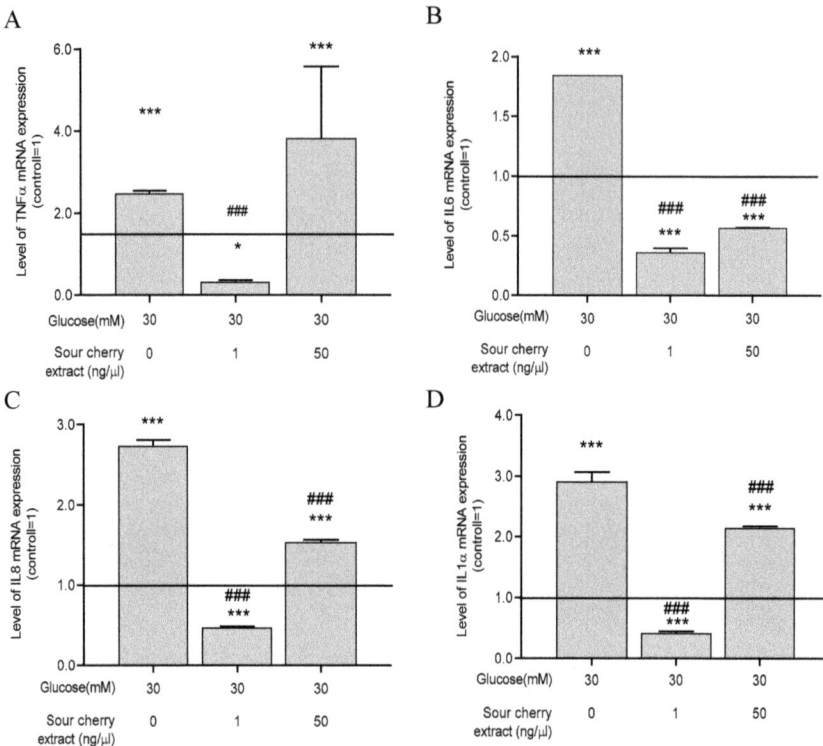

Figure 3. The anti-inflammatory action of anthocyanin-rich sour cherry extract. qPCR analyses of gene expression of tumor necrosis factor-alpha (TNF-α) (**A**), interleukin-6 (IL-6) (**B**), interleukin-8 (IL-8) (**C**), and interleukin-1α (IL-1α) (**D**) on HUVECs following the indicated seven days of simultaneous treatment. Data are presented using the ΔΔCT method regarding glyceraldehyde-3-phosphate dehydrogenase (GAPDH)-normalized mRNA expressions of the untreated control (100%, solid line) with normoglycemia (5 mM) mean ± SD of two independent determinations. * and *** mark significant ($p < 0.05$ and $p < 0.001$, respectively) differences as indicated compared to the untreated control with normoglycemia (5 mM). ### marks significant ($p < 0.001$) differences as indicated compared to the untreated control with hyperglycemia (30 mM).

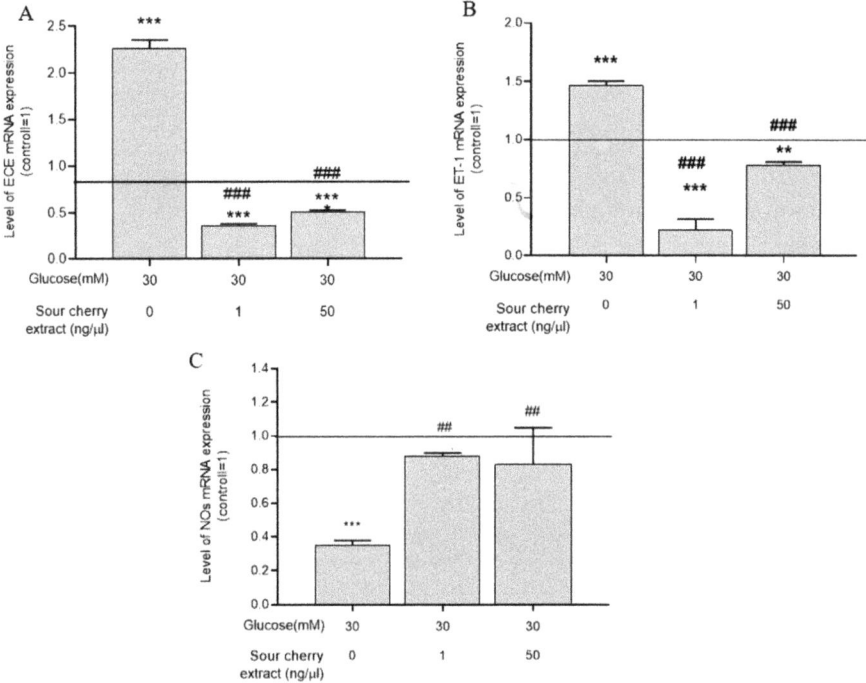

Figure 4. Vasorelaxant effect of anthocyanin-rich sour cherry extract. qPCR analyses of gene expression of endothelin-converting enzyme-1 (ECE-1) (**A**), endothelin-1 (ET-1) (**B**), and nitric oxide synthase (NOS) (**C**) on HUVECs following the indicated seven days of simultaneous treatment. Data are presented using the ΔΔCT method regarding GAPDH-normalized mRNA expressions of the untreated control (100%, solid line) with normoglycemia (5 mm) mean ± SD of two independent determinations. ** and *** mark significant ($p < 0.01$ and $p < 0.001$, respectively) differences as indicated compared to the untreated control with normoglycemia (5 mM). ## and ### mark significant ($p < 0.01$ and $p < 0.001$, respectively) differences as indicated compared to the untreated control with hyperglycemia (30 mM).

In parallel, the expression of NOS, which is responsible for vasodilation, was significantly decreased. Anthocyanin-rich sour cherry extract was able to increase the gene expression of NOS.

4. Discussion

In our current experimental design, hyperglycemia-induced endothelial dysfunction was investigated. Before evaluating hyperglycemia-induced endothelial changes, we examined the combined effect of the hyperglycemic environment and anthocyanin-rich cherry extract. To monitor the negative effects of possible cross reactions, the viability of HUVECs was assessed. The combined use of anthocyanin-rich cherry extract and high glucose concentration did not show a cytotoxic effect, even after 48 h. We further examined hyperglycemia-induced endothelial changes by evaluating inflammatory response, oxidative stress, and damaged endothelium-dependent vasodilation. Anthocyanin-rich sour cherry extract was able to eliminate, in a concentration-dependent manner, hyperglycemia-induced ROS production in HUVECs, thereby alleviating oxidative stress. The investigated extract also alleviated hyperglycemia-induced increased expression of proinflammatory cytokines, indicating its immunomodulatory effects. Furthermore, hyperglycemia-induced impaired vasodilation processes were studied. The extract was able to improve endothelium-dependent vasorelaxation in hyperglycemic environments, pointing to its possible vasorelaxant effects.

Hyperglycemia-induced tissue damage and consequent oxidative stress and inflammatory processes, forming a vicious circle, play a pivotal role in the pathogenesis of the vascular complication of T2D [12]. The radical scavenging capacity of anthocyanins has been described in several studies [17,31,32]. Consistent with these studies, the investigated extract has a potent antioxidant effect. However, anthocyanin-rich sour cherry extract at a concentration of 50 ng/μL also significantly reduced ROS compared to the normoglycemia. Increased presence of antioxidants can also result in adverse effects [33]. Therefore, in further experiments, an upper limit should be determined that does not yet cause the phenomenon of antioxidant loading.

To obtain more comprehensive details about the inflammatory processes caused by hyperglycemia, we examined the expression of TNF-α, IL-6, IL-8, and IL-1α. By detecting changes in the gene expression level of our chosen cytokines, the state of the inflammatory profile of cells caused by hyperglycemia can be inferred relatively accurately. While IL-6 is involved in T cell differentiation and B cell stimulation and plays a central role in activating and maintaining inflammatory response, IL-8 is involved in the chemotaxis of neutrophil granulocytes. IL-1α is one of the strongest indicators of immune response to oxidative stress. TNF-α is the central coordinator in mediating cell survival and inflammatory response [34]. Anthocyanin-rich sour cherry extract was able to reduce hyperglycemia-induced overexpression of the investigated genes. Interestingly, lower concentration of anthocyanin-rich sour cherry extract elicited a stronger suppressive effect compared to higher concentration. Although no precise explanation can be given for this, it can be concluded from the literature that some flavonoids are able to activate some receptors at low concentrations, while they exert a desensitizing effect at high concentrations [35]. We assume that increased expression of TNF-α upon treatment at a concentration of 50 ng/μL is the result of this desensitizing effect. To clarify this issue, the signaling pathways of the TNF-α receptor with different concentrations of anthocyanin-rich sour cherry extract should be investigated. Considering our results are limited to PCR assays, further studies are needed in which the signaling pathways of the TNF-α receptor are investigated using Western blot analysis or in-cell ELISA. Moreover, as the extract at a concentration of 50 ng/μL had higher antioxidant capacity but lower immunomodulatory activity compared to 1 ng/μL, the positive effect of anthocyanin-rich sour cherry extract is not only and exclusively due to its antioxidant capacity.

Under hyperglycemic conditions, endothelium-dependent vasorelaxation processes are impaired [36]. One of the main hallmarks of hyperglycemia-induced endothelial dysfunction is the decrease of bioavailable NO [37]. Anthocyanins have been reported to increase the expression of NOS and decrease the expression of various genes responsible for vasoconstriction, including ET-1 [38]. Therefore, we examined the effect of anthocyanin-rich extract on the expression of NO synthase and ET-1 as well as the enzyme producing its active form under hyperglycemic conditions. Our results showed that anthocyanin-rich sour cherry extract was able to improve hyperglycemia-induced damage by enhancing endothelium-dependent vasodilation.

Collectively, in this study, we examined the effect of anthocyanin-rich extract of Hungarian sour cherry on hyperglycemia-induced endothelial dysfunction. The investigated extract has a strong immunomodulatory, antioxidative, and potent vasorelaxant effect. Although further investigations are needed to elucidate the mechanisms of action, our results suggest that Hungarian sour cherry, which is rich in anthocyanins, may have therapeutic potential in diseases associated with endothelial dysfunction, including T2D. Sour cherry can be a component of a diet that supports the prevention and treatment of T2D.

Author Contributions: J.R., A.M. and A.B. conceived and designed the experiments. A.M., A.B., M.É.F., A.A.R. and M.P. performed the experiments. A.M., A.B., A.K.-N., L.S. and J.L. analyzed the data. A.M., A.B. and J.R. wrote the paper. All authors have read and agreed to the published version of the manuscript.

Funding: This research received no external funding.

Acknowledgments: The work is supported by the GINOP-2.2.1-15-2017-00079 project. This project is cofinanced by the European Union and the European Social Fund. The authors would like to acknowledge the help of the Hungarian Academy of Sciences—University of Debrecen (HAS-UD) Vascular Biology and Myocardial Pathophysiology Research Group, Faculty of Medicine, Nephrology Division, Debrecen, Hungary—for the human umbilical vein endothelial cell isolation.

Conflicts of Interest: The authors declare no conflict of interest.

References

1. WHO Director-General Addresses US Department of Health and Human Services. Available online: https://www.who.int/dg/speeches/detail/who-director-general-addresses-us-department-of-health-and-human-services (accessed on 25 August 2020).
2. International Diabetes Federation—Facts & Figures. Available online: https://idf.org/aboutdiabetes/what-is-diabetes/factsfigures.html?fbclid=IwAR38xQdGZ6WrThzPIwgmfTZrmyN9lXvKEITWYWji0M3Q12ZvhAoPt1yMoc0 (accessed on 25 August 2020).
3. American Diabetes Association. Diagnosis and classification of diabetes mellitus. *Diabetes Care* **2010**, *33*, S62–S69. [CrossRef] [PubMed]
4. Tan, S.Y.; Mei Wong, J.L.; Sim, Y.J.; Wong, S.S.; Mohamed Elhassan, S.A.; Tan, S.H.; Ling Lim, G.P.; Rong Tay, N.W.; Annan, N.C.; Bhattamisra, S.K.; et al. Type 1 and 2 diabetes mellitus: A review on current treatment approach and gene therapy as potential intervention. *Diabetes Metab. Syndr.* **2019**, *13*, 364–372. [CrossRef] [PubMed]
5. Kibel, A.; Selthofer-Relatic, K.; Drenjancevic, I.; Bacun, T.; Bosnjak, I.; Kibel, D.; Gros, M. Coronary microvascular dysfunction in diabetes mellitus. *J. Int. Med. Res.* **2017**, *45*, 1901–1929. [CrossRef] [PubMed]
6. Brownlee, M. The pathobiology of diabetic complications: A unifying mechanism. *Diabetes* **2005**, *54*, 1615–1625. [CrossRef] [PubMed]
7. Hussain, T.; Tan, B.; Yin, Y.; Blachier, F.; Tossou, M.C.B.; Rahu, N. Oxidative stress and inflammation: What polyphenols can do for us? *Oxidative Med. Cell. Longev.* **2016**, *2016*, 7432797. [CrossRef] [PubMed]
8. Suryavanshi, S.V.; Kulkarni, Y.A. NF-κβ: A potential target in the management of vascular complications of diabetes. *Front. Pharmacol.* **2017**, *8*, 798. [CrossRef] [PubMed]
9. Yada, T.; Shimokawa, H.; Tachibana, H. Endothelium-dependent hyperpolarization-mediated vasodilatation compensates nitric oxide-mediated endothelial dysfunction during ischemia in diabetes-induced canine coronary collateral microcirculation in vivo. *Microcirculation* **2018**, *25*, e12456. [CrossRef]
10. Rapoport, R. Acute nitric oxide synthase inhibition and endothelin-1-dependent arterial pressure elevation. *Front. Pharmacol.* **2014**, *5*, 5. [CrossRef]
11. Ortmann, J.; Nett, P.C.; Celeiro, J.; Traupe, T.; Tornillo, L.; Hofmann-Lehmann, R.; Haas, E.; Frank, B.; Terraciano, L.M.; Barton, M. Endothelin inhibition delays onset of hyperglycemia and associated vascular injury in type I diabetes: Evidence for endothelin release by pancreatic islet β-cells. *Biochem. Biophys. Res. Commun.* **2005**, *334*, 689–695. [CrossRef]
12. Hadi, H.A.; Suwaidi, J.A. Endothelial dysfunction in diabetes mellitus. *Vasc. Health Risk Manag.* **2007**, *3*, 853–876.
13. Kalani, M. The importance of endothelin-1 for microvascular dysfunction in diabetes. *Vasc. Health Risk Manag.* **2008**, *4*, 1061–1068. [CrossRef] [PubMed]
14. Matsumoto, T.; Yoshiyama, S.; Kobayashi, T.; Kamata, K. Mechanisms underlying enhanced contractile response to endothelin-1 in diabetic rat basilar artery. *Peptides* **2004**, *25*, 1985–1994. [CrossRef]
15. Czemplik, M.; Kulma, A.; Wang, Y.F.; Szopa, J. Therapeutic strategies of plant-derived compounds for diabetes via regulation of monocyte chemoattractant protein-1. *Curr. Med. Chem.* **2017**, *24*, 1453–1468. [CrossRef] [PubMed]
16. Fairlie-Jones, L.; Davison, K.; Fromentin, E.; Hill, A.M. The effect of anthocyanin-rich foods or extracts on vascular function in adults: A systematic review and meta-analysis of randomised controlled trials. *Nutrients* **2017**, *9*, 908. [CrossRef]
17. Khoo, H.E.; Azlan, A.; Tang, S.T.; Lim, S.M. Anthocyanidins and anthocyanins: Colored pigments as food, pharmaceutical ingredients, and the potential health benefits. *Food Nutr. Res.* **2017**, *61*, 1361779. [CrossRef] [PubMed]

18. Reyes, B.A.S.; Dufourt, E.C.; Ross, J.; Warner, M.J.; Tanquilut, N.C.; Leung, A.B. Chapter 4—Selected phyto and marine bioactive compounds: Alternatives for the treatment of type 2 diabetes. In *Studies in Natural Products Chemistry*; Rahman, A.-U., Ed.; Elsevier: Amsterdam, The Netherlands, 2018; Volume 55, pp. 111–143.
19. Wojdyło, A.; Nowicka, P.; Carbonell-Barrachina, Á.A.; Hernández, F. Phenolic compounds, antioxidant and antidiabetic activity of different cultivars of *Ficus carica* L. fruits. *J. Funct. Foods* **2016**, *25*, 421–432. [CrossRef]
20. Nizamutdinova, I.T.; Jin, Y.C.; Chung, J.I.; Shin, S.C.; Lee, S.J.; Seo, H.G.; Lee, J.H.; Chang, K.C.; Kim, H.J. The anti-diabetic effect of anthocyanins in streptozotocin-induced diabetic rats through glucose transporter 4 regulation and prevention of insulin resistance and pancreatic apoptosis. *Mol. Nutr. Food Res.* **2009**, *53*, 1419–1429. [CrossRef]
21. Stull, A.J.; Cash, K.C.; Johnson, W.D.; Champagne, C.M.; Cefalu, W.T. Bioactives in blueberries improve insulin sensitivity in obese, insulin-resistant men and women. *J. Nutr.* **2010**, *140*, 1764–1768. [CrossRef]
22. El Assar, M.; Angulo, J.; Vallejo, S.; Peiró, C.; Sánchez-Ferrer, C.F.; Rodríguez-Mañas, L. Mechanisms involved in the aging-induced vascular dysfunction. *Front. Physiol.* **2012**, *3*, 132. [CrossRef]
23. Nemes, A.; Szőllősi, E.; Stündl, L.; Biró, A.; Homoki, J.R.; Szarvas, M.M.; Balogh, P.; Cziáky, Z.; Remenyik, J. Determination of flavonoid and proanthocyanidin profile of Hungarian sour cherry. *Molecules* **2018**, *23*, 3278. [CrossRef]
24. Biró, A.; Markovics, A.; Fazekas, M.É.; Fidler, G.; Szalóki, G.; Paholcsek, M.; Lukács, J.; Stündl, L.; Remenyik, J. Allithiamine alleviates hyperglycaemia-induced endothelial dysfunction. *Nutrients* **2020**, *12*, 1690. [CrossRef]
25. Biro, A.; Markovich, A.; Homoki, J.R.; Szőllősi, E.; Hegedűs, C.; Tarapcsák, S.; Lukács, J.; Stündl, L.; Remenyik, J. Anthocyanin-rich sour cherry extract attenuates the lipopolysaccharide-induced endothelial inflammatory response. *Molecules* **2019**, *24*, 3427. [CrossRef]
26. Kay, C.D.; Pereira-Caro, G.; Ludwig, I.A.; Clifford, M.N.; Crozier, A. Anthocyanins and flavanones are more bioavailable than previously perceived: A review of recent evidence. *Annu. Rev. Food Sci. Technol.* **2017**, *8*, 155–180. [CrossRef]
27. Oláh, A.; Markovics, A.; Szabó-Papp, J.; Szabó, P.T.; Stott, C.; Zouboulis, C.C.; Bíró, T. Differential effectiveness of selected non-psychotropic phytocannabinoids on human sebocyte functions implicates their introduction in dry/seborrhoeic skin and acne treatment. *Exp. Dermatol.* **2016**, *25*, 701–707. [CrossRef]
28. Cásedas, G.; Les, F.; Gómez-Serranillos, M.P.; Smith, C.; López, V. Anthocyanin profile, antioxidant activity and enzyme inhibiting properties of blueberry and cranberry juices: A comparative study. *Food Funct.* **2017**, *8*, 4187–4193. [CrossRef]
29. Kaur, R.; Kaur, M.; Singh, J. Endothelial dysfunction and platelet hyperactivity in type 2 diabetes mellitus: Molecular insights and therapeutic strategies. *Cardiovasc. Diabetol.* **2018**, *17*, 1–17. [CrossRef]
30. Shi, Y.; Vanhoutte, P.M. Macro-and microvascular endothelial dysfunction in diabetes. *J. Diabetes* **2017**, *9*, 434–449. [CrossRef]
31. Szymanowska, U.; Baraniak, B. Antioxidant and potentially anti-inflammatory activity of anthocyanin fractions from pomace obtained from enzymatically treated raspberries. *Antioxidants* **2019**, *8*, 299. [CrossRef]
32. Kähkönen, M.P.; Heinonen, M. Antioxidant activity of anthocyanins and their aglycons. *J. Agric. Food Chem.* **2003**, *51*, 628–633. [CrossRef]
33. Salehi, B.; Martorell, M.; Arbiser, J.L.; Sureda, A.; Martins, N.; Maurya, P.K.; Sharifi-Rad, M.; Kumar, P.; Sharifi-Rad, J. Antioxidants: Positive or negative actors? *Biomolecules* **2018**, *8*, 124. [CrossRef] [PubMed]
34. Kany, S.; Vollrath, J.T.; Relja, B. Cytokines in inflammatory disease. *Int. J. Mol. Sci.* **2019**, *20*, 6008. [CrossRef]
35. Warner, E.F.; Smith, M.J.; Zhang, Q.; Raheem, K.S.; O'Hagan, D.; O'Connell, M.A.; Kay, C.D. Signatures of anthocyanin metabolites identified in humans inhibit biomarkers of vascular inflammation in human endothelial cells. *Mol. Nutr. Food Res.* **2017**, *61*. [CrossRef] [PubMed]
36. Brouwers, O.; Niessen, P.M.; Haenen, G.; Miyata, T.; Brownlee, M.; Stehouwer, C.D.; De Mey, J.G.; Schalkwijk, C.G. Hyperglycaemia-induced impairment of endothelium-dependent vasorelaxation in rat mesenteric arteries is mediated by intracellular methylglyoxal levels in a pathway dependent on oxidative stress. *Diabetologia* **2010**, *53*, 989–1000. [CrossRef]

37. Tessari, P.; Cecchet, D.; Cosma, A.; Vettore, M.; Coracina, A.; Millioni, R.; Iori, E.; Puricelli, L.; Avogaro, A.; Vedovato, M. Nitric oxide synthesis is reduced in subjects with type 2 diabetes and nephropathy. *Diabetes* **2010**, *59*, 2152–2159. [CrossRef] [PubMed]
38. Lazzè, M.C.; Pizzala, R.; Perucca, P.; Cazzalini, O.; Savio, M.; Forti, L.; Vannini, V.; Bianchi, L. Anthocyanidins decrease endothelin-1 production and increase endothelial nitric oxide synthase in human endothelial cells. *Mol. Nutr. Food Res.* **2006**, *50*, 44–51. [CrossRef] [PubMed]

Publisher's Note: MDPI stays neutral with regard to jurisdictional claims in published maps and institutional affiliations.

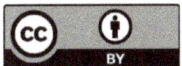 © 2020 by the authors. Licensee MDPI, Basel, Switzerland. This article is an open access article distributed under the terms and conditions of the Creative Commons Attribution (CC BY) license (http://creativecommons.org/licenses/by/4.0/).

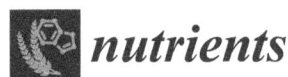

Article

Association between Intake of Energy and Macronutrients and Memory Impairment Severity in US Older Adults, National Health and Nutrition Examination Survey 2011–2014

Qinran Liu [1,†], Jianjun Guo [2,*,†], Liang Hu [3], Nicola Veronese [4], Lee Smith [5], Lin Yang [6,7] and Chao Cao [8]

1. Department of Public Health Sciences, University of Miami Miller School of Medicine, Miami, FL 33136, USA; liu.q@miami.edu
2. Sports and Medicine Integration Center, Capital University of Physical Education and Sports, Beijing 100191, China
3. Department of Sport and Exercise Science, Zhejiang University, Hangzhou 310027, China; lianghu@zju.edu.cn
4. Department of Internal Medicine and Geriatrics, University of Palermo, 90133 Palermo, Italy; ilmannato@gmail.com
5. The Cambridge Centre for Sport and Exercise Sciences, Anglia Ruskin University, Cambridge CB1 1PT, UK; Lee.Smith@anglia.ac.uk
6. Department of Cancer Epidemiology and Prevention Research, Cancer Care Alberta, Alberta Health Services, Calgary, AB T2S 3C3, Canada; lin.yang@albertahealthservices.ca
7. Departments of Oncology and Community Health Sciences, Cumming School of Medicine, University of Calgary, Calgary, AB T2N 4N2, Canada
8. Program in Physical Therapy, Washington University School of Medicine, St Louis, MO 63110, USA; caochao@wustl.edu
* Correspondence: guojianjun@cupes.edu.cn
† Contributed equally and shared first authorship.

Received: 29 October 2020; Accepted: 19 November 2020; Published: 20 November 2020

Abstract: Without a cure, dementia affects about 50 million people worldwide. Understanding the effects of dietary habits, a key lifestyle behavior, on memory impairment is critical to inform early behavioral modification to delay further memory loss and progression to dementia. We examined the associations of total energy intake and energy intake from macronutrients with memory impairment among older US adults using data from the nationally representative National Health and Nutrition Examination Survey study 2011–2014. A total of 3623 participants aged ≥60 years were analyzed. Comparing to those with low total energy intake, individuals with high intake were more likely to have severe memory impairment (OR: 1.52, 95% CI: 1.15 to 2.02; p_{trend} = 0.005). Specifically, higher energy intake from carbohydrate (OR: 1.59, 95% CI: 1.12 to 2.26) and sugar (OR: 1.54, 95% CI: 1.11 to 2.16) were both significantly associated with the presence of memory impairment. Additionally, higher energy intake from fat, carbohydrate and sugar were significantly associated with more server memory impairment (fat: p_{trend} = 0.04; carbohydrate: p_{trend} = 0.03; sugar: p_{trend} = 0.02). High energy intake, either total or from carbohydrates, fat or sugar, is associated with memory impairment severity in the older US population. No such association was found in energy intake from protein.

Keywords: energy intake; memory impairment; carbohydrates; sugar; older adults

1. Introduction

Dementia is a syndrome characterized as deterioration in cognitive function, memory loss, and problems controlling emotions [1]. Worldwide, about 50 million people were diagnosed with dementia and there are nearly 10 million new cases every year [2]. The true burden of dementia is likely to be higher due to the lack of a single diagnostic test for dementia and its subtypes [3]. Alzheimer's disease (AD) is the most common cause of dementia [4], affecting an estimate of 44 million individuals. AD is also the sixth-leading cause of death [5], costing the healthcare system up to $277 billion in the United States in 2018 [6]. Although the disease progression of AD varies from person to person, it is typically associated with a decline in cognitive and functional abilities [7]. Emerging data suggest that memory impairment might be an early sign of AD. Prospective studies found subject memory impairment was commonly reported among individuals years before they developed AD and dementia [8,9]. Even without the presence of dementia, the perception of memory problems is associated with negative outcomes of individual and societal significance. In addition, the severity of memory impairment was negatively associated with quality of life and various health outcomes [10–12]. As there is currently no cure for dementia, developing accessible preventive strategies is an urgent but unmet need [13]. Therefore, it is critical to explore the effects of lifestyle factors including dietary habits on memory impairment, as early behavioral modification may delay further memory loss and disease progression.

The important role of nutrition has been recognized in the prevention of cognitive decline, dementia and AD. Observational studies have identified the protective effects of several dietary components, including antioxidants, n-3 polyunsaturated fatty acids, and B vitamins on cognitive function [14]. A meta-analysis also summarized evidence from longitudinal studies and clinical trials and revealed that higher adherence to healthy eating patterns, such as the Mediterranean diet, was associated with better cognitive function and a lower risk of AD [15,16]. Several randomized clinical trials indicated that well-nourished calorie restriction had a myriad of benefits, including metabolic health, aging-associated biomarkers, and quality of life [17–20], whereas metabolic syndrome negatively impacts cognitive performance and brain structure [21]. However, limited research focuses on the impact of energy intake from each macronutrient (i.e., carbohydrates, protein, fat) on cognitive outcomes. Some observational studies suggested a higher intake of calories was associated with a high risk of developing AD or dementia but reported inconsistent findings on specific energy sources. Specifically, Luchsinger et al. found that a higher intake of calories and fats but not carbohydrates was associated with a higher risk of AD in individuals carrying the apolipoprotein E ϵ 4 [22]. In contrast, Roberts and his colleagues reported caloric intake from carbohydrates and but not fat and protein increased the risk of mild cognitive impairment or dementia [23]. Nevertheless, comprehensive studies are needed to address the effects of total caloric intake and macronutrient intake, on the presence and severity of memory impairment at the population level, as well as within population subgroups defined by several sociodemographic and behavioral factors.

To address these knowledge gaps, we examined the associations of total energy intake and energy intake from carbohydrates, protein, and fat with memory impairment among older US adults using a nationally representative sample.

2. Materials and Methods

2.1. Study Population

The National Health and Nutrition Examination Survey (NHANES) study is a series of cross-sectional nationally representative health examinations conducted by the National Center for Health Statistics. Since 1999, the NHANES collects data using complex, stratified, multistage, clustered samples to estimate the prevalence of the health, nutritional status and potential disease risk factors among the civilian noninstitutionalized US population in 2-year cycles [24]. Each survey participant completed a written informed consent, a household interview, and a physical examination at a Mobile Examination Center

(MEC). We extracted and aggregated data on sociodemographic characteristics, measured weight and height, lifestyle behavior, medical condition among adults aged 65 and older in 2 waves, 2011–2012 and 2013–2014, due to the availability of memory impairment data.

2.2. Assessment of Exposure

The NHANES 24-h dietary recall was developed by the National Cancer Institute (NCI) and provided validated information on the amount in grams of each food and beverage consumed during the 24-h period prior to the interview [25]. Additionally, the NHANE dietary interview component, called What We Eat in American, is conducted as a partnership between the U.S. Department of Agriculture (USDA) and the U.S. Department of Health and Human Services (DHHS). Under this partnership, DHHS' National Center for Health Statistics (NCHS) is responsible for the survey sample design and all aspects of data collection and USDA's Food Surveys. The first interview was conducted in-person by a trained interviewer in the MEC. The 24-h dietary recall is administered using a proxy interview or an interpreter if needed (e.g., participants who cannot recall their dietary information due to cognitive impairment) [25]. Daily total and nutrient specific energy intake (calories) were extracted from foods and beverages documented in the total Nutrient intakes files, including total calorie intake, total intake of carbohydrate, protein, fat, sugar, saturated fatty acid, monounsaturated fatty acid and polyunsaturated fatty acid. Sex-specific tertile categories were applied for each source of energy intake. The Low group was defined as the first tertile, the moderate group was defined as the second tertile category; and the high group was defined as the third tertile category.

2.3. Outcome Measures

Identification of the memory impairment and severity were acquired from the medical condition questionnaire by trained interviewers using the Computer-Assisted Personal Interviewing system [7,26]. Participants were asked "During the past 7 days, how often have you had trouble remembering where you put things like keys or wallet?" The response options included "never", "about once", "two or three times", "nearly every day" and "several times a day". This ordinal variable was used to reflect memory impairment severity. The participants who responded "never" were categorized as no memory impairment, otherwise as to any memory impairment. This measurement was used in the previous literature to evaluate the early sign of memory impairment (Table 1) [7].

Table 1. The Severity of Memory Impairment Using NHANES 2011–2014 Memory Question.

Value Description	Memory Impairment Severity Classification
Never	None
About once	Early-stage
Two or three times	
Nearly every day	Late-stage
Several times a day	

2.4. Socio-Demographic Characteristics and Lifestyle Behaviors

Self-reported sociodemographic characteristics included age, sex, race/ethnicity (non-Hispanic white, non-Hispanic black, Hispanic, and others), family income-to-poverty ratio (<1.3 [lowest income], $1.3 \leq 3.5$, ≥ 3.5 [highest income]), and educational level (less than high school, high school, and above high school) [27,28]. Participants' weight and height were measured during the physical examination following standard procedures. Body mass index (BMI) was calculated as weight in kilograms divided by height in meters squared and categorize into three groups (<25 kg/m^2, 25.0–29.9 kg/m^2, $\geq$30 kg/m^2). Leisure-time physical activity status was defined by engaging in no (inactive) or any (active) moderate or vigorous recreational physical activity over the past 30 days [29]. The Healthy Eating Index-2010 (HEI-2010, derived from 24-h dietary recall interviews). HEI-2010 indicates the overall dietary quality with a score ranged from 0 (worst-quality diet) to 100 (best-quality diet) [30].

2.5. Chronic Condition

Hypertension was determined by participants receiving a diagnosis from a health professional, or NHANES measured blood pressure ≥130 mm Hg systolic or ≥80 mm Hg diastolic [31]. Hypercholesterolemia was determined by participants receiving a diagnosis from a health professional or NHANES measured total cholesterol level ≥6.2 mmol/L (240 mg/dL) [32]. Cardiovascular disease was identified through participants self-reported ever being diagnosed with conditions such as congestive heart failure, angina, heart attack, or coronary heart disease. Participants were considered as having cancer by self-reported having ever been told by a physician that they had such conditions. Diabetes was defined by self-reporting having been told by a physician that they had diabetes or reporting currently taking insulin to treat diabetes [33].

2.6. Statistical Analysis

All analyses followed the NHANES analytical guideline. Survey analysis procedures were used to account for the complex survey design to ensure nationally representative estimates [24]. We conducted a descriptive analysis to assess participants' characteristics according to whether they have memory impairment. Weighted means (standard error) were calculated for continuous variables, and weighted frequency percentages were calculated for categorical variables. The t-test and chi-square tests were conducted to examine the difference across participants' characteristics as appropriate.

Then, the associations between different sources of calorie intake (including total energy intake, energy intake from carbohydrate, protein, fat, total sugar, total saturated fatty acid, total monounsaturated fatty acid and total polyunsaturated fatty acid) and the memory impairment (no vs. any) were assessed using weighted logistic regression, respectively Multivariable logistic regression models were adjusted for age, sex, race/ethnicity, education attainment, and family poverty ratio, physical activity, alcohol intake, BMI, body weight, smoking status, hypertension, hypercholesterolemia, family history of diabetes, history of CVD, and history of cancer. In addition, the associations between energy intake (total and nutrient specific) and memory impairment severity using an ordinal variable ("never", "about once", "two or three times", "nearly every day" and "several times a day") were investigated using multivariable-adjusted ordinal logistic regression models, respectively Only one individual dietary component was included in each regression model.

All statistical analyses were conducted using STATA, version 15.1 (StataCorp, College Station, TX, USA). All statistical significance was set at $p < 0.05$. p values were not adjusted for multiple tests and should be interpreted as exploratory analyses.

3. Results

A total of 3623 participants aged ≥60 years were included in the analysis. Characteristics of the participants are presented according to memory impairment status in Table 2. Of participants, 20.6% and 7.7% have any kind of memory impairment and late-stage memory impairment, respectively. Female participants (24.6%) had higher prevalence of memory impairment compared to males (15.9%) ($p < 0.001$). Non-Hispanic and Hispanic individuals were more likely to have memory impairment compared to non-Hispanic whites and others ($p = 0.001$). The prevalence of memory impairment was significantly higher among participants with CVD history (25.2% vs. 19.3%, $p = 0.008$). Additionally, participants who were physically inactive (22.7%), had lower education level (<high school: 27.2%), and lower poverty ratio (<1.3: 24.8%) were more likely to have memory impairment comparing to participants who were physically active (17.9%) ($p = 0.012$), had higher education level (high school: 22.8%, >high school: 17.7%, $p = 0.001$), and higher poverty ratio (1/3 ≤ 3.5: 21.2%, ≥3.5: 17.4%, $p = 0.015$).

Table 2. Characteristics of the US Adults ≥60 years According to Memory Impairment, NHANES 2011–2014 [a].

	Memory Impairment		p Value
	No	Any	
N	2802	821	
Weighted N	47,243,167	12,303,530	
Age, y	69.2 (0.3)	71.5 (0.4)	<0.001
Sex			
Male	84.1	15.9	<0.001
Female	75.4	24.6	
Race/ethnicity			
Non-Hispanic white	80.1	19.9	
Non-Hispanic black	79.6	20.4	0.001
Hispanic	70.4	29.6	
Other	80.6	19.4	
Family poverty ratio			
<1.3	75.2	24.8	
1.3 ≤ 3.5	78.9	21.2	0.019
≤3.5	82.6	17.4	
Education			
<High school	72.8	27.2	
High school	77.2	22.8	0.001
>High school	82.3	17.7	
Body mass index [b], kg/m^2			
<25	76.1	23.9	
25 ≤ 30	81.0	19.0	0.106
≥30	80.5	19.5	
Leisure-time physical activity [c]			
Inactive	77.3	22.7	0.012
Active	82.1	17.9	
Cardiovascular Disease			
No	80.7	19.3	0.008
Yes	74.8	25.2	
Cancer			
No	79.3	20.7	0.873
Yes	79.6	20.4	
Diabetes			
No	79.8	20.2	0.379
Yes	77.6	22.4	
Healthy Eating Index-2010	58.7 (0.5)	57.9 (0.9)	0.348

[a] All estimates were weighted to be nationally representative. [b] Weight status was defined by body mass index (BMI = weight(kg)/height(m)^2). [c] Leisure-time physical activity level was defined by engaging in no (inactive) or any (active) moderate or vigorous recreational physical activity over the past 30 days.

The associations between energy intake (total and macronutrient-specific) and memory impairment are shown in Table 3. Individuals with high total energy intake were more likely to report severe memory impairment compared to those with low total energy intake (OR: 1.52, 95% CI: 1.15 to 2.12; p for trend = 0.005). With respect to specific macronutrients, a dose-response relationship was observed between energy intake from carbohydrates and the presence (p for trend = 0.01) and the severity level (p for trend = 0.03) of memory impairment. Additionally, high energy intake from fat is associated with memory impairment severity (p for trend = 0.04). There was no statistically significant association observed between energy intake from protein and memory impairment. In addition, high energy intake from sugar intake was significantly associated with memory impairment (OR: 1.54, 95% CI: 1.11 to 2.16) and severity of memory impairment (OR: 1.52, 95% CI: 1.12 to 2.09) (Table 4). In addition, high energy intake from total saturated fatty acid was associated with memory impairment severity (p for trend = 0.02). Finally, the associations of energy intake from carbohydrate, protein, and fat with memory impairment were consistent across each subgroup, such as sex, race/ethnicity, physical activity, weight status, smoke status, and chronic diseases (Figures 1–3).

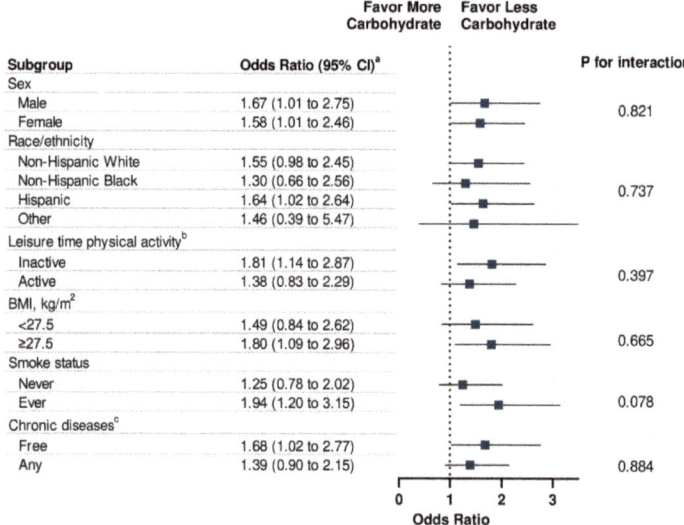

Figure 1. Stratification Analysis on Association Between Energy Intake from Carbohydrate and Memory Impairment Among US Adults ≥60 years, NHANES 2011–2014. [a] Multivariable models were adjusted for age, sex, race/ethnicity, education attainment, and family poverty ratio, physical activity, HEI-2010, alcohol intake, BMI, Body Weight, smoking status, hypertension, hypercholesterolemia, family history of diabetes, history of CVD, and history of cancer. [b] Leisure-time physical activity level was defined by engaging in no (inactive) or any (active) moderate or vigorous recreational physical activity over the past 30 days. [c] Chronic Diseases included diabetes, CVD, and Cancer.

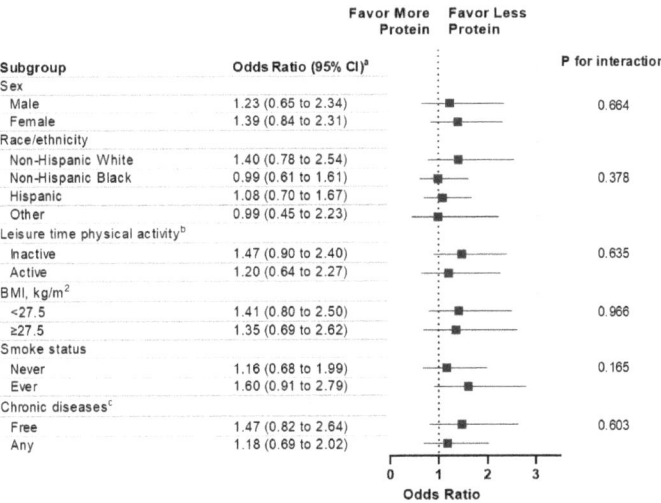

Figure 2. Stratification Analysis on Association Between Energy Intake from Protein and Memory Impairment Among US Adults ≥60 years, NHANES 2011–2014. [a] Multivariable models were adjusted for age, sex, race/ethnicity, education attainment, and family poverty ratio, physical activity, HEI-2010, alcohol intake, BMI, Body Weight, smoking status, hypertension, hypercholesterolemia, family history of diabetes, history of CVD, and history of cancer. [b] Leisure-time physical activity level was defined by engaging in no (inactive) or any (active) moderate or vigorous recreational physical activity over the past 30 days. [c] Chronic Diseases included diabetes, CVD, and Cancer.

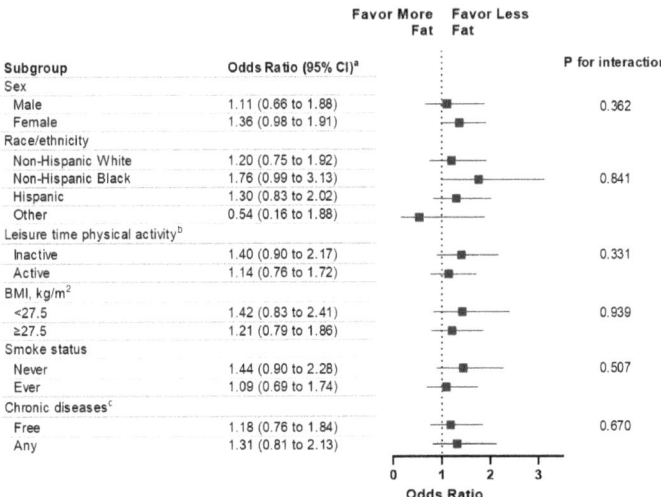

Figure 3. Stratification Analysis on Association Between Energy Intake from Fat and Memory Impairment Among US Adults ≥60 years, NHANES 2011–2014. [a] Multivariable models were adjusted for age, sex, race/ethnicity, education attainment, and family poverty ratio, physical activity, HEI-2010, alcohol intake, BMI, Body Weight, smoking status, hypertension, hypercholesterolemia, family history of diabetes, history of CVD, and history of cancer. [b] Leisure-time physical activity level was defined by engaging in no (inactive) or any (active) moderate or vigorous recreational physical activity over the past 30 days. [c] Chronic Diseases included diabetes, CVD, and Cancer.

Table 3. Multivariable-adjusted Association of Source Specific Energy Intake and Memory Severity Impairment Among US Adults ≥60 years, NHANES 2011–2014 [a].

	Source of Calorie Intake [b]			
	Total	Carbohydrate	Protein	Fat
Memory Impairment [c]				
Energy Intake				
Low	1 [Reference]	1 [Reference]	1 [Reference]	1 [Reference]
Moderate	1.10 (0.79 to 1.52)	1.34 (0.98 to 1.85)	1.03 (0.71 to 1.50)	1.23 (0.86 to 1.77)
High	1.46 (1.00 to 2.12)	1.59 (1.12 to 2.26)	1.35 (0.88 to 2.06)	1.26 (0.90 to 1.76)
p for trend	0.055	0.01	0.15	0.17
Memory Impairment Severity [d]				
Energy Intake				
Low	1 [Reference]	1 [Reference]	1 [Reference]	1 [Reference]
Moderate	1.19 (0.95 to 1.49)	1.16 (0.88 to 1.54)	1.10 (0.78 to 1.54)	1.16 (0.84 to 1.59)
High	1.52 (1.15 to 2.02)	1.40 (1.04 to 1.88)	1.39 (0.95 to 2.02)	1.33 (1.01 to 1.76)
p for trend	0.005	0.03	0.08	0.04

[a] Multivariable models were adjusted for age, sex, race/ethnicity, education attainment, and family poverty ratio, physical activity, Healthy Eating Index-2010, alcohol intake, BMI, Body Weight, smoking status, hypertension, hypercholesterolemia, family history of diabetes, history of CVD, and history of cancer. [b] Sex-specific tertile categories were applied for each source of energy intake. The Low group was defined as the first tertile, the moderate group was defined as the second tertile category; and the high group was defined as the third tertile category. Only one source of energy intake was included in each model. [c] Binary outcome (No vs. Any memory Impairment) was used in the multivariable-adjusted logistic regression models. [d] Ordinal outcome ("never", "about once", "two or three times", "nearly every day" and "several times a day") was used in the multivariable-adjusted ordinal logistic regression models.

Table 4. Multivariable-adjusted Association of Source-Specific Energy Intake and Memory Impairment Among US Adults ≥60 years, NHANES 2011–2014 [a].

	Source of Calorie Intake [b]			
	Sugar	Total Saturated Fatty Acid	Total Monounsaturated Fatty Acid	Total Polyunsaturated Fatty Acid
Memory Impairment [c]				
Energy Intake				
Low	1 [Reference]	1 [Reference]	1 [Reference]	1 [Reference]
Moderate	1.43 (1.04 to 1.96)	1.35 (0.95 to 1.92)	1.14 (0.85 to 1.54)	1.15 (0.80 to 1.64)
High	1.54 (1.06 to 2.24)	1.31 (0.97 to 1.78)	1.23 (0.91 to 1.67)	1.34 (0.94 to 1.92)
p for trend	0.02	0.07	0.17	0.09
Memory Impairment Severity [d]				
Energy Intake				
Low	1 [Reference]	1 [Reference]	1 [Reference]	1 [Reference]
Moderate	1.37 (1.04 to 1.80)	1.13 (0.85 to 1.49)	1.20 (0.93 to 1.55)	1.14 (0.86 to 1.50)
High	1.42 (1.05 to 1.92)	1.40 (1.07 to 1.84)	1.31 (0.98 to 1.75)	1.26 (0.96 to 1.66)
p for trend	0.02	0.02	0.07	0.10

[a] Multivariable models were adjusted for age, sex, race/ethnicity, education attainment, and family poverty ratio, physical activity, Healthy Eating Index-2010, alcohol intake, BMI, Body Weight, smoking status, hypertension, hypercholesterolemia, family history of diabetes, history of CVD, and history of cancer. [b] Sex-specific tertile categories were applied for each source of energy intake. The Low group was defined as the first tertile, the moderate group was defined as the second tertile category; and the high group was defined as the third tertile category. Only one source of energy intake was included in each model. [c] Binary outcome (No vs. Any memory Impairment) was used in the multivariable-adjusted logistic regression models. [d] Ordinal outcome ("never", "about once", "two or three times", "nearly every day" and "several times a day") was used in the multivariable-adjusted ordinal logistic regression models.

4. Discussion

In this large representative sample of US older adults, higher total energy intake was associated with higher memory impairment severity, after adjusting for an array of potential confounders including sociodemographic characteristics, lifestyle factors, and chronic conditions. Specifically, energy intake from carbohydrate was associated with memory impairment. This association kept consistent across sex, race/ethnicity, physical activity level, weight status, smoke status, and chronic diseases. However, energy intake from neither protein nor fat was related to memory impairment. Further exploratory results suggested that more energy intake from sugar was significantly associated with a higher likelihood of memory impairment.

Our study extended the previous evidence on the association of total and macronutrient-specific energy intake with memory impairment at the population level. Findings from the present analyses were in line with previous studies that investigated a limited number of macronutrients in a smaller sample. Specifically, a prospective study followed up with 980 individuals free of dementia at baseline for 4 years. Comparing to lower energy intake, higher calorie and fat intake were associated with a 2-fold increased risk of AD among individuals with the apolipoprotein E ∈4 allele but not among those without the apolipoprotein E ∈4 allele [22]. Another prospective cohort of 937 elderly adults with a median age of 79.5 found a dietary pattern with relatively high caloric intake from carbohydrates and low caloric intake from fat and proteins was linked with a higher risk of mild cognitive impairment or dementia [23]. A cross-sectional study found that the dietary pattern with a high percentage of energy intake from fat and protein, and low-energy intake from carbohydrate was associated with impaired cognitive function in 661 Chinese young adults [34]. The present association between sugar intake and memory impairment agreed with previous findings that habitual sugar intake appeared to be associated with poor cognitive function [35]. However, evidence on the effects of energy intake on memory impairment is lacking among adults at early stages, because previous studies enrolled most participants at very advanced ages (around 80 years). Our findings extended previous evidence to the early age stage of older adults (≥60 years) at the population level. Meanwhile, our stratification analyses indicated that the present association was consistent across different subpopulation, such as sex, race/ethnicity, physical activity level, weight status, and chronic diseases.

Several potential biological pathways could explain the negative association between energy intake and memory function. Animal studies found that a high-calorie diet could induce the activation of an inflammatory response (e.g., increased in reactive astrocytes and interleukin1-β) and oxidative stress (e.g., reactive oxygen species and lipid peroxidation), as well as reducing the number of neurons in the temporal cortex and hippocampus, which contribute to neurodegeneration and memory impairments [18]. A theoretical model was proposed that excessive energy intake leads to increased oxidative stress, impaired protein degradation, and elevated inflammation, which may negatively impact synaptic plasticity and neurogenesis and cause cognitive deficits and AD [36]. Specifically, some research indicated that high sugar consumption causes inflammation in the brain, leading to hippocampal-dependent memory problems [37], whereas such negative effects may be reversed by reducing sugar intake and supplementing with omega-3 fatty acids and curcumin [38]. In addition, excess caloric intake could alter the brain's reward system and result in a progressive addiction to foods that are low-nutrient but rich in sugar. Lenoir and colleagues demonstrated that intense sweetness could surpass cocaine reward, even in drug-sensitized and -addicted individuals [39]. Added sugar intake was associated with a wide range of health problems, such as cardiovascular diseases and diabetes, which are both linked to neurodegeneration and cognitive decline [40].

The 2015–2020 Dietary Guideline for Americans encourages individuals to adhere to a healthy eating pattern across the lifespan. The guideline highlighted the importance of consuming less than 10% of total calories from added sugars each day and reducing the consumption of sugar-sweetened beverages such as soft drinks, which has contributed to the high prevalence of obesity in the United States [41]. Our findings provided additional evidence supporting the benefits of a healthy diet in cognition and memory function. Furthermore, further research is needed to confirm the causal relationship between energy intake and memory impairment.

A clear strength of this study is the use of a large representative sample of the older US population to generalize the findings at the population level. This study is not without limitations. First, the 24-h dietary call interview may cause recall bias. However, data on participants who cannot recall their dietary information were to be collected from their proxies (e.g., caregivers). In addition, the dietary data were comprehensively reviewed by the trained NHANES staff to avoid potential inaccurate data. Second, the memory impairment was not diagnosed by an expert evaluating the Clinical Dementia Rating Scale. However, in the present study, using an early indicator of memory impairment based on structured questions during the in-person interview may provide valuable evidence on preventive strategies. Third, due to the nature of the study design, the causality cannot be determined. Indeed, longitudinal studies using repeated-measurement and clinical trials are further needed to investigate the effect of macronutrient energy intake on memory deterioration changes in a long-term period.

5. Conclusions

In conclusion, energy intake is significantly associated with worsened memory impairment severity in the older US population. In particular, the energy intake from carbohydrates and fat, but not protein, is linked to memory impairment. These findings provide evidence on the potential cognitive benefits of healthy eating patterns for preventing AD and dementia, and highlight the need of developing strategies for promoting a healthy diet among older adults, especially for those at risk of memory impairment.

Author Contributions: Conceptualization, Q.L., J.G. and C.C.; methodology, C.C.; software, C.C.; validation, Q.L., J.G. and C.C.; formal analysis, Q.L., J.G. and C.C.; investigation, Q.L., J.G. and C.C.; resources, C.C.; data curation, C.C.; writing—original draft preparation, Q.L., J.G. and C.C.; writing—review and editing, L.H., N.V., L.S., and L.Y.; visualization, C.C.; supervision, C.C.; project administration, C.C.; funding acquisition, J.G. All authors have read and agreed to the published version of the manuscript.

Funding: Jianjun Guo is supported by Key Project of the Beijing Municipal Education Commission (2020).

Conflicts of Interest: The authors have no conflicts to disclose.

References

1. Center for Disease Control and Prevention. What Is Dementia? Available online: https://www.cdc.gov/aging/dementia/index.html (accessed on 25 June 2020).
2. Alzheimer's Association. 2020 Alzheimer's disease facts and figures. *Alzheimer's Dement.* **2020**, *16*, 391–460. [CrossRef] [PubMed]
3. Rossor, M.N.; Fox, N.C.; Mummery, C.J.; Schott, J.M.; Warren, J.D. The diagnosis of young-onset dementia. *Lancet Neurol.* **2010**, *9*, 793–806. [CrossRef]
4. World Health Organization. Dementia. Available online: https://www.who.int/news-room/fact-sheets/detail/dementia (accessed on 25 June 2020).
5. Center for Disease Control and Prevention. Leading Causes of Death. Available online: https://www.cdc.gov/nchs/fastats/leading-causes-of-death.htm (accessed on 25 June 2020).
6. Alzheimer's Association. 2018 Alzheimer's disease facts and figures. *Alzheimer's Dement.* **2018**, *14*, 367–429. [CrossRef]
7. Aigbogun, M.S.; Stellhorn, R.; Krasa, H.; Kostic, D. Severity of memory impairment in the elderly: Association with health care resource use and functional limitations in the United States. *Alzheimer's Dement.* **2017**, *8*, 51–59. [CrossRef] [PubMed]
8. Jessen, F.; Wiese, B.; Bachmann, C.; Eifflaender-Gorfer, S.; Haller, F.; Kölsch, H.; Luck, T.; Mösch, E.; van den Bussche, H.; Wagner, M.; et al. Prediction of Dementia by Subjective Memory Impairment: Effects of Severity and Temporal Association With Cognitive Impairment. *Arch. Gen. Psychiatry* **2010**, *67*, 414–422. [CrossRef]

9. Mitchell, A.J.; Beaumont, H.; Ferguson, D.; Yadegarfar, M.; Stubbs, B. Risk of dementia and mild cognitive impairment in older people with subjective memory complaints: Meta-analysis. *Acta Psychiatr. Scand.* **2014**, *130*, 439–451. [CrossRef]
10. Reisberg, B.; Shulman, M.B.; Torossian, C.; Leng, L.; Zhu, W. Outcome over seven years of healthy adults with and without subjective cognitive impairment. *Alzheimer's Dement.* **2010**, *6*, 11–24. [CrossRef]
11. Pressler, S.J.; Subramanian, U.; Kareken, D.; Perkins, S.M.; Gradus-Pizlo, I.; Sauvé, M.J.; Ding, Y.; Kim, J.; Sloan, R.; Jaynes, H.; et al. Cognitive deficits and health-related quality of life in chronic heart failure. *J. Cardiovasc. Nurs.* **2010**, *25*, 189–198. [CrossRef]
12. Pan, C.-W.; Wang, X.; Ma, Q.; Sun, H.-P.; Xu, Y.; Wang, P. Cognitive dysfunction and health-related quality of life among older Chinese. *Sci. Rep.* **2015**, *5*, 17301. [CrossRef]
13. Cummings, J.; Aisen, P.S.; DuBois, B.; Frölich, L.; Jack, C.R.; Jones, R.W.; Morris, J.C.; Raskin, J.; Dowsett, S.A.; Scheltens, P. Drug development in Alzheimer's disease: The path to 2025. *Alzheimer's Res. Ther.* **2016**, *8*, 39. [CrossRef]
14. Smith, P.J.; Blumenthal, J.A. Dietary Factors and Cognitive Decline. *J. Prev. Alzheimers Dis.* **2016**, *3*, 53–64. [CrossRef] [PubMed]
15. Van den Brink, A.C.; Brouwer-Brolsma, E.M.; Berendsen, A.A.M.; van de Rest, O. The Mediterranean, Dietary Approaches to Stop Hypertension (DASH), and Mediterranean-DASH Intervention for Neurodegenerative Delay (MIND) Diets Are Associated with Less Cognitive Decline and a Lower Risk of Alzheimer's Disease—A Review. *Adv. Nutr. (Bethesda Md.)* **2019**, *10*, 1040–1065. [CrossRef] [PubMed]
16. Smyth, A.; Dehghan, M.; Donnell, M.; Anderson, C.; Teo, K.; Gao, P.; Sleight, P.; Dagenais, G.; Probstfield, J.L.; Mente, A.; et al. Healthy eating and reduced risk of cognitive decline. *Neurology* **2015**, *84*, 2258–2265. [CrossRef] [PubMed]
17. Xu, B.-L.; Wang, R.; Ma, L.-N.; Dong, W.; Zhao, Z.-W.; Zhang, J.-S.; Wang, Y.-L.; Zhang, X. Effects of Caloric Intake on Learning and Memory Function in Juvenile C57BL/6J Mice. *BioMed Res. Int.* **2015**, *2015*, 759803. [CrossRef]
18. Treviño, S.; Aguilar-Alonso, P.; Flores Hernandez, J.A.; Brambila, E.; Guevara, J.; Flores, G.; Lopez-Lopez, G.; Muñoz-Arenas, G.; Morales-Medina, J.C.; Toxqui, V.; et al. A high calorie diet causes memory loss, metabolic syndrome and oxidative stress into hippocampus and temporal cortex of rats. *Synapse* **2015**, *69*, 421–433. [CrossRef]
19. Redman, L.M.; Smith, S.R.; Burton, J.H.; Martin, C.K.; Il'yasova, D.; Ravussin, E. Metabolic Slowing and Reduced Oxidative Damage with Sustained Caloric Restriction Support the Rate of Living and Oxidative Damage Theories of Aging. *Cell Metab.* **2018**, *27*, 805–815.e4. [CrossRef]
20. Most, J.; Tosti, V.; Redman, L.M.; Fontana, L. Calorie restriction in humans: An update. *Ageing Res. Rev.* **2017**, *39*, 36–45. [CrossRef]
21. Yates, K.F.; Sweat, V.; Yau, P.L.; Turchiano, M.M.; Convit, A. Impact of metabolic syndrome on cognition and brain: A selected review of the literature. *Arterioscler. Thromb. Vasc. Biol.* **2012**, *32*, 2060–2067. [CrossRef]
22. Luchsinger, J.A.; Tang, M.-X.; Shea, S.; Mayeux, R. Caloric Intake and the Risk of Alzheimer Disease. *Arch. Neurol.* **2002**, *59*, 1258–1263. [CrossRef]
23. Roberts, R.O.; Roberts, L.A.; Geda, Y.E.; Cha, R.H.; Pankratz, V.S.; O'Connor, H.M.; Knopman, D.S.; Petersen, R.C. Relative intake of macronutrients impacts risk of mild cognitive impairment or dementia. *J. Alzheimers Dis.* **2012**, *32*, 329–339. [CrossRef]
24. Cao, C.; Liu, Q.; Abufaraj, M.; Han, Y.; Xu, T.; Waldhoer, T.; Shariat, S.F.; Li, S.; Yang, L.; Smith, L. Regular Coffee Consumption Is Associated with Lower Regional Adiposity Measured by DXA among US Women. *J. Nutr.* **2020**, *150*, 1909–1915. [CrossRef] [PubMed]
25. Raper, N. An overview of USDA's Dietary Intake Data System. *J. Food Compos. Anal.* **2004**, *17*, 545–555. [CrossRef]
26. Centers for Disease Control and Prevention. NHANES 2013-2014 Questionnaire Data Overview. Available online: https://wwwn.cdc.gov/nchs/nhanes/ContinuousNhanes/OverviewQuex.aspx?BeginYear=2013 (accessed on 25 June 2020).
27. Yang, L.; Cao, C.; Kantor, E.D.; Nguyen, L.H.; Zheng, X.; Park, Y.; Giovannucci, E.L.; Matthews, C.E.; Colditz, G.A.; Cao, Y. Trends in Sedentary Behavior Among the US Population, 2001–2016. *JAMA* **2019**, *321*, 1587–1597. [CrossRef] [PubMed]

28. Cao, C.; Hu, L.; Xu, T.; Liu, Q.; Koyanagi, A.; Yang, L.; Carvalho, A.F.; Cavazos-Rehg, P.A.; Smith, L. Prevalence, correlates and misperception of depression symptoms in the United States, NHANES 2015–2018. *J. Affect. Disord.* **2020**, *269*, 51–57. [CrossRef] [PubMed]
29. Roberts, J.; Liu, Q.; Cao, C.; Jackson, S.E.; Zong, X.; Meyer, G.A.; Yang, L.; Cade, W.T.; Zheng, X.; López-Sánchez, G.F.; et al. Association of Hot Tea Consumption with Regional Adiposity Measured by Dual-Energy X-ray Absorptiometry in NHANES 2003–2006. *Obesity* **2020**, *28*, 445–451. [CrossRef]
30. Guenther, P.M.; Casavale, K.O.; Reedy, J.; Kirkpatrick, S.I.; Hiza, H.A.; Kuczynski, K.J.; Kahle, L.L.; Krebs-Smith, S.M. Update of the Healthy Eating Index: HEI-2010. *J. Acad. Nutr. Diet.* **2013**, *113*, 569–580. [CrossRef]
31. Whelton Paul, K.; Carey Robert, M.; Aronow Wilbert, S.; Casey Donald, E.; Collins Karen, J.; Dennison Himmelfarb, C.; DePalma Sondra, M.; Gidding, S.; Jamerson Kenneth, A.; Jones Daniel, W.; et al. 2017 ACC/AHA/AAPA/ABC/ACPM/AGS/APhA/ASH/ASPC/NMA/PCNA Guideline for the Prevention, Detection, Evaluation, and Management of High Blood Pressure in Adults: A Report of the American College of Cardiology/American Heart Association Task Force on Clinical Practice Guidelines. *Hypertension* **2018**, *71*, e13–e115. [CrossRef]
32. Gregg, E.W.; Cheng, Y.J.; Cadwell, B.L.; Imperatore, G.; Williams, D.E.; Flegal, K.M.; Narayan, K.M.; Williamson, D.F. Secular trends in cardiovascular disease risk factors according to body mass index in US adults. *JAMA* **2005**, *293*, 1868–1874. [CrossRef]
33. Cao, C.; Yang, L.; Cade, W.T.; Racette, S.B.; Park, Y.; Cao, Y.; Friedenreich, C.M.; Hamer, M.; Stamatakis, E.; Smith, L. Cardiorespiratory Fitness Is Associated with Early Death Among Healthy Young and Middle-aged Baby Boomers and Generation Xers. *Am. J. Med.* **2020**, *133*, 961–968.e3. [CrossRef]
34. Ding, B.; Xiao, R.; Ma, W.; Zhao, L.; Bi, Y.; Zhang, Y. The association between macronutrient intake and cognition in individuals aged under 65 in China: A cross-sectional study. *BMJ Open* **2018**, *8*, e018573. [CrossRef]
35. Chong, C.P.; Shahar, S.; Haron, H.; Din, N.C. Habitual sugar intake and cognitive impairment among multi-ethnic Malaysian older adults. *Clin. Interv. Aging* **2019**, *14*, 1331–1342. [CrossRef] [PubMed]
36. Mattson, M.P. The impact of dietary energy intake on cognitive aging. *Front. Aging Neurosci.* **2010**, *2*, 5. [CrossRef] [PubMed]
37. Beilharz, J.E.; Maniam, J.; Morris, M.J. Short-term exposure to a diet high in fat and sugar, or liquid sugar, selectively impairs hippocampal-dependent memory, with differential impacts on inflammation. *Behav. Brain Res.* **2016**, *306*, 1–7. [CrossRef] [PubMed]
38. Beilharz, J.E.; Maniam, J.; Morris, M.J. Diet-Induced Cognitive Deficits: The Role of Fat and Sugar, Potential Mechanisms and Nutritional Interventions. *Nutrients* **2015**, *7*, 6719–6738. [CrossRef] [PubMed]
39. Lenoir, M.; Serre, F.; Cantin, L.; Ahmed, S.H. Intense Sweetness Surpasses Cocaine Reward. *PLoS ONE* **2007**, *2*, e698. [CrossRef]
40. Zilliox, L.A.; Chadrasekaran, K.; Kwan, J.Y.; Russell, J.W. Diabetes and Cognitive Impairment. *Curr. Diabetes Rep.* **2016**, *16*, 87. [CrossRef]
41. US Department of Health and Human Services; US Department of Agriculture. *2015-2020 Dietary Guidelines for Americans*, 8th ed.; US Department of Health and Human Services: Washington, DC, USA, 2015. Available online: http://www.health.gov/DietaryGuidelines (accessed on 16 November 2020).

Publisher's Note: MDPI stays neutral with regard to jurisdictional claims in published maps and institutional affiliations.

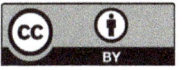

© 2020 by the authors. Licensee MDPI, Basel, Switzerland. This article is an open access article distributed under the terms and conditions of the Creative Commons Attribution (CC BY) license (http://creativecommons.org/licenses/by/4.0/).

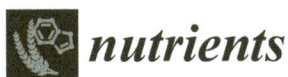

Article

Effects of Nutrient Intake on Diagnostic Measures of Sarcopenia among Arab Men: A Cross-Sectional Study

Maha H. Alhussain [1,*], Shaea Alkahtani [2], Osama Aljuhani [3] and Syed Shahid Habib [4]

1. Department of Food Science and Nutrition, College of Food and Agriculture Sciences, King Saud University, Riyadh 11451, Saudi Arabia
2. Department of Exercise Physiology, College of Sport Sciences and Physical Activity, King Saud University, Riyadh 11451, Saudi Arabia; shalkahtani@ksu.edu.sa
3. Department of Physical Education, College of Sport Sciences and Physical Activity, King Saud University, Riyadh 11451, Saudi Arabia; oaljuhani@ksu.edu.sa
4. Department of Physiology, College of Medicine, King Saud University, Riyadh 11451, Saudi Arabia; sshahid@ksu.edu.sa
* Correspondence: mhussien@ksu.edu.sa; Tel.: +966-14670000

Abstract: Sarcopenia is a major public health condition and is, therefore, of great clinical interest. However, the role of nutrient intake in sarcopenia is unclear. We examined the associations between nutrient intake and diagnostic measures of sarcopenia, including low muscle mass (appendicular lean mass (ALM) divided by height squared, ALM/h^2) and strength (hand-grip strength, HGS) among Arab men. This cross-sectional study included 441 men aged 46.8 ± 15.98 years. Habitual nutrient intake was assessed using a food frequency questionnaire (FFQ). Participants were classified according to different ALM/h^2 and HGS reference values. Participants with normal muscle mass, defined by an ALM/h^2 cutoff of <8.68 kg/m^2 (−1 standard deviation (SD) <reference values Arab men), had greater daily energy, protein and fat intake, and percentage of energy from protein and fat ($p < 0.01$). Conversely, normal muscle mass was associated with a lower percentage of energy from carbohydrates (CHO) ($p < 0.001$). Regarding muscle strength, participants with HGS above 42 kg (median HGS of Arab men) had higher daily energy and protein and fat intake, but a lower percentage of energy from CHO and a lower intake of total omega-3 fatty acids ($p < 0.05$). Individuals with normal muscle mass and high HGS have greater daily energy, protein, and fat intake and a lower percentage of energy from CHO compared to sarcopenic individuals.

Keywords: sarcopenia; muscle mass; muscle strength; nutrition; food frequency questionnaire

1. Introduction

Aging is an inevitable phenomenon associated with progressive changes in body composition and a gradual decline in muscle mass [1,2]. The term sarcopenia, first introduced by Rosenberg, is used to describe this age-related loss of muscle mass [3]. In 2010, the European Working Group on Sarcopenia in Older People (EWGSOP) developed a consensus set of diagnostic criteria for sarcopenia based on low muscle mass, determined by appendicular lean mass (ALM), combined with low muscle function, determined by handgrip strength (HGS) and/or gait speed. The EWGSOP also recommended using appropriate measurements and cutoff points as references for sarcopenia diagnosis [4]. In 2018, the Second European Working Group on Sarcopenia in Older People (EWGSOP2) [5] revised the original recommendations and used low muscle strength as the primary diagnostic measure of sarcopenia. Low muscle strength is better than mass at predicting adverse health outcomes [6–8].

Although overt sarcopenia is more pronounced in older adults, the development of sarcopenia begins during middle age (40–50 years old) in some individuals [9]. Sarcopenia is of great clinical interest because it predicts frailty, disability, decreased quality of life, loss

Citation: Alhussain, M.H.; Alkahtani, S.; Aljuhani, O.; Habib, S.S. Effects of Nutrient Intake on Diagnostic Measures of Sarcopenia among Arab Men: A Cross-Sectional Study. Nutrients 2021, 13, 114. https://doi.org/10.3390/nu13010114

Received: 11 December 2020
Accepted: 28 December 2020
Published: 30 December 2020

Publisher's Note: MDPI stays neutral with regard to jurisdictional claims in published maps and institutional affiliations.

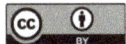

Copyright: © 2020 by the authors. Licensee MDPI, Basel, Switzerland. This article is an open access article distributed under the terms and conditions of the Creative Commons Attribution (CC BY) license (https://creativecommons.org/licenses/by/4.0/).

of independent living, and mortality [10–12]. Furthermore, at the societal level, sarcopenia leads to increased health care costs [13]. Accordingly, the need to understand more about its etiology is of immediate interest. The onset and progression of sarcopenia can be accelerated by numerous factors, including chronic diseases and lifestyle behaviors like physical inactivity and poor diet [14]. Physical activity is often cited as a modifiable lifestyle factor that is negatively associated with low muscle mass and strength [15,16]. However, the role of nutrient intake in sarcopenia has not been thoroughly investigated. Several studies link adequate intake of single nutrients, such as protein and omega-3 fatty acids, to improvements in muscle mass and strength in older adults [17–19]. Micronutrients have also been linked to muscle mass and strength, including vitamin D, vitamin E, calcium (Ca), and magnesium (Mg) [20–26]. In addition to inadequate intake of certain nutrients, the total energy intake and percentage contribution of energy from macronutrients may influence the risk for sarcopenia. A study by Park et al. [20] reported that sarcopenia is inversely correlated with total energy, protein, and carbohydrates (CHO) intake in older adults. Another recent study by Beaudart et al. [26] concluded that sarcopenic individuals seem to consume significantly reduced amounts of total energy, proteins, and fat compared with nonsarcopenic individuals.

Few population-based studies have investigated the association between nutrient intake and diagnostic measures of sarcopenia [27]. To address this gap in extant literature, more investigation is required to enhance the evidence for dietary recommendations to prevent or delay the development of sarcopenia. Thus, the primary aim of this study was to examine the associations between dietary nutrient intake and diagnostic measures of sarcopenia, muscle mass (ALM by bio-impedance analyzer (BIA)) and muscle strength (HGS), in Arab men in Riyadh, Saudi Arabia. The associations of anthropometry and body composition with muscle mass and strength were also assessed.

2. Materials and Methods

2.1. Participants

A total of 441 participants were recruited via a poster advertisement sent to Community Development Commissions of Riyadh districts and posted on social media platforms. Inclusion requirements included male sex, aged 18–85 years, BMI ≤ 40 kg/m^2, Saudi or Arab Riyadh residents, and the ability to move independently. Exclusion criteria included professional athletes, cardiovascular diseases, musculoskeletal diseases, cerebrovascular accidents, chronic obstructive pulmonary disease, cancer, and dementia. Using G*Power [28] calculation, power analysis was calculated for actual power = 0.948 using the effect size of HGS = 0.75.

The study was conducted according to the guidelines established by the Declaration of Helsinki and the study was approved by the institutional review board (IRB) of King Saud University (IRB No. E-18-3381). Informed written consent was obtained from all participants before study enrollment.

2.2. Study Design

The community-based, descriptive, cross-sectional study was conducted between October 2018 and June 2019. After an initial telephone interview, potentially eligible participants were invited to selected sites for data collection. Data were collected at different sites depending on the participant age. For men aged under 40 years, data were collected at the Exercise Physiology Unit, College of Sport Sciences and Physical Activity, King Saud University, Riyadh, Saudi Arabia. For men aged 40 and over, data were collected at seven Community Development Commissions located in the north, south, east, and central districts of Riyadh. Participants arrived early in the morning (~8:00 A.M.) after fasting overnight (at least 8 h) and were given detailed information about the study. Eligible participants had anthropometry and body composition measured. They were then asked to complete a validated food frequency questionnaire (FFQ) to assess their typical food intake.

2.3. Measurements

2.3.1. Anthropometry

Weight, height, and waist circumference (WC) were measured using standardized protocols [29]. Weight was measured to the nearest 0.1 kg using a calibrated, digital scale (PD100 ProDoc, Detecto Scale, Cardinal, Webb City, MO, USA); participants wore light clothing and no shoes. Height was measured to the nearest 0.1 cm using a stadiometer (Seca 213, Seca GmbH & Co., Hamburg, Germany) without shoes and with participants in a freestanding position. WC was measured to the nearest 0.1 cm in a horizontal plane at the level of the midpoint between the lower margin of the last rib and the crest of the ileum when the subject stood with feet 25–30 cm apart using a flexible non-stretch tape. Body mass index (BMI) was calculated (weight (kg)/height^2 (m)).

2.3.2. Body Composition

Body composition was assessed using a multi-frequency Tanita MC-980MA BIA (Tanita Corporation, Tokyo, Japan), according to the manufacturer's guidelines. This analyzer was designed to measure the body composition in segmental parts of the whole body, including arms, legs, and the trunk area. The measurement procedure requires the subject to stand in bare feet on the metal plates of the analyzer and hold a pair of handgrips, one in each hand. The bio-impedance component of the measurements took approximately 30 seconds per participant and output was printed. Absolute body fat, body fat %, and muscle mass were obtained from these analyses.

2.3.3. Diagnostic Measures of Sarcopenia

Muscle Mass

ALM was used to calculate the ratio of total lean arm and leg mass [30] to the squared height (ALM/h^2). Based on EWGSOP2 recommendations [5], muscle mass was considered low if ALM/h^2 < 7.0 kg/m^2 which indicates a predictor of sarcopenia. A local cutoff value for ALM/h^2 (−1 standard deviation (SD) <reference values young Arab men; 8.68 kg/m^2) [31] was also used in this study to identify people with low muscle mass.

Muscle Strength

The muscle strength was measured using a handgrip test. HGS (maximum voluntary contractions) was measured twice using a standardized protocol [32] with a manual spring dynamometer (Baseline®Smedley Spring Dynamometers, Fabrication enterprises Inc., NY, USA). Participants were instructed to hold the dynamometer in their dominant hand with the arm stretched parallel to the body while standing upright. The best performance (in kg) was considered the maximum grip strength used for further analysis.

Based on HGS values, participants were divided into three groups: a low HGS group (<27 kg; EWGSOP2 cutoff [5]); a second group with HGS > 42 kg, which was the median HGS of 471 Arab men [31]; and a third group with HGS ranging from 27 to 42 kg, which is higher than the risk of low HGS (≥27 kg) but < 50% in the same population (≤42 kg).

2.3.4. Nutrient Intake Assessments

Dietary intake was assessed using a self-administered FFQ, designed and validated to measure participants' habitual diet over the previous 12 months [33]. The questionnaire was developed in the Arabic language. A list of 140 common Saudi food items was included in the questionnaire, where a closed-ended approach was used. Participants were asked to indicate the average consumption frequency of each FFQ item using nine frequency categories as follows: never or less than once a month, 1–3 per month, once a week, 2–4 per week, 5–6 per week, once a day, 2–3 per day, 4–5 per day, and more than 6 per day. The portion sizes were described and supported by household measures. Participants completed the FFQ in paper or electronic format and a trained dietitian reviewed the questionnaire. Exclusions were made due to invalid or incompletely filled FFQs.

Nutritional intakes of energy, CHO, protein, fat, total omega-3 fatty acids (sum of a-linolenic acid (ALA), eicosapentaenoic acid (EPA), docosapentaenoic acid (DPA), and docosahexaenoic acid (DHA)), vitamin D, vitamin E, Ca, and Mg were assessed. These nutrients were chosen based on previous studies demonstrating associations between these nutrients and sarcopenia [34–38]. Average daily energy and nutrient intakes were calculated using the U.S. Department of Agriculture (USDA) software (Edition 27, 2014, Beltsville, MD, USA) and the Nutribase software (Edition 11, 2014, CyberSoft, Inc, Phoenix, AZ, USA), which utilizes food macronutrients and micronutrients. Additionally, for Saudi traditional food, an Arabic food analysis program was used (1st version, 2007).

2.4. Statistical Analysis

All statistical tests were completed using IBM SPSS Statistics version 23 (IBM Corp., Armonk, NY, USA). Data were checked for normality using the Kolmogorov–Smirnov test and the appropriate transformations were applied for non-normally distributed data. Data are presented as a mean ± SD for normally distributed variables and median (Q1–Q3) for non-normally distributed variables. Independent *t*-test and Mann–Whitney U test were used to compare mean or median differences in normal and low ALM/h^2 groups.

One-way ANOVA was used to compare mean differences in HGS groups. When an overall statistically significant difference in group means was shown, Tukey's post hoc test was performed to confirm where the differences occurred between groups. Pearson correlation coefficient analyses were performed to study the relationships between ALM/h^2 or HGS and each parameter. Correlations were classified as weak if $r < 0.5$, moderate if $r \geq 0.5$ to < 0.8, strong if $r \geq 0.8$, and perfect if $r = 1$ [39]. Multiple regressions were used to calculate the correlation between ALM/h^2 or HGS and each category (age and anthropometry (height, body weight, BMI and WC), body composition (body fat, fat mass, and muscle mass), and nutrient intake (energy, CHO [%], CHO [g/day], protein [%], protein [g/day], fat [%], fat [g/day], total omega-3 fatty acids, vitamin D, vitamin E, Ca, and Mg)) and to calculate R^2 to study the effect of each category on ALM/h^2 or HGS. Stepwise procedures were used in the multiple regression analysis to determine the significant variables that affect ALM/h^2 or HGS in each category. Age-specific subgroup sensitivity analyses were performed for both ALM/h^2 and HGS for participants aged over 65 years. Statistical significance was set at <0.05 for all statistical tests.

3. Results

3.1. Participant Characteristics

Of the 500 participants enrolled in the study, 30 participants withdrew (no longer interested in study participation), 470 participants completed the study, 29 participants were excluded due to incomplete or invalid nutritional data (FFQ), and 441 participants were included in the final analysis. Participants who were missing values for HGS were excluded only from the HGS comparisons (Figure 1). General characteristics and nutrient intake of the study participants are summarized in Table 1.

3.2. Between-Group Differences

Table 2 displays the differences between the normal and low ALM/h^2 groups (mean ± SD ALM/h^2: 8.98 ± 1.21 kg/m^2 and 6.37 ± 0.69 kg/m^2, respectively) with regard to general characteristics and nutrient intake. Using the EWGSOP2 cutoff, low muscle mass was observed in 4.8% of the participants. Participants with low muscle mass were significantly older and had lower BMI, lower fat mass, lower muscle mass, and lower HGS (*t*-test, $p < 0.05$). No other significant differences were observed between participants with low muscle mass and those with normal muscle mass, including nutrient intake. According to the local cutoff, participants with low muscle mass (46% of the participants) were older, taller, and had lower BMI, WC, body fat %, muscle mass, and HGS (*t*-test, $p < 0.01$). In terms of nutrient intake, those with low muscle mass differed in their total energy intake, CHO (as a percentage of energy intake; energy%), protein (g/day), protein (energy%), fat (g/day), and fat (energy%) compared with those with normal muscle mass (*t*-test, $p < 0.05$). However, no significant differences were observed in other nutrient intakes.

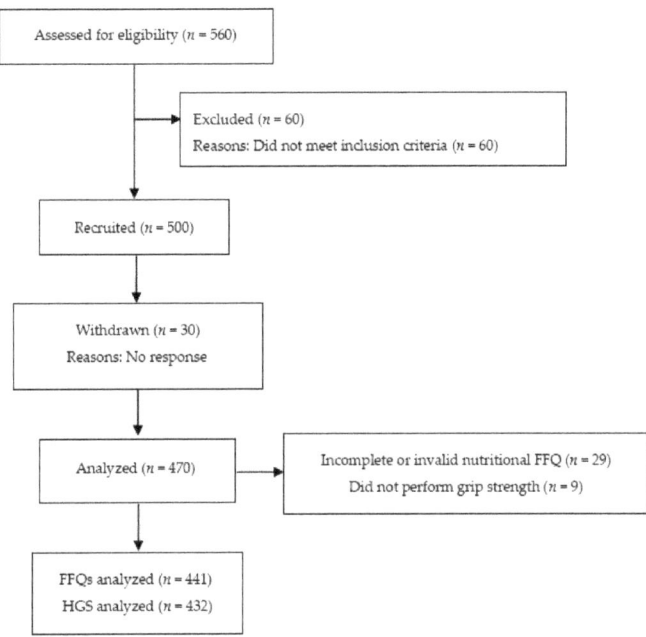

Figure 1. Flow chart of enrollment for the study.

Table 1. General characteristics and nutrient intake of study participants [1].

Parameters	Total ($n = 441$)
Age (year)	46.80 ± 15.98
Height (cm)	168.40 ± 6.90
Body weight (kg)	81.12 ± 15.55
BMI (kg/m^2)	28.59 ± 5.08
WC (cm)	92.59 ± 20.46
Body fat (%)	27.41 ± 7.45
Fat mass (kg)	23.41 ± 9.81
Muscle mass (kg)	55.08 ± 8.00
ALM/h^2 (kg/m^2)	8.86 ± 1.32
HGS (kg)	39.31 ± 8.91
Energy (kcal/day)	2327.84 ± 679.59
CHO (g/day)	293.03 ± 80.57
CHO (energy%)	51.47 ± 11.46
Protein (g/day)	140.14 ± 104.64
Protein (energy%)	22.62 ± 11.07
Fat (g/day)	66.31 ± 31.79
Fat (energy%)	25.90 ± 10.09
Total omega-3 fatty acids (g/day)	0.10 ± 0.07
Vitamin D (ug/day)	2.89 ± 2.04
Vitamin E (mg/day)	3.53 ± 2.22
Ca (mg/day)	393.67 ± 175.80
Mg (mg/day)	66.72 ± 37.77

[1] Data are presented as mean ± SD. Abbreviations: BMI, body mass index; WC, waist circumference; ALM, appendicular lean mass; HGS, handgrip strength; CHO, carbohydrate; Ca, calcium; Mg, magnesium.

Table 2. General characteristics and nutrient intake of study participants based on different ALM/h^2 reference values [1].

Parameters	EWGSOP2			−1 SD < Reference Values Arab Men		
	Normal (ALM/h^2 ≥ 7.0 kg/m^2)	Low (ALM/h^2 < 7.0 kg/m^2)	p-Value [2]	Normal (ALM/h^2 ≥ 8.68 kg/m^2)	Low (ALM/h^2 < 8.68 kg/m^2)	p-Value [2]
n (432)	420	21		238	203	
Age (year)	49 (32–60)	62 (47–67.5)	0.002	42.91 ± 14.46	51.37 ± 16.49	<0.001
Height (cm)	168.45 ± 6.92	167.39 ± 6.51	0.493	169.21 ± 6.98	167.45 ± 6.70	0.008
Body weight (kg)	81.98 ± 15.22	63.93 ± 11.79	<0.001	89.04 ± 14.89	71.84 ± 10.30	<0.001
BMI (kg/m^2)	28.87 ± 4.94	22.90 ± 4.37	<0.001	31.08 ± 4.77	25.66 ± 3.68	<0.001
WC (cm)	95.5 (85–105)	92 (76–98)	0.090	95.81 ± 20.86	88.78 ± 19.26	<0.001
Body fat (%)	27.41 ± 7.18	27.48 ± 11.85	0.979	28.46 ± 6.86	26.18 ± 7.93	<0.001
Fat mass (kg)	23.36 ± 9.69	18.75 ± 11.44	0.035	26.31 ± 10.15	19.42 ± 7.95	<0.001
Muscle mass (kg)	55.69 ± 7.65	42.74 ± 3.74	<0.001	59.73 ± 6.33	49.62 ± 6.08	<0.001
HGS (kg)	39.75 ± 8.76	30.57 ± 7.29	0.003	42.35 ± 8.15	35.68 ± 8.41	<0.001
Energy (kcal/day)	2322.71 ± 680.47	2430.39 ± 669.55	0.479	2415.16 ± 713.87	2225.46 ± 623.35	0.003
CHO (g/day)	291.82 ± 80.37	317.23 ± 82.84	0.159	290.16 ± 79.52	296.40 ± 81.85	0.418
CHO (energy%)	51.39 ± 11.48	53.14 ± 11.11	0.493	49.27 ± 11.35	54.05 ± 11.06	<0.001
Protein (g/day)	139.60 ± 104.32	150.94 ± 113.12	0.629	151.63 ± 113.82	126.67 ± 91.19	0.011
Protein (energy%)	22.62 ± 11.09	22.67 ± 11.52	0.985	23.58 ± 11.71	21.50 ± 10.24	0.047
Fat (g/day)	66.33 ± 32.05	61.97 ± 26.47	0.540	72.00 ± 34.80	59.24 ± 26.32	<0.001
Fat (energy%)	25 (18–32)	19 (16–28)	0.214	27.11 ± 10.29	24.47 ± 9.71	0.006
Total omega-3 fatty acids (g/day)	0.10 ± 0.07	0.10 ± 0.05	0.899	0.10 ± 0.07	0.10 ± 0.07	0.336
Vitamin D (ug/day)	2.86 ± 2.02	3.39 ± 2.41	0.247	2.80 ± 2.04	2.99 ± 2.04	0.314
Vitamin E (mg/day)	3.25 (1.66–4.89)	3.48 (2.15–4.69)	0.427	3.37 ± 2.30	3.73 ± 2.1	0.093
Ca (mg/day)	396.57 ± 177.51	335.76 ± 126.77	0.122	399.37 ± 184.58	386.99 ± 165.12	0.462
Mg (mg/day)	55.09 (41.24–81.17)	45.67 (40.33–97.38)	0.725	68.09 ± 38.12	65.11 ± 37.38	0.410

[1] Data are presented as mean ± SD or median (Q1–Q3). [2] p-value significant < 0.05. p-value tested by unpaired t-test to compare mean differences or nonparametric Mann–Whitney U to compare median differences. Abbreviations: EWGSOP2, Second European Working Group on Sarcopenia in Older People; BMI, body mass index; WC, waist circumference; ALM, appendicular lean mass; HGS, handgrip strength; CHO, carbohydrate; Ca, calcium; Mg, magnesium.

The general characteristics and nutrient intake of participants with and without low muscle strength according to HGS using different reference values are shown in Table 3. The percentages of participants who had HGS < 27 kg, 27–42 kg, and above 42 kg were 8.1% (mean ± SD HGS: 22.31 ± 3.49 kg), 54.7% (mean ± SD HGS: 35.70 ± 4.13 kg), and 37% (mean ± SD HGS: 48.37 ± 4.62 kg), respectively. There were significant differences between the three groups with respect to age, height, body weight, BMI, muscle mass, and ALM/h^2 (one-way ANOVA, p < 0.01). As shown in Table 3, participants with HGS < 27 kg were the oldest and shortest and had the lowest body weight, muscle mass, and ALM/h^2. Regarding nutrient intake, there were significant differences between the three groups in total energy intake, CHO (energy%), protein (g/day), fat (g/day), and total omega-3 fatty acids (one-way ANOVA, p < 0.05). Participants who had HGS > 42 kg had higher total energy, protein (g/day), and fat (g/day) intakes compared with participants with HGS between 27 and 42 kg. Additionally, the highest intake of total omega-3 fatty acids was observed in participants with HGS < 27 kg. There were no significant differences among the three groups in micronutrient intake.

3.3. Correlation Analysis

Pearson's correlations between ALM/h^2 and HGS and each parameter are shown in Table 4. Significant positive correlations were observed between ALM/h^2 and anthropometry, body composition, protein (g/day), protein (energy%), and fat (g/day). ALM/h^2 and muscle mass had the strongest correlation (strong correlation). Significant negative correlations were also observed between ALM/h^2 and age and CHO (energy%). Conversely, no significant correlations were found between ALM/h^2 and CHO (g/day), fat (energy%), and micronutrients. Multiple regression analyses (Figure 2) showed that body composition explained 86.9% (R^2) of the variance in ALM/h^2. Muscle mass and body fat percentage contributed to this variance, as determined by a stepwise procedure. Age and anthropometric measurements explained 71.3% (R^2) of the variance in ALM/h^2, while dietary intake explained 45.0% (R^2) of the variance in ALM/h^2. Age, BMI, WC, body weight, energy (kcal/day), CHO (energy%), protein (g/day), and fat (energy%) contributed to this variance. Age-specific subgroup sensitivity analyses were performed for ALM/h^2 for participants aged over 65 years and RUC = 0.730 ((0.664–0.796) 95%CI, ($p < 0.001$)) was observed.

HGS was positively correlated with height, weight, BMI, fat mass, muscle mass, energy (kcal/day), protein (g/day), and protein (energy%). However, these correlations were weak and the only moderate correlation was observed between HGS and muscle mass. Weak negative correlations were found between HGS and age, body fat%, CHO (energy%), and total omega-3 fatty acids. HGS did not significantly correlate with the other parameters. According to a multiple regression analysis (Figure 3), age and anthropometric measurements accounted for 36% of the HGS variance. The results from the stepwise regression analysis revealed that age, body weight, and height contributed to this variance. Body composition with contribution of body fat percentage accounted for 34.7% (R^2) of the HGS variance. Nutrient intake contributed to 14.6% (R^2) of the variance in HGS, and energy (kcal/day), CHO (energy%), and fat (g/day) contributed to this variance. Age-specific subgroup sensitivity analyses were performed for HGS for participants aged over 65 years; RUC = 0.839 ((0.0.783–0.895) 95%CI, $p < 0.001$)) was detected.

Table 3. General characteristics and nutrient intake of study participants based on different HGS reference values [1].

Parameters	HGS (kg)			p-Value [2]
	<27 kg	27–42 kg	>42 kg	
n (441)	35	237	160	
Age (year)	63.49 ± 14.76(ab) [3]	48.84 ± 15.51(ac)	40.11 ± 13.12(bc)	<0.001
Height (cm)	164.06 ± 5.80(a)	166.64 ± 6.37(b)	172.01 ± 6.25(ab)	<0.001
Body weight (kg)	71.83 ± 12.69(ab)	78.33 ± 13.81(ac)	87.28 ± 16.34(bc)	<0.001
BMI (kg/m^2)	88.06 ± 25.02	93.06 ± 19.55	93.06 ± 20.76	0.384
WC (cm)	26.79 ± 5.04(a)	28.21 ± 4.72(b)	29.51 ± 5.37(ab)	0.004
Body fat (%)	27.96 ± 8.80	27.90 ± 7.15	26.44 ± 7.44	0.139
Fat mass (kg)	20.79 ± 9.40	22.61 ± 9.03	24.33 ± 10.72	0.079
Muscle mass (kg)	48.86 ± 7.34(ab)	52.96 ± 7.22(ac)	59.67 ± 7.05(bc)	<0.001
ALM/h^2 (kg/m^2)	7.73 ± 1.16(ab)	8.6578 ± 1.22(ac)	9.4188 ± 1.27(bc)	<0.001
Energy (kcal/day)	2259.76 ± 535.90	2252.57 ± 612.69(a)	2467.23 ± 787.04(a)	<0.001
CHO (g/day)	291.42 ± 81.12	290.74 ± 77.68	297.69 ± 84.45	0.693
CHO (energy%)	52.17 ± 11.56	52.69 ± 11.12(a)	49.49 ± 11.71(a)	0.022
Protein (g/day)	130.84 ± 93.82	130.29 ± 92.48(a)	159.16 ± 122.36(a)	0.023
Protein (energy%)	21.77 ± 10.50	22.03 ± 10.87	23.89 ± 11.56	0.230
Fat (g/day)	63.41 ± 27.57	63.16 ± 32.67(a)	71.09 ± 31.26(a)	0.046
Fat (energy%)	26.14 ± 11.07	25.27 ± 10.22	26.57 ± 9.52	0.442
Total omega-3 fatty acids (g/day)	0.13 ± 0.14(ab)	0.01 ± 0.06(ac)	0.10 ± 0.06(bc)	0.018
Vitamin D (ug/day)	3.33 ± 2.09	3.01 ± 2.15	2.69 ± 1.87	0.141
Vitamin E (mg/day)	3.56 ± 1.82	3.39 ± 2.03	3.71 ± 2.57	0.383
Ca (mg/day)	424.21 ± 155.74	395.38 ± 169.80	383.66 ± 183.80	0.444
Mg (mg/day)	67.68 ± 40.75	65.67 ± 37.46	67.40 ± 37.33	0.886

[1] Data presented as mean ± SD. [2] p-value significant < 0.05, tested by one-way ANOVA. [3] The same letter for two groups means that there is a significant difference using Tukey's post hoc test. Abbreviations: HGS, handgrip strength; BMI, body mass index; WC, waist circumference; ALM, appendicular lean mass; CHO, carbohydrate; Ca, calcium; Mg, magnesium.

Table 4. Pearson's correlation coefficient of ALM/h^2 and HGS with general characteristics and nutrient intake.

Parameters	ALM/h^2 (n = 441)		HGS (kg) (n = 432)	
	Pearson Correlation	p-Value [1]	Pearson Correlation	p-Value
Age (year)	−0.31	<0.001	−0.45	<0.001
Height (cm)	0.11	0.018	0.44	<0.001
Body weight (kg)	0.74	<0.001	0.37	<0.001
BMI (kg/m^2)	0.28	<0.001	0.05	0.338
WC (cm)	0.74	<0.001	0.19	<0.001
Body fat (%)	0.23	<0.001	−0.12	0.016
Fat mass (kg)	0.50	<0.001	0.12	0.017
Muscle mass (kg)	0.80	<0.001	0.53	<0.001
Energy (kcal/day)	0.17	<0.001	0.12	0.014
CHO (g/day)	−0.04	0.419	0.01	0.829
CHO (energy%)	−0.24	<0.001	−0.13	0.007
Protein (g/day)	0.18	<0.001	0.12	0.009
Protein (energy%)	0.17	<0.001	0.09	0.040
Fat (g/day)	0.18	<0.001	0.09	0.075
Fat (energy%)	0.07	0.117	0.04	0.445
Total omega-3 fatty acids (g/day)	−0.02	0.622	−0.09	0.041
Vitamin D (ug/day)	−0.05	0.258	−0.12	0.015
Vitamin E (mg/day)	−0.08	0.102	0.07	0.177
Ca (mg/day)	0.03	0.565	−0.04	0.388
Mg (mg/day)	0.05	0.323	0.00	0.988

[1] p-value significant < 0.05. Abbreviations: ALM, appendicular lean mass; HGS, handgrip strength; BMI, body mass index; WC, waist circumference; CHO, carbohydrate; Ca, calcium; Mg, magnesium.

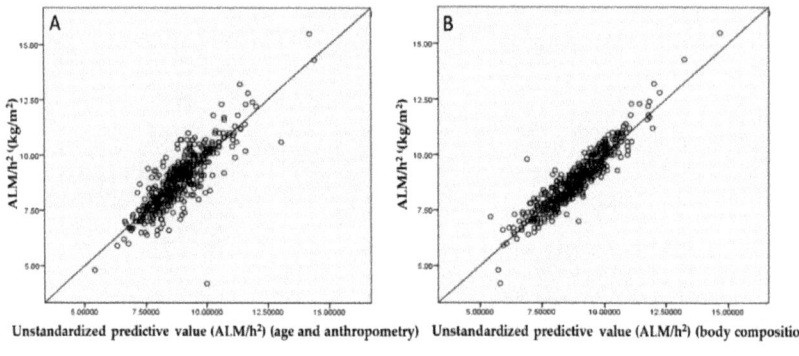

Figure 2. Multiple regression analyses between ALM/h^2 and age and anthropometry ((**A**) R^2 = 0.869), body composition ((**B**) R^2 = 0.713), and nutrient intake ((**C**) R^2 = 0.450). (n = 441). Abbreviations: ALM, appendicular lean mass.

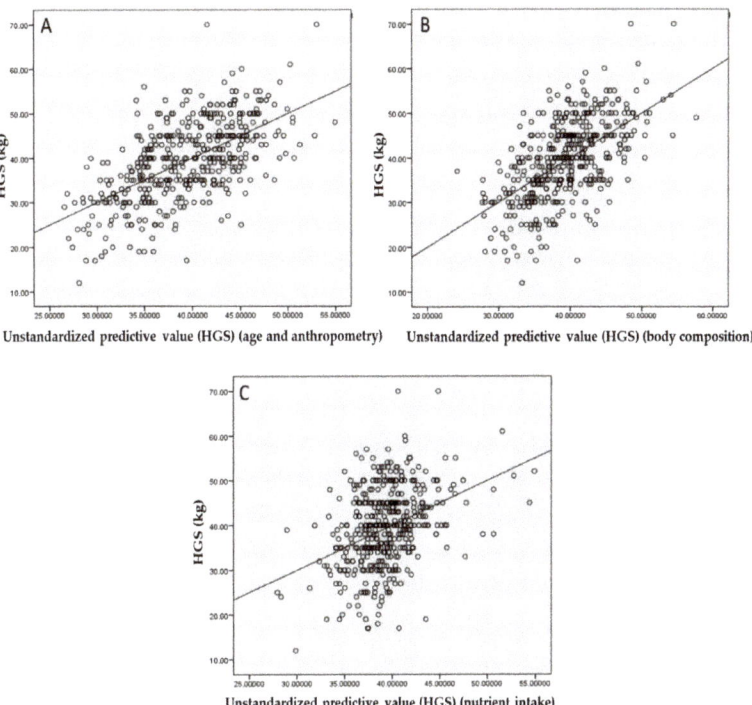

Figure 3. Multiple regression analyses between HGS and age and anthropometry ((**A**) R^2 = 0.360), body composition ((**B**) R^2 = 0.347), and nutrient intake ((**C**) R^2 = 0.146). (n= 432). Abbreviations: HGS, handgrip strength.

4. Discussion

In the present study, we investigated the associations between muscle mass and strength with dietary nutrient intake, anthropometry, and body composition in Arab men. Participants were defined as having low muscle mass and strength using international (EWGSOP2) and local cutoffs for ALM/h^2 and HGS. Our results showed that participants with normal muscle mass, as defined by a local cutoff of ALM/h^2, had greater daily energy, protein, and fat intakes (g/day) and that a greater percentage of their energy came from protein and fat (energy%). Conversely, normal muscle mass was associated with a lower percentage of energy from CHO (energy%). Regarding muscle strength, participants with HGS above 42 kg had higher daily energy, protein, and fat intakes (g/day). On the other hand, a lower percentage of energy from CHO (energy%) was found in participants with HGS above 42 kg and, surprisingly, these participants had a lower intake of total omega-3 fatty acids (g/day).

In agreement with our energy intake findings, several studies have demonstrated that energy intake is associated with sarcopenia and muscle mass [40,41]. Reduced energy intake causes a reduction in protein synthesis [42]. The differences in energy intake in the present study can be explained by the significantly younger age of participants with higher ALM/h^2 and HGS. A gradual decline in energy intake in old age has been reported [43–45]. This can be caused by aging processes, including physiological changes, the presence of diseases, and the use of medications. Age-related decline in energy intake is accompanied by a reduction in the percentage of energy from fat, whereas the contribution of CHO to energy intake increases [45,46]. In the present study, similar results were observed in ALM/h^2 groups when the local cutoff of ALM/h^2 was used. Additionally, the contribution of CHO to energy intake was the lowest in participants with HGS above 42 kg. These findings suggest that the percentage of energy from macronutrients may have important effects on muscle mass and strength maintenance with advancing age.

Increasing protein intake has been proposed as an important pillar of sarcopenia treatment [47,48]. Insufficient protein intake can contribute to loss of muscle mass and strength due to chronic disruption in the balance between muscle protein synthesis and degradation [49]. In the current study, a significant difference in protein intake (g/day) was observed within muscle mass and strength groups. Comparable results were found in previous studies [26,50] in which a lower intake of protein was reported in sarcopenic versus nonsarcopenic older adults. We also observed a greater intake of fat (g/day) in groups with normal muscle mass and HGS above 42 kg compared with other groups. Low fat intake can be a result of low daily energy intake. Thus, monitoring fat intake may be important. In the current study, multiple regression analyses indicated that among the dietary nutrient intakes considered, energy (kcal/day), CHO (energy%), and fat (g/day) accounted for the variance in ALM/h^2 and energy (kcal/day), CHO (energy%), protein (g/day), and fat (energy%) explained the variance in HGS.

We found an inverse association between total omega-3 fatty acids (g/day) and muscle strength. This finding does not strengthen the emerging hypothesis that the intake of total omega-3 fatty acids is positively associated with muscle strength in older men [37]. This discrepancy might be due to differences in the techniques used to assess muscle strength. The relationship between the intake of omega-3 fatty acids and sarcopenia, as reflected by direct measures of muscle mass and strength, needs further investigation. In the current study, no differences in either vitamins or minerals among the muscle mass and strength groups were observed. Although vitamin D is the most researched vitamin that has been hypothesized to play a role in sarcopenia, there is currently little evidence to link the dietary intake of vitamin D with sarcopenia [50,51]. Pharmacological doses of vitamin D have been used in many interventional studies concerning sarcopenia [49]. Further, vitamin D status is typically assessed as 25-hydroxy vitamin D (25(OH)D) in blood, as it reflects the sum of vitamin D from dietary intake and sunlight exposure. In general, the association between dietary micronutrients and muscle mass and strength may be stronger than measured by the FFQ. More work is warranted to elucidate the potential benefits of micronutrient intake to prevent sarcopenia and support healthy aging.

Low muscle mass among study participants was more prevalent when classifying participants into low and normal muscle mass groups based on the local cutoff of ALM/h^2 compared with the international one. We found that neither daily energy intake nor nutrient intake differed significantly between muscle mass groups when considering the international cutoff. This might be explained by the relatively small number of participants in the low muscle mass group when defined by the international cutoff.

The association between increasing age and sarcopenia has been well established. The same association between age and muscle mass and strength was observed in this study. We also found that height, body weight, and BMI were positively associated with muscle mass and strength. This result is in line with a previous study carried out in older adults [50]. The associations between muscle mass (kg) and ALM/h^2 or HGS in this study were unsurprising, given the fact that sarcopenia is characterized by loss of muscle mass and strength. In addition to the loss of muscle mass and strength, sarcopenia can be characterized by an increase in fat mass, which has been defined as sarcopenic obesity [52]. In the present study, however, lower fat mass (kg) was associated with lower ALM/h^2. If energy intake is inadequate to meet requirements, muscle and fat are catabolized to provide energy [42].

In the current study, nutrient intake was assessed using a self-administered FFQ. FFQ is a common dietary assessment approach because it is easy to apply, retrospective (i.e., capturing usual intake over an extended period of time), and relatively cheap. However, this method has some limitations, including that the food lists are not comprehensive and are highly reliant on memory and conceptual skills. Despite of these limitations, it has been reported that applying an FFQ approach to assess the nutrient intake of healthy older adults might be applicable [53]. No strong evidence exists that older adults provide less valid self-reports using FFQs compared with younger adults [53].

Body composition including muscle mass was estimated in our study by BIA technique. This technique measures muscle mass indirectly based on whole-body electrical conductivity. Previous studies that validate the accuracy of BIA against dual-energy x-ray absorptiometry (DEXA) as reference standards have demonstrated contradictory findings. However, according to EWGSOP [4,5], BIA can be considered as a portable alternative to DEXA. The current study has several strengths. To the best of our knowledge, this was the first study to investigate the associations between dietary nutrient intake and sarcopenia, muscle mass, and strength in Arab men. This is particularly important because most sarcopenia studies are from eastern Asia and further sarcopenia research in western Asia has been recommended [54]. Moreover, noticeable muscle mass and strength declines may occur as early as 45 years of age [9]. Therefore, this study examined sarcopenia progression in adults aged 18 years and above. However, like all studies, this study has some limitations. No causal relationship can be obtained from this study because of its cross-sectional design. Nutrient intake was evaluated by FFQs over the previous 12 months and this may be subject to recall bias. Hence, measurement errors may attenuate associations between intakes and outcome measurements. Only the nutrients that were reported to be associated with muscle mass and strength in previous studies were examined in this study. The results refer only to nutrient intake from food sources; however, dietary supplements may have been consumed. We did not measure the biochemical nutrients in the blood, which are effective markers to evaluate the nutrient status. Finally, some covariables were not included in the analyses (such as physical activity that can influence muscle mass and strength).

5. Conclusions

Individuals with normal muscle mass and high HGS have greater daily energy, protein, and fat intake and a lower percentage of energy from CHO compared with sarcopenic participants. Our findings highlight the potentially important role of energy intake and composition as well as macronutrient intake in sarcopenia and healthy aging. Manipulating CHO, fat, and protein intakes may ameliorate the progression of sarcopenia with age. Further work is needed to improve our understanding of the effects of whole dietary nutrient intake on sarcopenia among both adult men and adult women.

Author Contributions: Conceptualization, M.H.A., S.A., O.A. and S.S.H.; methodology, M.H.A., S.A., O.A. and S.S.H.; validation, M.H.A.; formal analysis, M.H.A.; investigation, M.H.A., S.A., O.A. and S.S.H.; re-sources, S.A.; data curation, M.H.A., S.A., O.A. and S.S.H.; writing—original draft preparation, M.H.A.; writing—review and editing, M.H.A., S.A., O.A. and S.S.H.; visualization, M.H.A., and S.A.; project administration, S.A.; funding acquisition, M.H.A., S.A., O.A. and S.S.H. All authors have read and agreed to the published version of the manuscript.

Funding: This research was funded by a grant from the Research Group Program (RG-1439-82), Deanship of Scientific Research, King Saud University, Riyadh, Saudi Arabia.

Institutional Review Board Statement: The study was conducted according to the guidelines of the Declaration of Helsinki, and approved by the Institutional Review Board (IRB) of King Saud University (protocol code. E-18-3381, 08 January 2019).

Informed Consent Statement: Informed consent was obtained from all subjects involved in the study.

Data Availability Statement: The datasets used in the current study are available from the corresponding author on reasonable request.

Acknowledgments: The authors would like to thank the study participants whose participation made this study possible. We also thank the Research Support and Services Unit of the Deanship of Scientific Research at King Saud University for their technical support.

Conflicts of Interest: The authors declare no conflict of interest.

References

1. Prentice, A.M.; Jebb, S.A. Beyond body mass index. *Obes. Rev.* **2001**, *2*, 141–147. [CrossRef]
2. Buffa, R.; Floris, G.U.; Putzu, P.F.; Marini, E. Body composition variations in ageing. *Coll. Antropol.* **2011**, *35*, 259–265.
3. Rosenberg, I.H. Sarcopenia: Origins and clinical relevance. *J. Nutr.* **1997**, *127*, 990S–991S. [CrossRef]
4. Cruz-Jentoft, A. European Working Group on Sarcopenia in Older People: Sarcopenia: European consensus on definition and diagnosis. Report of the European Workikgn Group on Sarcopenia in Older People. *Age Ageing* **2010**, *39*, 412–423. [CrossRef] [PubMed]
5. Cruz-Jentoft, A.J.; Bahat, G.; Bauer, J.; Boirie, Y.; Bruyère, O.; Cederholm, T.; Cooper, C.; Landi, F.; Rolland, Y.; Sayer, A.A. Sarcopenia: Revised European consensus on definition and diagnosis. *Age Ageing* **2019**, *48*, 16–31. [CrossRef] [PubMed]
6. Kim, Y.H.; Kim, K.-I.; Paik, N.-J.; Kim, K.-W.; Jang, H.C.; Lim, J.-Y. Muscle strength: A better index of low physical performance than muscle mass in older adults. *Geriatr. Gerontol. Int.* **2016**, *16*, 577–585. [CrossRef] [PubMed]
7. Ibrahim, K.; May, C.; Patel, H.P.; Baxter, M.; Sayer, A.A.; Roberts, H. A feasibility study of implementing grip strength measurement into routine hospital practice (GRImP): Study protocol. *Pilot Feasibility Stud.* **2016**, *2*, 27. [CrossRef]
8. Schaap, L.A.; van Schoor, N.M.; Lips, P.; Visser, M. Associations of Sarcopenia Definitions, and Their Components, With the Incidence of Recurrent Falling and Fractures: The Longitudinal Aging Study Amsterdam. *J. Gerontol. A Biol. Sci. Med. Sci.* **2017**, *73*, 1199–1204. [CrossRef]
9. Frontera, W.R.; Hughes, V.A.; Fielding, R.A.; Fiatarone, M.A.; Evans, W.J.; Roubenoff, R. Aging of skeletal muscle: A 12-yr longitudinal study. *J. Appl. Physiol.* **2000**, *88*, 1321–1326. [CrossRef]
10. Janssen, I.; Heymsfield, S.B.; Ross, R. Low relative skeletal muscle mass (sarcopenia) in older persons is associated with functional impairment and physical disability. *J. Am. Geriatr. Soc.* **2002**, *50*, 889–896. [CrossRef]
11. Landi, F.; Cruz-Jentoft, A.J.; Liperoti, R.; Russo, A.; Giovannini, S.; Tosato, M.; Capoluongo, E.; Bernabei, R.; Onder, G. Sarcopenia and mortality risk in frail older persons aged 80 years and older: Results from ilSIRENTE study. *Age Ageing* **2013**, *42*, 203–209. [CrossRef] [PubMed]
12. McLean, R.R.; Shardell, M.D.; Alley, D.E.; Cawthon, P.M.; Fragala, M.S.; Harris, T.B.; Kenny, A.M.; Peters, K.W.; Ferrucci, L.; Guralnik, J.M.; et al. Criteria for Clinically Relevant Weakness and Low Lean Mass and Their Longitudinal Association With Incident Mobility Impairment and Mortality: The Foundation for the National Institutes of Health (FNIH) Sarcopenia Project. *J. Gerontol. A Biol. Sci. Med. Sci.* **2014**, *69*, 576–583. [CrossRef] [PubMed]
13. Janssen, I.; Shepard, D.S.; Katzmarzyk, P.T.; Roubenoff, R. The Healthcare Costs of Sarcopenia in the United States. *J. Am. Geriatr. Soc.* **2004**, *52*, 80–85. [CrossRef] [PubMed]
14. Cruz-Jentoft, A.J.; Landi, F.; Topinková, E.; Michel, J.-P. Understanding sarcopenia as a geriatric syndrome. *Curr. Opin. Clin. Nutr. Metab. Care* **2010**, *13*, 1–7. [CrossRef]
15. Montero-Fernández, N.; Serra-Rexach, J.A. Role of exercise on sarcopenia in the elderly. *Eur. J. Phys. Rehabil. Med.* **2013**, *49*, 131–143.
16. Landi, F.; Marzetti, E.; Martone, A.M.; Bernabei, R.; Onder, G. Exercise as a remedy for sarcopenia. *Curr. Opin. Clin. Nutr. Metab. Care* **2014**, *17*, 25–31. [CrossRef]
17. Deer, R.R.; Volpi, E. Protein intake and muscle function in older adults. *Curr. Opin. Clin. Nutr. Metab. Care* **2015**, *18*, 248–253. [CrossRef]
18. Landi, F.; Calvani, R.; Tosato, M.; Martone, A.M.; Ortolani, E.; Savera, G.; D'Angelo, E.; Sisto, A.; Marzetti, E. Protein intake and muscle health in old age: From biological plausibility to clinical evidence. *Nutrients* **2016**, *8*, 295. [CrossRef]
19. Smith, G.I.; Julliand, S.; Reeds, D.N.; Sinacore, D.R.; Klein, S.; Mittendorfer, B. Fish oil–derived n−3 PUFA therapy increases muscle mass and function in healthy older adults1. *Am. J. Clin. Nutr.* **2015**, *102*, 115–122. [CrossRef]
20. Park, S.; Ham, J.-O.; Lee, B.-K. A positive association of vitamin D deficiency and sarcopenia in 50 year old women, but not men. *Clin. Nutr.* **2014**, *33*, 900–905. [CrossRef]
21. Kim, M.K.; Baek, K.H.; Song, K.-H.; Il Kang, M.; Park, C.Y.; Lee, W.Y.; Oh, K.W. Vitamin D Deficiency Is Associated with Sarcopenia in Older Koreans, Regardless of Obesity: The Fourth Korea National Health and Nutrition Examination Surveys (KNHANES IV) 2009. *J. Clin. Endocrinol. Metab.* **2011**, *96*, 3250–3256. [CrossRef] [PubMed]
22. Kim, J.-S.; Wilson, J.M.; Lee, S.-R. Dietary implications on mechanisms of sarcopenia: Roles of protein, amino acids and antioxidants. *J. Nutr. Biochem.* **2010**, *21*, 1–13. [CrossRef]
23. Khor, S.C.; Abdul Karim, N.; Wan Ngah, W.Z.; Mohd Yusof, Y.A.; Makpol, S. Vitamin E in Sarcopenia: Current Evidences on Its Role in Prevention and Treatment. *Oxid. Med. Cell. Longev.* **2014**, *2014*, 914853. [CrossRef] [PubMed]
24. van Dronkelaar, C.; van Velzen, A.; Abdelrazek, M.; van der Steen, A.; Weijs, P.J.M.; Tieland, M. Minerals and Sarcopenia; The Role of Calcium, Iron, Magnesium, Phosphorus, Potassium, Selenium, Sodium, and Zinc on Muscle Mass, Muscle Strength, and Physical Performance in Older Adults: A Systematic Review. *J. Am. Med. Dir. Assoc.* **2018**, *19*, 6–11.e13. [CrossRef] [PubMed]
25. Dominguez, L.J.; Barbagallo, M.; Lauretani, F.; Bandinelli, S.; Bos, A.; Corsi, A.M.; Simonsick, E.M.; Ferrucci, L. Magnesium and muscle performance in older persons: The InCHIANTI study. *Am. J. Clin. Nutr.* **2006**, *84*, 419–426. [CrossRef] [PubMed]
26. Beaudart, C.; Locquet, M.; Touvier, M.; Reginster, J.-Y.; Bruyère, O. Association between dietary nutrient intake and sarcopenia in the SarcoPhAge study. *Aging Clin. Exp. Res.* **2019**, *31*, 815–824. [CrossRef] [PubMed]

27. Scott, D.; Blizzard, L.; Fell, J.; Giles, G.; Jones, G. Associations between dietary nutrient intake and muscle mass and strength in community-dwelling older adults: The Tasmanian Older Adult Cohort study. *J. Am. Geriatr. Soc.* **2010**, *58*, 2129–2134. [CrossRef] [PubMed]
28. Faul, F.; Erdfelder, E.; Lang, A.G.; Buchner, A. G* Power 3: A flexible statistical power analysis program for the social, behavioral, and biomedical sciences. *Behav. Res. Methods* **2007**, *39*, 175–191. [CrossRef]
29. Lohman, T.G.; Roche, A.F.; Martorell, R. *Anthropometric Standardization Reference Manual*; Human kinetics books Champaign: Champaign, IL, USA, 1988; Volume 177.
30. Heymsfield, S.B.; Smith, R.; Aulet, M.; Bensen, B.; Lichtman, S.; Wang, J.; Pierson, R.N., Jr. Appendicular skeletal muscle mass: Measurement by dual-photon absorptiometry. *Am. J. Clin. Nutr.* **1990**, *52*, 214–218. [CrossRef]
31. Alkahtani, S.A. A cross-sectional study on sarcopenia using different methods: Reference values for healthy Saudi young men. *BMC Musculoskelet. Disord.* **2017**, *18*, 119. [CrossRef]
32. Roberts, H.C.; Denison, H.J.; Martin, H.J.; Patel, H.P.; Syddall, H.; Cooper, C.; Sayer, A.A. A review of the measurement of grip strength in clinical and epidemiological studies: Towards a standardised approach. *Age Ageing* **2011**, *40*, 423–429. [CrossRef] [PubMed]
33. Gosadi, I.M.; Alatar, A.A.; Otayf, M.M.; AlJahani, D.M.; Ghabbani, H.M.; AlRajban, W.A.; Alrsheed, A.M.; Al-Nasser, K.A. Development of a Saudi Food Frequency Questionnaire and testing its reliability and validity. *Saudi Med. J.* **2017**, *38*, 636–641. [CrossRef] [PubMed]
34. Calvani, R.; Miccheli, A.; Landi, F.; Bossola, M.; Cesari, M.; Leeuwenburgh, C.; Sieber, C.C.; Bernabei, R.; Marzetti, E. Current nutritional recommendations and novel dietary strategies to manage sarcopenia. *J. Frailty Aging* **2013**, *2*, 38–53. [PubMed]
35. Houston, D.K.; Nicklas, B.J.; Ding, J.; Harris, T.B.; Tylavsky, F.A.; Newman, A.B.; Lee, J.S.; Sahyoun, N.R.; Visser, M.; Kritchevsky, S.B. Dietary protein intake is associated with lean mass change in older, community-dwelling adults: The Health, Aging, and Body Composition (Health ABC) Study. *Am. J. Clin. Nutr.* **2008**, *87*, 150–155. [CrossRef] [PubMed]
36. Bradlee, M.L.; Mustafa, J.; Singer, M.R.; Moore, L.L. High-Protein Foods and Physical Activity Protect Against Age-Related Muscle Loss and Functional Decline. *J. Gerontol. A Biol. Sci. Med. Sci.* **2017**, *73*, 88–94. [CrossRef]
37. Rossato, L.T.; de Branco, F.M.S.; Azeredo, C.M.; Rinaldi, A.E.M.; de Oliveira, E.P. Association between omega-3 fatty acids intake and muscle strength in older adults: A study from National Health and Nutrition Examination Survey (NHANES) 1999–2002. *Clin. Nutr.* **2020**, *39*, 3434–3441. [CrossRef]
38. Semba, R.D.; Blaum, C.; Guralnik, J.M.; Moncrief, D.T.; Ricks, M.O.; Fried, L.P. Carotenoid and vitamin E status are associated with indicators of sarcopenia among older women living in the community. *Aging Clin. Exp. Res.* **2003**, *15*, 482–487. [CrossRef]
39. Zou, K.H.; Tuncali, K.; Silverman, S.G. Correlation and Simple Linear Regression. *Radiology* **2003**, *227*, 617–628. [CrossRef]
40. Cameron, J.D.; Sigal, R.J.; Kenny, G.P.; Alberga, A.S.; Prud'homme, D.; Phillips, P.; Doucette, S.; Goldfield, G. Body composition and energy intake—skeletal muscle mass is the strongest predictor of food intake in obese adolescents: The HEARTY trial. *Appl. Physiol. Nutr. Metab.* **2016**, *41*, 611–617. [CrossRef]
41. Okamura, T.; Miki, A.; Hashimoto, Y.; Kaji, A.; Sakai, R.; Osaka, T.; Hamaguchi, M.; Yamazaki, M.; Fukui, M. Shortage of energy intake rather than protein intake is associated with sarcopenia in elderly patients with type 2 diabetes: A cross-sectional study of the KAMOGAWA-DM cohort. *J. Diabetes* **2019**, *11*, 477–483. [CrossRef]
42. Newman, A.B.; Lee, J.S.; Visser, M.; Goodpaster, B.H.; Kritchevsky, S.B.; Tylavsky, F.A.; Nevitt, M.; Harris, T.B. Weight change and the conservation of lean mass in old age: The Health, Aging and Body Composition Study. *Am. J. Clin. Nutr.* **2005**, *82*, 872–878. [CrossRef]
43. Risonar, M.G.D.; Rayco-Solon, P.; Ribaya-Mercado, J.D.; Solon, J.A.A.; Cabalda, A.B.; Tengco, L.W.; Solon, F.S. Physical activity, energy requirements, and adequacy of dietary intakes of older persons in a rural Filipino community. *Nutr. J.* **2009**, *8*, 19. [CrossRef] [PubMed]
44. Jungjohann, S.M.; Lührmann, P.M.; Bender, R.; Blettner, M.; Neuhäuser-Berthold, M. Eight-year trends in food, energy and macronutrient intake in a sample of elderly German subjects. *Br. J. Nutr.* **2005**, *93*, 361–378. [CrossRef] [PubMed]
45. De Groot, C.; Van Staveren, W.; De Graaf, C. Determinants of macronutrient intake in elderly people. *Eur. J. Clin. Nutr.* **2000**, *54*, S70–S76. [CrossRef] [PubMed]
46. Morley, J.E. Anorexia of aging: Physiologic and pathologic. *Am. J. Clin. Nutr.* **1997**, *66*, 760–773. [CrossRef]
47. Bauer, J.; Biolo, G.; Cederholm, T.; Cesari, M.; Cruz-Jentoft, A.J.; Morley, J.E.; Phillips, S.; Sieber, C.; Stehle, P.; Teta, D. Evidence-based recommendations for optimal dietary protein intake in older people: A position paper from the PROT-AGE Study Group. *J. Am. Med. Dir. Assoc.* **2013**, *14*, 542–559. [CrossRef]
48. Morley, J.E.; Argiles, J.M.; Evans, W.J.; Bhasin, S.; Cella, D.; Deutz, N.E.; Doehner, W.; Fearon, K.C.; Ferrucci, L.; Hellerstein, M.K. Nutritional recommendations for the management of sarcopenia. *J. Am. Med. Dir. Assoc.* **2010**, *11*, 391–396. [CrossRef]
49. Cruz-Jentoft, A.J.; Kiesswetter, E.; Drey, M.; Sieber, C.C. Nutrition, frailty, and sarcopenia. *Aging Clin. Exp. Res.* **2017**, *29*, 43–48. [CrossRef]
50. ter Borg, S.; de Groot, L.C.P.G.M.; Mijnarends, D.M.; de Vries, J.H.M.; Verlaan, S.; Meijboom, S.; Luiking, Y.C.; Schols, J.M.G.A. Differences in Nutrient Intake and Biochemical Nutrient Status Between Sarcopenic and Nonsarcopenic Older Adults—Results From the Maastricht Sarcopenia Study. *J. Am. Med. Dir. Assoc.* **2016**, *17*, 393–401. [CrossRef]

51. Dupuy, C.; Lauwers-Cances, V.; Van Kan, G.A.; Gillette, S.; Schott, A.-M.; Beauchet, O.; Annweiler, C.; Vellas, B.; Rolland, Y. Dietary vitamin D intake and muscle mass in older women. Results from a cross-sectional analysis of the EPIDOS study. *J. Nutr. Health Aging* **2013**, *17*, 119–124. [CrossRef]
52. Baumgartner, R.N. Body composition in healthy aging. *Ann. N. Y. Acad. Sci.* **2000**, *904*, 437–448. [CrossRef] [PubMed]
53. De Vries, J.; De Groot, L.; Van Staveren, W. Dietary assessment in elderly people: Experiences gained from studies in the Netherlands. *Eur. J. Clin. Nutr.* **2009**, *63*, S69–S74. [CrossRef] [PubMed]
54. Arai, H.; Akishita, M.; Chen, L.-K. Growing research on sarcopenia in Asia. *Geriatr. Gerontol. Int.* **2014**, *14*, 1–7. [CrossRef] [PubMed]

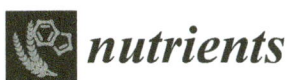

Article

Dietary Patterns and Frailty in Older Korean Adults: Results from the Korean Frailty and Aging Cohort Study

Jinhee Kim [1,2], Yunhwan Lee [1,2,*], Chang Won Won [3], Mi Kyung Kim [4], Seunghee Kye [5], Jee-Seon Shim [6,7], Seungkook Ki [1,2] and Ji-hye Yun [1,2]

1. Department of Preventive Medicine and Public Health, Ajou University School of Medicine, 164 World cup-ro, Youngtong-gu, Suwon 16499, Korea; jhkim06@ajou.ac.kr (J.K.); donquixote@outlook.com (S.K.); dream10307@naver.com (J.-h.Y.)
2. Institute on Aging, Ajou University Medical Center, 164 World cup-ro, Youngtong-gu, Suwon 16499, Korea
3. Elderly Frailty Research Center, Department of Family Medicine, College of Medicine, Kyung Hee University, 23 Kyung Hee Dae-ro, Dongdaemun-gu, Seoul 02447, Korea; chunwon@khmc.or.kr
4. Department of Preventive Medicine, College of Medicine, Hanyang University, 222 Wangsimni-ro, Seongdong-gu, Seoul 04763, Korea; kmkkim@hanyang.ac.kr
5. Nutrition Education, Graduate School of Education, Gachon University, 1342 Seongnamdae-ro, Sujeong-gu, Seongnam 13120, Korea; shkye2@gmail.com
6. Cardiovascular and Metabolic Diseases Etiology Research Center, Yonsei University College of Medicine, 50-1 Yonsei-ro, Seodaemun-gu, Seoul 03722, Korea; SHIMJS@yuhs.ac
7. Department of Preventive Medicine, Yonsei University College of Medicine, 50-1 Yonsei-ro, Seodaemun-gu, Seoul 03722, Korea
* Correspondence: yhlee@ajou.ac.kr; Tel.: +82-31-219-5085; Fax: +82-31-219-5084

Abstract: There are few studies on dietary patterns and frailty in Asians, and the results are controversial. Therefore, this study examined the association between dietary patterns and frailty in older Korean adults using the Korean Frailty and Aging Cohort Study (KFACS). The sample consisted of 511 subjects, aged 70–84 years, community-dwelling older people from the KFACS. Dietary data were obtained from the baseline study (2016–2017) using two nonconsecutive 24-h dietary recalls, and dietary patterns were extracted using reduced rank regression. Frailty was measured by a modified version of the Fried Frailty Phenotype (FFP) in both the baseline (2016) and the first follow-up study (2018). A logistic regression analysis was used to examine the association between dietary patterns and frailty status in 2018. The "meat, fish, and vegetables" pattern was inversely associated with pre-frailty (OR = 0.41, 95% CI = 0.21–0.81, p for trend = 0.009) and exhaustion (OR = 0.41, 95% CI = 0.20–0.85, p for trend = 0.020). The "milk" pattern was not significantly associated with frailty status or the FFP components. In conclusion, a dietary pattern with a high consumption of meat, fish, and vegetables was associated with a lower likelihood of pre-frailty.

Keywords: dietary patterns; reduced rank regression; frailty; community-dwelling older people

Citation: Kim, J.; Lee, Y.; Won, C.W.; Kim, M.K.; Kye, S.; Shim, J.-S.; Ki, S.; Yun, J.-h. Dietary Patterns and Frailty in Older Korean Adults: Results from the Korean Frailty and Aging Cohort Study. *Nutrients* 2021, 13, 601. https://doi.org/10.3390/nu13020601

Academic Editor: Emiliana Giacomello

Received: 11 December 2020
Accepted: 8 February 2021
Published: 12 February 2021

Publisher's Note: MDPI stays neutral with regard to jurisdictional claims in published maps and institutional affiliations.

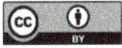

Copyright: © 2021 by the authors. Licensee MDPI, Basel, Switzerland. This article is an open access article distributed under the terms and conditions of the Creative Commons Attribution (CC BY) license (https://creativecommons.org/licenses/by/4.0/).

1. Introduction

Frailty is a condition whereby decreased homeostatic reserves result in adverse reactions to stress, as a result of age-related decline in many physiological systems [1]. In older adults, frailty leads to poor health outcomes such as impaired cognitive function, falls, fracture, physical disability, hospitalization, and mortality [1]. With rising healthcare costs and increases in the life expectancy of older people with frailty [2], prevention of frailty is crucial for successful aging.

Among the modifiable risk factors associated with frailty, the role of diet has been examined for frailty prevention [3]. Previous studies have mainly focused on specific single nutrients or foods, and they reported that vegetables, fruits, whole grains, and low-fat dairy products are inversely related to frailty [3]. However, people eat meals that contain a combination of nutrients and a variety of foods. Nutrients and foods create interactions within the body that can affect health outcomes; therefore, identifying dietary patterns may be more beneficial for preventing frailty [4]. In Western countries, a recent meta-analysis showed that the Mediterranean diet, a priori-defined dietary pattern, is associated with reduced incidence of frailty in older people [5]. Various a posteriori dietary patterns [4] have been derived using principal component analysis, factor analysis, or cluster analysis, and their association with frailty has been investigated [6–8]; however, previous results from studies on diets in Western countries are different from those relating to the Asian diet. Moreover, although a few studies [9–11] have examined the relationship between dietary patterns and frailty in Asian countries, the results are controversial.

Therefore, we examined the association between dietary patterns extracted using reduced rank regression (RRR) and frailty in older Korean community-dwelling residents. RRR reduces the dimensions of the predictor variables and maximizes the variation of the response variables, reflecting both a priori-defined and posteriori-derived dietary patterns [12].

2. Materials and Methods

2.1. Study Population

Data were retrieved from the Korean Frailty and Aging Cohort study [13]. The subjects were enrolled according to age- and gender-specific strata from South Korean, community-dwelling older people, aged 70–84 years. Baseline surveys were conducted from May to November 2016 across eight university-affiliated hospitals and two public health centers (n = 1559). Dietary intake was examined during home visits on two nonconsecutive days for a sub-cohort study including two-thirds of the baseline subjects from September 2016 to November 2017. The first follow-up surveys were conducted from March to December 2018. The study was performed following the tenets of the Helsinki Declaration, and it was approved by the Institutional Review Board of Ajou University Hospital (AJIRB-SBR-SUR-20-356). Written informed consent was obtained from all subjects. Of the 580 who completed all evaluations, those with missing values (n = 69) for educational level, marital status, smoking, number of physician-diagnosed chronic diseases, depression index, and cognitive function were excluded. The final analytical sample included 511 subjects.

2.2. Assessment of Dietary Intake

Dietary data were obtained from the baseline surveys (2016–2017) using two non-consecutive 24-h dietary recalls, which were carried out by trained interviewers during home visits over 3–10 month intervals. Bowls, plates, and food pictures, developed by the National Institutes of Health (NIH) and the Korea Disease Control and Prevention Agency (KDCA), were used to estimate portion size. Trained interviewers examined the names and amount of food consumed, the types of meals, and eating locations of the previous day. Food and nutrient intakes were calculated using the 24-h recall dietary assessment system of the NIH and KDCA based on the National Rural Living Science Institute database [14]. Individual foods were grouped into 22 food groups based on similar nutritional content and characteristics [14].

2.3. Assessment of Frailty

Frailty status was measured by a modified version of the Fried Frailty Phenotype (FFP) [15] in both the baseline (2016) and the first follow-up survey (2018). It contains five components: weight loss (unintentional, 4.5 kg or more in the previous year), self-reported exhaustion (felt that everything was an effort or that one could not get going ≥ 3 times a week), low physical activity, measured by the International Physical Activity Questionnaire Short Form (Korean version) [16] (<494.65 kcal/week for men, < 283.50 kcal/week for women) [17], low grip strength (Takei dynamometer, with body mass index (BMI) < 22.0 then $\leq$ 25.4 kg, 22.0 $\leq$ BMI $\leq$ 23.9 then $\leq$ 27.1 kg, 24.0 $\leq$ BMI $\leq$ 25.9 then $\leq$ 27.8 kg, BMI $\geq$ 26.0 then $\leq$ 28.5 kg for men, and BMI < 23.0 then $\leq$ 16.8 kg, 23.0 $\leq$ BMI $\leq$ 24.9 then $\leq$ 17.6 kg, 25.0 $\leq$ BMI $\leq$ 26.9 then $\leq$ 17.8 kg, BMI $\geq$ 27.0 then $\leq$ 17.7 kg for women) [13], and slow gait speed (if height ≤ 165.0 cm then ≤ 0.93 m/sec and if height > 165.0 cm then ≤ 0.98 m/sec for men, and if height ≤ 152.0 cm then ≤ 0.85 m/sec and if height > 152.0 cm then ≤ 0.93 m/sec for women) [13]. Each component was assigned a score of 1 (if present) or 0 (if absent). Frailty scores ranged from 0 to 5, and frailty status was categorized as robust (0), pre-frail (1–2), and frail (3–5). We used the frailty incidence data (excluding the subjects classified as frail in 2016), the remaining subjects' frailty status in 2018 was measured, and these were included in the analysis.

2.4. Covariates

Baseline data (2016) were used for covariates. Age, gender, education, and marital status were included for demographic characteristics. Body mass index was calculated as kg/m^2. Physician-diagnosed chronic diseases included imbalances of the circulatory system, musculoskeletal system and its connective tissue, respiratory, digestive, endocrine, nervous, and urogenital systems as well as neoplasms, and diseases were classified as 0, 1, and ≥2. The number of prescription drug treatments was categorized as < 4 and ≥ 4. The Korean version of the Short Form Geriatric Depression Scale (SGDS-K) [18] was used as a depression index (depression ≥ 8 points), and the Mini-Mental State Examination in the Korean version of the CERAD Assessment Packet (MMSE-KC) [19] was used as a cognitive function index (normal ≥ 24 points). Falls (experience of falling over in the past year) were also included. Smoking, dietary supplement use, and energy intake were included for health behaviors.

2.5. Statistical Analysis

The dietary patterns were extracted using RRR, and the RRR method is described elsewhere [12]. Briefly, the purpose of this approach is to reduce the dimension of the predictor variables (food groups) and maximize the variation of the response variables (usually nutrients or biomarkers) that are hypothesized to be associated with the outcome. Intake of protein and vitamin D have been associated with frailty in a previous study [3] and these were selected as responses for RRR. Two dietary patterns were extracted using RRR from 22 food groups. The relationship between the food groups and the dietary patterns was designated by factor loadings. Food groups with factor loadings ≥0.2 were considered positive contributors to the patterns, and foods with factor loadings up to −0.2 were negative contributors to the patterns. Dietary pattern scores were classified into tertiles.

The relationships between the dietary pattern and subject characteristics or between frailty status and subject characteristics were analyzed using the analysis of variance and post-hoc tests, chi-square tests and were presented as the mean ± standard deviation or a number (percentage). After adjusting for covariates, a multinomial logistic regression analysis was used for the association between dietary patterns and frailty, and a logistic regression analysis was used for the association between dietary patterns and the individual FFP. p-values for trend were also estimated according to the dietary pattern tertiles. The odds ratio (OR) and 95% confidence interval (CI) were calculated. We also added the results of the analysis using a continuous variable (dietary pattern scores divided by standard deviation). The p-values reported were two-sided, and the significance level was set at <0.05. All statistical analyses were conducted using SAS version 9.4 (SAS Institute, Inc., Cary, NC, USA).

3. Results

Two dietary patterns were obtained using RRR with factor loadings for each food group (Table 1). The first dietary pattern, labeled the "meat, fish, and vegetables" pattern, was characterized by high consumption of meat, fish, vegetables, rice, poultry, oils and fats, sugars and sweets, and seasonings. The second pattern, labeled as the "milk" pattern, was characterized by high consumption of milk and dairy products, fish, eggs, and nuts and seeds, and low consumption of noodles and dumplings, meat, poultry, beans, and seasonings. The two dietary patterns combined explained 13.7% of the total variation in the food group consumption and 64.2% of the variation in the response variables (protein and vitamin D).

Table 1. Factor loading values derived by reduced rank regression [a] (n = 511).

Food Groups	Meat, Fish, and Vegetables Pattern	Milk Pattern
Rice	**0.24**	−0.16
Rice cakes	−0.04	−0.08
Other grains	0.01	−0.12
Noodles & dumplings	0.10	**−0.24**
Flour & bread	0.12	0.07
Potatoes & starches	0.08	−0.08
Meat	**0.35**	**−0.36**
Poultry	**0.22**	**−0.24**
Fish	**0.41**	**0.30**
Eggs	0.17	**0.26**
Beans	0.17	**−0.20**
Shellfish	0.10	0.07
Nuts & seeds	0.18	**0.23**
Vegetables	**0.37**	−0.09
Kimchi	0.18	−0.18
Fruits	0.07	−0.01
Milk & dairy products	0.13	**0.55**
Oils & fats	**0.21**	0.01
Sugars & sweets	**0.25**	0.02
Beverages	0.10	−0.01
Alcohol	0.06	−0.19
Seasonings	**0.41**	**−0.23**
Explained variation (%)		
Food groups	8.3	5.4
Responses	51.2	13.0

[a] Factor loadings with absolute values ≥ 0.20 are shown in bold.

The study subjects had an average age of 75.9 ± 4.0 years, and 50.5% were women. Of the subjects, 43.1%, 50.7%, and 6.3% were robust, pre-frail, and frail, respectively, in 2018 (data not shown). The relationship between the dietary pattern score and subject characteristics is shown in Table 2. For the "meat, fish, and vegetables" pattern, subjects in the highest tertile of the dietary pattern score were more likely men, highly educated, married, and they were less likely to have physician-diagnosed chronic diseases. They also had lower depression scores (SGDS-K ≥ 8 points), higher normal cognitive function (MMSE-KC ≥ 24 points), and had higher energy intake than those in the lowest tertile. For the "milk" pattern, gender, education, dietary supplement use, and energy intake were significantly different among the tertiles of dietary pattern scores.

The relationship between frailty status and subject characteristics is shown in Table 3. Compared with those who were robust, frail subjects tended to be older, women, less educated, not married, with more physician-diagnosed chronic diseases, and had received more prescription drug treatments. They also had higher depression scores (SGDS-K ≥ 8 points), lower normal cognitive function (MMSE-KC ≥ 24 points), and had less energy intake.

Table 4 shows the association between the dietary pattern score and frailty. In the "meat, fish, and vegetables" pattern, subjects in the highest tertile of the dietary pattern score were less likely to have pre-frailty compared to those subjects in the lowest tertile, after adjusting for covariates (OR = 0.41, 95% CI = 0.21–0.81, p for trend = 0.009). Subjects in the highest tertile of the dietary pattern score were less likely to have frailty compared to those subjects in the lowest tertile (unadjusted) (OR = 0.14, 95% CI = 0.04–0.43, p for trend <0.001), but the significant association disappeared after adjusting for covariates. In regard to the individual components of the FFP, the increasing tertiles of the dietary pattern score were inversely associated with exhaustion (OR = 0.41, 95% CI = 0.20–0.85,

p for trend = 0.020). The "milk" pattern was not significantly associated with either the frailty status or the individual components of the FFP criteria. In addition, the result of the relationship between the continuous change in the dietary pattern scores (dietary pattern scores divided by the standard deviation) and frailty status was similar to the above.

Table 2. Relationship between tertiles of dietary pattern scores and subject characteristics (n = 511).

Characteristics	Meat, Fish, and Vegetables Pattern				Milk Pattern			
	Tertile 1 (n = 170)	Tertile 2 (n = 171)	Tertile 3 (n = 170)	p-Value [a]	Tertile 1 (n = 170)	Tertile 2 (n = 171)	Tertile 3 (n = 170)	p-Value [a]
Dietary Pattern Score	−1.12 ± 0.38	−0.08 ± 0.27	1.20 ± 0.86		−1.05 ± 0.56	−0.07 ± 0.20	1.12 ± 0.66	
Age (years)				0.512				0.682
70–74	61 (35.9)	71 (41.5)	77 (45.3)		76 (44.7)	69 (40.4)	64 (37.6)	
75–79	64 (37.6)	61 (35.7)	56 (32.9)		55 (32.4)	64 (37.4)	62 (36.5)	
80–84	45 (26.5)	39 (22.8)	37 (21.8)		39 (22.9)	38 (22.2)	44 (25.9)	
Gender				**<0.001**				**0.001**
Men	42 (24.7)	90 (52.6)	121 (71.2)		102 (60.0)	68 (39.8)	83 (48.8)	
Women	128 (75.3)	81 (47.4)	49 (28.8)		68 (40.0)	103 (60.2)	87 (51.2)	
Education				**<0.001**				**<0.001**
Elementary school	110 (64.7)	65 (38.0)	46 (27.1)		71 (41.8)	95 (55.6)	55 (32.4)	
Higher than elementary school	660 (35.3)	106 (62.0)	124 (72.9)		99 (58.2)	76 (44.4)	115 (67.6)	
Marital status				**<0.001**				0.168
Married	98 (57.6)	120 (70.2)	133 (78.2)		126 (74.1)	114 (66.7)	111 (65.3)	
Others	72 (42.4)	51 (29.8)	37 (21.8)		44 (25.9)	57 (33.3)	59 (34.7)	
Body mass index (Kg/m^2)	24.4 ± 2.8	24.5 ± 2.7	24.4 ± 3.0	0.856	24.3 ± 2.8	24.3 ± 2.9	24.8 ± 2.7	0.224
Number of physician-diagnosed chronic diseases				**0.004**				0.475
0	38 (22.4)	57 (33.3)	71 (41.8)		61 (35.9)	49 (28.7)	56 (32.9)	
1	81 (47.6)	70 (40.9)	65 (38.2)		64 (37.6)	81 (47.4)	71 (41.8)	
≥2	51 (30.0)	44 (25.7)	34 (20.0)		45 (26.5)	41 (24.0)	43 (25.3)	
Number of prescription drug treatments				0.425				0.551
<4	87 (51.2)	94 (55.0)	99 (58.2)		98 (57.6)	94 (55.0)	88 (51.8)	
≥4	83 (48.8)	77 (45.0)	71 (41.8)		72 (42.4)	77 (45.0)	82 (48.2)	
SGDS-K				**0.001**				0.191
<8	137 (80.6)	154 (90.1)	159 (93.5)		155 (91.2)	145 (84.8)	150 (88.2)	
≥8	33 (19.4)	17 (9.9)	11 (6.5)		15 (8.8)	26 (15.2)	20 (11.8)	
MMSE-KC				**0.001**				0.419
<24	36 (21.2)	27 (15.8)	12 (7.1)		27 (15.9)	28 (16.4)	20 (11.8)	
≥24	134 (78.8)	144 (84.2)	158 (92.9)		143 (84.1)	143 (83.6)	150 (88.2)	
Falls				0.398				0.246
Yes	30 (17.6)	32 (18.7)	23 (13.5)		24 (14.1)	35 (20.5)	26 (15.3)	
No	140 (82.4)	139 (81.3)	147 (86.5)		146 (85.9)	136 (79.5)	144 (84.7)	
Smoking				0.766				0.618
Never or former	162 (95.3)	162 (94.7)	159 (93.5)		160 (94.1)	160 (93.6)	163 (95.9)	
Current	8 (4.7)	9 (5.3)	11 (6.5)		10 (5.9)	11 (6.4)	7 (4.1)	
Dietary supplement use				0.102				**0.001**
Yes	98 (57.6)	102 (59.6)	116 (68.2)		92 (54.1)	100 (58.5)	124 (72.9)	
No	72 (42.4)	69 (40.4)	54 (31.8)		78 (45.9)	71 (41.5)	46 (27.1)	
Energy intake (Kcal/day)	1134.0 ± 249.2 *	1420.1 ± 265.6 **	1797.7 ± 375.9 ***	**<0.001**	1595.5 ± 428.4 *	1365.3 ± 354.9 **	1391.3 ± 393.9 **	**<0.001**

Values are mean ± standard deviation or number (percentage). [a] Analysis of variance (*, **, ***: Results of post-hoc tests) for continuous variables and chi-square test for categorical variables. Abbreviation: SGDS-K-Korean version of the Short Form Geriatric Depression Scale [18]; MMSE-KC-Mini-Mental State Examination in the Korean version of the CERAD Assessment Packet [19]. We marked significant p-values in bold.

Table 3. Relationship between frailty status and subject characteristics ($n = 511$).

Characteristics	Frailty Status			p-Value [a]
	Robust (n = 220)	Pre-Frail (n = 259)	Frail (n = 32)	
Age (years)				<0.001
70–74	117 (53.2)	89 (34.4)	3 (9.4)	
75–79	67 (30.5)	102 (39.4)	12 (37.5)	
80–84	36 (16.4)	68 (26.3)	17 (53.1)	
Gender				0.008
Men	122 (55.5)	122 (47.1)	9 (28.1)	
Women	98 (44.5)	137 (52.9)	23 (71.9)	
Education				0.006
Elementary school	79 (35.9)	123 (47.5)	19 (59.4)	
Higher than elementary school	141 (64.1)	136 (52.5)	13 (40.6)	
Marital status				0.017
Married	165 (75.0)	168 (64.9)	18 (56.3)	
Others	55 (25.0)	91 (35.1)	14 (43.8)	
Body mass index (Kg/m^2)	24.4 ± 2.7	24.4 ± 2.9	24.8 ± 3.0	0.755
Number of physician-diagnosed chronic diseases				0.004
0	87 (39.5)	73 (28.2)	6 (18.8)	
1	91 (41.4)	113 (43.6)	12 (37.5)	
≥2	42 (19.1)	73 (28.2)	14 (43.8)	
Number of prescription drug treatments				<0.001
<4	140 (63.6)	133 (51.4)	7 (21.9)	
≥4	80 (36.4)	126 (48.6)	25 (78.1)	
SGDS-K				<0.001
<8	210 (95.5)	213 (82.2)	27 (84.4)	
≥8	10 (4.5)	46 (17.8)	5 (15.6)	
MMSE-KC				0.001
<24	18 (8.2)	48 (18.5)	9 (28.1)	
≥24	202 (91.8)	211 (81.5)	23 (71.9)	
Falls				0.082
Yes	28 (12.7)	49 (18.9)	8 (25.0)	
No	192 (87.3)	210 (81.1)	24 (75.0)	
Smoking				0.227
Never or former	212 (96.4)	242 (93.4)	29 (90.6)	
Current	8 (3.6)	17 (6.6)	3 (9.4)	
Dietary supplement use				0.524
Yes	135 (61.4)	164 (63.3)	17 (53.1)	
No	85 (38.6)	95 (36.7)	15 (46.9)	
Energy intake (Kcal/day)	1519.3 ± 409.2 *	1421.8 ± 402.1 **	1209.8 ± 287.6 ***	<0.001

Values are mean ± standard deviation or number (percentage). [a] Analysis of variance (*, **, ***: Results of post-hoc tests) for continuous variables and chi-square test for categorical variables. Abbreviation: SGDS-K-Korean version of the Short Form Geriatric Depression Scale [18]; MMSE-KC-Mini-Mental State Examination in the Korean version of the CERAD Assessment Packet [19]. We marked significant p-values in bold.

Table 4. Odds ratio (OR) and 95% confidence interval (CI) for frailty and the Fried Frailty Phenotype according to dietary pattern scores [a] ($n = 511$).

	Crude OR								Adjusted OR [b]						
	Tertile 1	Tertile 2		Tertile 3		*p* for Trend	Dietary Pattern Scores (Changes/SD) [c]	*p*-Value	Tertile 2		Tertile 3		*p* for Trend	Dietary Pattern Scores (Changes/SD) [c]	*p*-Value
		OR	95% CI	OR	95% CI		OR		OR	95% CI	OR	95% CI		OR	
Meat, Fish, and Vegetables Pattern															
Frailty status															
Pre-frail vs. robust	1.00	0.87	0.55–1.37	0.41	0.26–0.65	**<0.001**	0.67	**<0.001**	0.98	0.57–1.67	0.41	0.21–0.81	**0.009**	0.61	**0.004**
Frail vs. robust	1.00	0.57	0.25–1.31	0.14	0.04–0.43	**<0.001**	0.41	**<0.001**	1.25	0.43–3.64	0.38	0.07–1.90	0.289	0.84	0.663
Fried Frailty Phenotype															
Unintentional weight loss	1.00	1.55	0.72–3.32	1.18	0.53–2.64	0.702	0.98	0.902	1.67	0.70–4.00	1.21	0.38–3.89	0.724	0.84	0.534
Exhaustion	1.00	0.59	0.38–0.93	0.32	0.20–0.53	**<0.001**	0.62	**<0.001**	0.77	0.45–1.31	0.41	0.20–0.85	**0.020**	0.62	**0.013**
Low physical activity	1.00	0.93	0.45–1.91	0.56	0.25–1.27	0.173	0.78	0.163	0.95	0.41–2.20	0.61	0.19–1.94	0.426	0.87	0.642
Low grip strength	1.00	1.18	0.74–1.88	0.47	0.28–0.81	**0.008**	0.67	**0.001**	1.59	0.89–2.83	0.79	0.36–1.73	0.667	0.90	0.592
Slow gait speed	1.00	0.74	0.42–1.31	0.45	0.24–0.85	**0.014**	0.68	**0.008**	0.97	0.49–1.95	0.69	0.26–1.80	0.484	0.88	0.594
Milk Pattern															
Frailty status															
Pre-frail vs. robust	1.00	1.30	0.84–2.02	0.89	0.58–1.39	0.551	0.89	0.222	1.02	0.63–1.67	0.73	0.45–1.19	0.192	0.83	0.065
Frail vs. robust	1.00	1.15	0.43–3.07	1.52	0.62–3.71	0.337	1.02	0.935	0.51	0.16–1.63	1.17	0.40–3.44	0.572	0.95	0.841
Fried Frailty Phenotype															
Unintentional weight loss	1.00	0.68	0.31–1.47	0.87	0.42–1.81	0.747	0.88	0.421	0.62	0.27–1.40	0.89	0.41–1.95	0.812	0.89	0.492
Exhaustion	1.00	1.35	0.85–2.16	1.26	0.79–2.01	0.379	1.02	0.866	0.96	0.57–1.62	1.07	0.63–1.81	0.772	0.95	0.659
Low physical activity	1.00	1.07	0.51–2.23	0.79	0.36–1.73	0.534	0.95	0.771	0.90	0.41–1.98	0.68	0.29–1.60	0.375	0.91	0.596
Low grip strength	1.00	1.52	0.92–2.51	1.44	0.87–2.39	0.192	1.04	0.672	1.39	0.79–2.43	1.32	0.74–2.33	0.396	0.99	0.906
Slow gait speed	1.00	0.86	0.46–1.59	1.05	0.58–1.90	0.841	1.00	0.998	0.65	0.33–1.30	1.02	0.52–2.00	0.847	1.01	0.975

[a] Multinomial logistic regression for frailty status, binomial logistic regression for the Fried Frailty Phenotype. [b] Adjusted for age, gender, education, marital status, body mass index, number of physician-diagnosed chronic diseases, number of prescription drug treatments, Korean version of the Short Form Geriatric Depression Scale [18], Mini-Mental State Examination in the Korean version of the CERAD Assessment Packet [19], falls, smoking, dietary supplement use, and energy intake. [c] Dietary pattern scores/standard deviation. We marked significant *p*-values in bold.

4. Discussion

In the current study, two dietary patterns were extracted using RRR. The "meat, fish, and vegetables" pattern was inversely associated with pre-frailty and exhaustion after adjustment for covariates. The "milk" pattern was not significantly associated with either the frailty status or the individual components of the FFP criteria.

To our knowledge, only three previous studies have investigated the association between dietary patterns and frailty in Asian populations [9–11]. A Chinese prospective study [9] showed that a "vegetable-fruit" dietary pattern was not related to frailty incidence. A Taiwanese cross-sectional study [10] reported that the RRR-derived dietary pattern, which included a high consumption of fruit, nuts and seeds, tea, vegetables, whole grains, shellfish, milk, and fish, was inversely associated with frailty. A Japanese prospective cohort study [11] showed that a "protein-rich" dietary pattern was negatively related to frailty while a "salt and pickles" pattern and "sugar and fat" pattern were positively related to frailty. In Western countries, most studies have examined the association between the Mediterranean diet (a priori-defined dietary pattern) and frailty. A recent meta-analysis showed that the Mediterranean diet was associated with lower frailty incidence [5]. While few studies have examined the association between a posteriori-derived dietary patterns and frailty, in a Spanish prospective study [6], "prudent" dietary patterns (high intake of olive oil and vegetables) were inversely associated with frailty incidence. In the Three-City Bordeaux Study [7], men in the "pasta" pattern and women in the "biscuits and snacking" pattern had higher rates of frailty than those in the "healthy" pattern (higher fish intake in men and higher fruits and vegetables intake in women). In the longitudinal results of the Rotterdam study [8], adherence to the "traditional" pattern (high in legumes, eggs and savory snacks) was associated with less frailty. The results of this current study are partially similar to those of the previous studies.

Several potential mechanisms related to dietary pattern and frailty have been suggested. Studies of nutrient intake and frailty have mainly focused on proteins, which stimulate muscle protein synthesis. The results have reported an inverse relationship between protein intake and frailty in older people [20,21]. In our study, higher consumption of protein-rich foods, such as meat, fish, and poultry were associated with reduced pre-frailty. Vitamin D is involved in frailty through two metabolic pathways, bone mineralization and muscle strength [3,22]. The antioxidant properties may delay the development of frailty by preventing oxidative stress [23]. Many studies have reported inverse associations between frailty and micro-nutrients such as carotenoids, vitamin C, vitamin E, and selenium [24,25]. Therefore, vegetables may contain antioxidative properties related to frailty prevention. The current study indicated that higher consumption of seasonings (mainly soy sauce, red pepper powder, Gochujang [fermented red pepper paste], Doenjang [soybean paste], table salt) was associated with lower pre-frailty. Although, we could not determine the mechanism by which these dietary factors reduce pre-frailty, the high consumption of seasonings involved a more balanced macronutrient composition than low consumption of seasonings [26], and this may have beneficial effect in preventing pre-frailty (Table S1).

The "meat, fish, and vegetables" pattern was not significantly associated with frailty after adjusting for covariates, which may be because of the low number of frail subjects (n = 32). A previous study reported that the consumption of dairy products may decrease frailty (mean intake of total dairy products: 306.3 g per day) [27]. However, in the current study, the "milk" pattern was not associated with frailty. The consumption of milk and dairy products was low (mean intake: 52.9 g per day, data not shown) and the low value of the explained variation for the "milk" pattern could partly explain the nonsignificant association with frailty status and FFP criteria.

This study has several potential limitations. First, dietary data were obtained using 24-h dietary recalls. This method cannot accurately reflect the usual dietary intake of study subjects. However, we examined the dietary intake for two nonconsecutive days and used the mean intake. Second, dietary patterns are highly related to the study population's diet. Therefore, the dietary patterns extracted from this study may not be generalizable to other populations, especially those of different cultures. Third, participants with cognitive impairment may be limited for 24-h dietary recalls and their estimation of intake may not be reliable. Fourth, although we included as many potential confounders as possible, residual confounding may remain. Lastly, although the current study focused on the relationship between physical frailty and dietary patterns, there are multidimensions of frailty and multidomain relevance of healthy behaviors related to frailty, so these should be considered in the future [28,29].

5. Conclusions

The "meat, fish, and vegetables" pattern was significantly associated with lower odds of pre-frailty. Our results suggest a potentially protective effect of a "protein-rich, vegetables" dietary pattern against frailty.

Supplementary Materials: The following are available online at http://www.mdpi.com/xxx/s1, Table S1: Macronutrient intake by tertiles of food group.

Author Contributions: Conceptualization, J.K., Y.L., C.W.W., and M.K.K.; methodology, J.K., S.K. (Seunghee Kye), and J.-S.S.; validation, S.K. (Seungkook Ki) and J.-h.Y.; formal analysis, J.K.; resources, M.K.K.; writing—original draft preparation, J.K.; writing—review & editing, Y.L.; supervision, Y.L., C.W.W., and M.K.K.; funding acquisition, C.W.W. All authors have read and agreed to the published version of the manuscript.

Funding: This work was supported by the Korea Health Technology R&D Project through the Korean Health Industry Development Institute (KHIDI), the Ministry of Health and Welfare, Republic of Korea (Grant Number: HI15C3153).

Institutional Review Board Statement: The study was performed following the tenets of the Helsinki Declaration, and it was approved by the Institutional Review Board of Ajou University Hospital (AJIRB-SBR-SUR-20-356).

Informed Consent Statement: Written informed consent was obtained from all subjects.

Conflicts of Interest: The authors declare no conflict of interest. The funders had no role in the design, execution, interpretation, or writing of the study.

References

1. Clegg, A.; Young, J.; Iliffe, S.; Rikkert, M.O.; Rockwood, K. Frailty in elderly people. *Lancet* **2013**, *381*, 752–762. [CrossRef]
2. Buckinx, F.; Rolland, Y.; Reginster, J.Y.; Ricour, C.; Petermans, J.; Bruyère, O. Burden of frailty in the elderly population: Perspectives for a public health challenge. *Arch. Public Health* **2015**, *73*, 19. [CrossRef]
3. Lorenzo-López, L.; Maseda, A.; de Labra, C.; Regueiro-Folgueira, L.; Rodríguez-Villamil, J.L.; Millán-Calenti, J.C. Nutritional determinants of frailty in older adults: A systematic review. *BMC Geriatr.* **2017**, *17*, 108. [CrossRef]
4. Hu, F.B. Dietary pattern analysis: A new direction in nutritional epidemiology. *Curr. Opin. Lipidol.* **2002**, *13*, 3–9. [CrossRef] [PubMed]
5. Kojima, G.; Avgerinou, C.; Iliffe, S.; Walters, K. Adherence to Mediterranean diet reduces incident frailty risk: Systematic review and meta-analysis. *J. Am. Geriatr. Soc.* **2018**, *66*, 783–788. [CrossRef]
6. León-Muñoz, L.M.; García-Esquinas, E.; López-García, E.; Banegas, J.R.; Rodríguez-Artalejo, F. Major dietary patterns and risk of frailty in older adults: A prospective cohort study. *BMC Med.* **2015**, *13*, 11. [CrossRef] [PubMed]
7. Pilleron, S.; Ajana, S.; Jutand, M.A.; Helmer, C.; Dartigues, J.F.; Samieri, C.; Féart, C. Dietary patterns and 12-year risk of frailty: Results from the three-city Bordeaux study. *J. Am. Med. Dir. Assoc.* **2017**, *18*, 169–175. [CrossRef]
8. De Haas, S.C.M.; de Jonge, E.A.L.; Voortman, T.; Graaff, J.S.; Franco, O.H.; Ikram, M.A.; Rivadeneira, F.; Kiefte-de Jong, J.C.; Schoufour, J.D. Dietary patterns and changes in frailty status: The Rotterdam study. *Eur. J. Nutr.* **2018**, *57*, 2365–2375. [CrossRef]
9. Chan, R.; Leung, J.; Woo, J. Dietary patterns and risk of frailty in Chinese community-dwelling older people in Hong Kong: A prospective cohort study. *Nutrients* **2015**, *7*, 7070–7084. [CrossRef] [PubMed]
10. Lo, Y.L.; Hsieh, Y.T.; Hsu, L.L.; Chuang, S.Y.; Chang, H.Y.; Hsu, C.C.; Chen, C.Y.; Pan, W.H. Dietary pattern associated with frailty: Results from Nutrition and Health Survey in Taiwan. *J. Am. Geriatr. Soc.* **2017**, *65*, 2009–2015. [CrossRef] [PubMed]
11. Huang, C.H.; Martins, B.A.; Okada, K.; Matsushita, E.; Uno, C.; Satake, S.; Kuzuya, M. A 3-year prospective cohort study of dietary patterns and frailty risk among community-dwelling older adults. *Clin. Nutr.* **2020**. online ahead of print. [CrossRef] [PubMed]

12. Hoffmann, K.; Schulze, M.B.; Schienkiewitz, A.; Nöthlings, U.; Boeing, H. Application of a new statistical method to derive dietary patterns in nutritional epidemiology. *Am. J. Epidemiol.* **2004**, *159*, 935–944. [CrossRef]
13. Won, C.W.; Lee, S.; Kim, J.; Chon, D.; Kim, S.; Kim, C.O.; Kim, M.K.; Cho, B.; Choi, K.M.; Roh, E.; et al. Korean frailty and aging cohort study (KFACS): Cohort profile. *BMJ Open* **2020**, *10*, e035573. [CrossRef] [PubMed]
14. National Rural Resources Development Institute. *Food Composition Table (1), Seventh Revision*; National Rural Resources Development Institute: Suwon, Korea, 2006; pp. 1–453.
15. Fried, L.P.; Tangen, C.M.; Walston, J.; Newman, A.B.; Hirsch, C.; Gottdiener, J.; Seeman, T.; Tracy, R.; Kop, W.J.; Burke, G.; et al. Frailty in older adults: Evidence for a phenotype. *J. Gerontol. Ser. A-Biol. Sci. Med. Sci.* **2001**, *56*, M146–M156. [CrossRef] [PubMed]
16. Oh, J.Y.; Yang, Y.J.; Kim, B.S.; Kang, J.H. Validity and reliability of Korean version of International Physical Activity Questionnaire (IPAQ) short form. *J. Korean Acad. Fam. Med.* **2007**, *28*, 532–541.
17. Keimyung University Industry Academic Cooperation Foundation; Ministry of Health and Welfare & Family. *2008 Living Profiles of Older People Survey*; Ministry of Health and Welfare & Family: Seoul, Korea, 2009; p. 636.
18. Cho, M.J.; Bae, J.N.; Suh, G.H.; Hahm, B.J.; Kim, J.K.; Lee, D.W.; Kang, M.H. Validation of Geriatric Depression Scale, Korean version (GDS) in the assessment of DSM-III-R major depression. *J. Korean Neuropsychiatr. Assoc.* **1999**, *38*, 48–63.
19. Lee, D.Y.; Lee, K.U.; Lee, J.H.; Kim, K.W.; Jhoo, J.H.; Kim, S.Y.; Yoon, J.C.; Woo, S.I.; Ha, J.; Woo, J.I. A normative study of the CERAD neuropsychological assessment battery in the Korean elderly. *J. Int. Neuropsychol. Soc.* **2004**, *10*, 72–81. [CrossRef]
20. Bartali, B.; Frongillo, E.A.; Bandinelli, S.; Lauretani, F.; Semba, R.D.; Fried, L.P.; Ferrucci, L. Low nutrient intake is an essential component of frailty in older persons. *J. Gerontol. Ser. A-Biol. Sci. Med. Sci.* **2006**, *61*, 589–593. [CrossRef]
21. Beasley, J.M.; LaCroix, A.Z.; Neuhouser, M.L.; Huang, Y.; Tinker, L.; Woods, N.; Michael, Y.; Curb, J.D.; Prentice, R.L. Protein intake and incident frailty in the Women's health initiative observational study. *J. Am. Geriatr. Soc.* **2010**, *58*, 1063–1071. [CrossRef]
22. Yannakoulia, M.; Ntanasi, E.; Anastasiou, C.A.; Scarmeas, N. Frailty and nutrition; from epidemiological and clinical evidence to potential mechanisms. *Metabolism* **2017**, *68*, 64–76. [CrossRef] [PubMed]
23. Kumawat, M.; Sharma, T.K.; Singh, I.; Singh, N.; Singh, S.K.; Ghalaut, V.S.; Shankar, V.; Vardey, S.K. Decrease in antioxidant status of plasma and erythrocytes from geriatric population. *Dis. Markers* **2012**, *33*, 303–308. [CrossRef]
24. Michelon, E.; Blaum, C.; Semba, R.D.; Xue, Q.L.; Ricks, M.O.; Fried, L.P. Vitamin and carotenoid status in older women: Associations with the frailty syndrome. *J. Gerontol. Ser. A-Biol. Sci. Med. Sci.* **2006**, *61*, 600–607. [CrossRef]
25. Semba, R.D.; Bartali, B.; Zhou, J.; Blaum, C.; Ko, C.W.; Fried, L.P. Low serum micronutrient concentrations predict frailty among older women living in the community. *J. Gerontol. Ser. A-Biol. Sci. Med. Sci.* **2006**, *61*, 594–599. [CrossRef] [PubMed]
26. Ministry of Health & Welfare; The Korean Nutrition Society. *Dietary Reference Intakes for Koreans 2015*; The Korean Nutrition Society: Seoul, Korea, 2016; p. 1050.
27. Lana, A.; Rodriguez-Artalejo, F.; Lopez-Garcia, E. Dairy consumption and risk of frailty in older adults: A prospective cohort study. *J. Am. Geriatr. Soc.* **2015**, *63*, 1852–1860. [CrossRef] [PubMed]
28. Cesari, M.; Gambassi, G.; Abellan van Kan, G.; Vellas, B. The frailty phenotype and the frailty index: Different instruments for different purposes. *Age Ageing* **2014**, *43*, 10–12. [CrossRef] [PubMed]
29. Jung, H.; Kim, M.; Lee, Y.; Won, C.W. Prevalence of physical frailty and its multidimensional risk factors in Korean community-dwelling older adults: Findings from Korean frailty and aging cohort study. *Int. J. Environ. Res. Public Health* **2020**, *17*, 7883. [CrossRef]

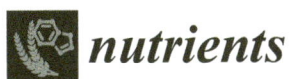

Article

Association of Adherence to the Mediterranean-Style Diet with Lower Frailty Index in Older Adults

Toshiko Tanaka [1,*], Sameera A. Talegawkar [2], Yichen Jin [2], Stephania Bandinelli [3] and Luigi Ferrucci [1]

[1] Longitudinal Study Section, Translation Gerontology Branch, National Institute on Aging, Baltimore, MD 21224, USA; FerrucciLu@grc.nia.nih.gov
[2] Department of Exercise and Nutrition Sciences, Milken Institute School of Public Health, The George Washington University, Washington, DC 20052, USA; stalega1@gwu.edu (S.A.T.); yjin@gwu.edu (Y.J.)
[3] Geriatric Unit, Azienda Sanitaria Toscana Centro, 50125 Firenze, Italy; stefania1.bandinelli@uslcentro.toscana.it
* Correspondence: tanakato@mail.nih.gov

Citation: Tanaka, T.; Talegawkar, S.A.; Jin, Y.; Bandinelli, S.; Ferrucci, L. Association of Adherence to the Mediterranean-Style Diet with Lower Frailty Index in Older Adults. *Nutrients* **2021**, *13*, 1129. https://doi.org/10.3390/nu13041129

Academic Editors: Emiliana Giacomello and Luana Toniolo

Received: 1 March 2021
Accepted: 24 March 2021
Published: 30 March 2021

Publisher's Note: MDPI stays neutral with regard to jurisdictional claims in published maps and institutional affiliations.

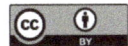

Copyright: © 2021 by the authors. Licensee MDPI, Basel, Switzerland. This article is an open access article distributed under the terms and conditions of the Creative Commons Attribution (CC BY) license (https://creativecommons.org/licenses/by/4.0/).

Abstract: Identifying modifying protective factors to promote healthy aging is of utmost public health importance. The frailty index (FI) reflects the accumulation of health deficits and is one widely used method to assess health trajectories in aging. Adherence to a Mediterranean-type diet (MTD) has been associated with favorable health trajectories. Therefore, this study explored whether adherence to a MTD is negatively associated with FI in the InCHIANTI study. Participants (*n* = 485) included individuals over 65 years of age at baseline with complete data over a follow-up period of 10 years. MTD was computed on a scale of 0–9 and categorized based on these scores into three groups of low (≤3), medium (4–5), and high (≥6) adherence. Being in a high or medium adherence group was associated with 0.03 and 0.013 unit lower FI scores over the follow-up period, compared to the low adherence group. In participants with a low FI at baseline, being in a high or medium MTD-adherence group had 0.004 and 0.005 unit/year slower progression of FI compared to the low adherence group. These study results support adherence to a MTD as a protective strategy to maintain a lower FI.

Keywords: Mediterranean diet; frailty index; trajectory

1. Introduction

As lifespan extends globally, there is a greater emphasis on improving health span. There are various metrics to evaluate "health" during the lifespan. It is generally recognized that the development of frailty is an important turning point in the trajectory of health in older persons. The frailty index (FI), a cumulative score of health deficits, is one of the most frequently used operational definitions of frailty [1,2]. The FI is calculated as a proportion of health deficits based on a varying (<30–70) number of variables reflecting symptoms, signs, diseases, and disabilities that accumulate over time. Although the variables included in the FI can vary from study to study, there is a strong rationale that they capture an important dimension of health in old age.

In the InCHIANTI study, an Italian prospective cohort study, the FI was operationalized using 42 variables that reflected age-related disease diagnosis, physical function, and cognitive health [3]. The FI at baseline was predictive of all-cause and cardiovascular disease mortality [3]. Similar associations between the FI and aging outcomes including major mobility disability [4], cardiovascular disease mortality [5], and all-cause mortality [6] have been reported in other cohort studies. These results show that the FI is an important indicator of health-span and identifying factors, particularly modifiable factors, that can improve FI is important.

Diet is one of the most important modifiable risk factors for various age-related conditions. A Mediterranean-type diet (MTD) that is characterized by higher daily intake of plant-based foods (vegetables, fruits, nuts, legumes, and cereals), fish, and monosaturated fats (primarily from olive oil), and lower intake of meats and saturated fats, with moderate intake of alcohol, has been associated with various aging conditions including cognitive decline [7], physical function [8,9], multimorbidity [10], and mortality [11]. We have previously shown that adherence to a MTD was associated with lower risk for the development of the frailty phenotype [12]. The frailty phenotype is another commonly studied frailty construct based on five criteria (unintentional weight loss, low grip strength, low energy, low walking speed, and low physical activity) that complements but is not identical to the FI. Thus, in this study, we examined the hypothesis that adherence to a MTD is associated with a lower FI in participants in the InCHIANTI study.

2. Materials and Methods

2.1. Study Population

The InCHIANTI study is a prospective cohort of older subjects living in the Chianti region in Tuscany, Italy. The primary aims of the study are to understand the factors contributing to mobility disability in aging. The details of the study have been described in detail [13]; in brief, subjects between 21 and 102 years of age (n = 1453) were recruited from the population registry of Greve in Chianti and Bagno a Ripoli at a participation rate of 90%. Participants were followed every three years from the baseline visit (1998–2000) to three follow-up visits. In the analysis, we included 825 participants over 65 at baseline with at least one follow-up visit. The study protocol was approved by the Italian National Institute of Research and, in the United States, the protocol was given an exemption status by the Office of Human Subject Research Protection (Exemption #11976).

2.2. Dietary Assessment and Mediterranean Diet Score Construction

At the baseline visit, dietary intake in the past year was assessed using a food frequency questionnaire (FFQ) adapted from the European Prospective Investigation on Cancer and Nutrition study, which was validated for use in the InCHIANTI study [14]. The Mediterranean-type diet score (MTD) was constructed using the algorithm developed by Trichopoulou et al. [15] as previously described [12]. Briefly, consumption of nine food groups was dichotomized using sex-specific median consumption as cutoffs. For "beneficial" foods (vegetables, legumes, fruits, cereal, fish, and a ratio of monounsaturated fats(MUFA):saturated fats(SFA)), consumption above the median was assigned a score of 1 and below the median was assigned a score of 0. Conversely, for detrimental foods (meat and dairy products), a score of 1 was assigned for consumption under the median and a score of 0 for consumption above the median. The median scores in men and women for each food group were as follows: 148.1 and 134.1 g (vegetables), 16 and 13.9 g (legumes), 273 and 261.8 g (fruits and nuts), 281.7 and 206.4 g (cereal), 23.6 and 20.4 g (fish), 1.5 and 1.4 (ratio of MUFA:SFA), 115.3 and 94.2 g (meat), and 153.4 and 173.6 g (dairy). For alcohol, a score of 1 was assigned to those who consumed between 10 and 50 g/d or 5 and 25 g/d in men and women respectively. Total MTD was derived as a sum of these scores and ranged from 0 (low adherence to a MTD) to 9 (maximal adherence). For analysis, the score was categorized into three groups as follows: low adherence (MTD $\leq$ 3), medium adherence (MTD 4–5), and high adherence (MTD $\geq$ 6). For all analyses, the low adherence group was used as a reference group.

2.3. Assessment of Frailty Index (FI)

The variable selection and operationalization of the FI in the InCHIANTI study were previously described [3]. In brief, 42 variables that represent health deficits and different functional domains were selected. These variables included major chronic medical conditions (hypertension, myocardial infarction, congestive heart failure, chronic liver disease, cancer, peripheral arterial disease, stroke, Parkinson's disease, diabetes, chronic lung disease, angina pectoris, and knee/hip arthritis) [16], difficulties with various activities of daily living (ADL) and instrumental ADL (IADL) [17,18], self-rated health, depressive symptoms (Center for Epidemiologic Studies Depression (CES-D) [19], subdomains of the Mini-Mental State Examination (MMSE) [20], self-reported weight loss, physical activity level in the past year, gait speed, and grip strength. An FI was calculated in participants with less than 20% of these 42 variables missing ($n = 12$). The FI was calculated as a ratio of the sum of all components to the total number of non-missing components and ranged from 0 to 1, reflecting having no deficits to having all deficits.

2.4. Measurement of Main Covariates

Clinical and demographic factors that were associated with the FI in univariate analyses were considered as covariates in the final analyses. Sociodemographic information such as age, sex, and years of education, was collected during a structured interview. Self-reported smoking status was categorized into three groups of never smokers, former smokers, or current smokers (within 3 years). Physical activity level in the past year was assessed using an interviewer-administered questionnaire [21]. A body mass index (BMI) was calculated as weight (kg) divided by squared height (meter). Plasma C-reactive protein (CRP) was measured using colorimetric competitive immunoassay (Roche Diagnostics, GmbH, Mannheim, Germany) and plasma IL-6 was measured using Bio-source cytoscreen ultrasensitivity kits. Plasma fatty acids omega-3 and omega-6 were measured using gas chromatography as previously described [22]. Plasma carotenoids, tocopherols, and MUFA were measured via high-performance liquid chromatography (HPLC) [23,24] and gas chromatography [22], respectively.

2.5. Statistical Analysis

Differences in baseline characteristics were tested using an analysis of variance for continuous variable and a chi-square for categorical variables. A cross-sectional analysis of adherence to the MTD and FI was assessed using linear regression using lm() function in R (version 3.6.2). An analysis of the longitudinal trajectories of FI was assessed using a linear mixed model with lmer() function from the lme4 package, using follow-up time as the time metric. Differences in trajectory (or slope) of the FI by MTD group were tested using an interaction term between the MTD group and follow-up time. For both cross-sectional and longitudinal analysis, the models were adjusted for age (at baseline), sex, study site (Greve or Bagno a Ripoli), total energy intake, smoking status, IL-6, CRP, BMI, years of education, and plasma levels of α-tocopherol, β-carotene, α-carotene, and monosaturated fatty acids (MUFA). To test whether association of MTD with FI trajectory differed by baseline FI, a stratified analysis was conducted in a sample split by the median baseline FI value. For all analyses, statistical significance was considered at $p \leq 0.05$. All analyses were conducted using R version 3.6.2.

3. Results

3.1. Association of Mediterranean-Type Diet with FI at Baseline

Compared to participants with follow-up data used in this analysis ($n = 825$), those who did not have follow-up data ($n = 180$) had profiles consistent with poorer health, including higher FI; older age; fewer years of education; lower MMSE; lower total energy intake; higher plasma concentrations of IL-6, CRP, and monounsaturated fatty acid (MUFA); and lower plasma concentrations of α-tocopherol, α-carotene, and β-carotene (Supplemental Table S1). At the baseline visit, the average age of participants with follow-up data was 73.5 years, and 56.1% were women (Table 1). FI ranged from 0.01 to 0.69 with a median value of 0.103. Participants with medium or high adherence to MTD were younger, had lower plasma CRP concentrations, greater total energy intake, and higher plasma b-carotene concentrations compared to the low adherence group. The highest percentage of women was in the medium adherence group, and the lowest percentage was found in the highest adherence group. No differences by MTD group were found for the study site; smoking status; BMI; years of education; MMSE score; and plasma concentrations of IL-6, α-tocopherol, and monosaturated fatty acids (MUFA). Those in the high adherence group had the lowest FI score, followed by the medium and low adherence group. When association was adjusted for covariates (age; sex; study site; total energy intake; years of education; smoking status; BMI; and plasma concentrations of MUFA, α-carotene, β-carotene, α-tocopherol, CRP, and IL-6) the association remained, with significant differences between the low and high adherence group (Figure 1).

To investigate which component had the strongest association with the FI, individual food groups were analyzed. In the unadjusted model, the consumption of vegetables and alcohol was significantly associated with the FI (Supplemental Table S2). In the fully adjusted model, alcohol consumption remained significantly inversely associated with the FI.

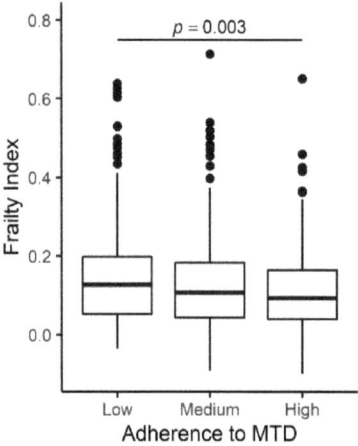

Figure 1. Association of adherence to a Mediterranean-type diet (MTD) at baseline. The boxplot displays the mean value of frailty index (FI) for subjects with low (MTD ≤ 3), medium (MTD 4–5), and high (MTD ≥ 6) adherence to a MTD. Significant differences were observed between low and high adherence group ($p = 0.0322$).

Table 1. Baseline demographic and clinical characteristics of InCHIANTI participants by adherence to the Mediterranean-type diet.

	All		Low Adherence		Medium Adherence		High Adherence		p *
	Mean/n	(SD/%)	Mean/n	(SD/%)	Mean/n	(SD/%)	Mean/n	(SD/%)	
n	825		235		357		233		
Age (y)	73.5	(6.4)	75.1	(7.0)	73.6	(6.5)	71.9	(5.2)	<0.001
Sex (%Female)	463	(56.1)	131	(55.7)	219	(61.3)	113	(48.5)	0.009
Site (%Bagno a Ripoli)	441	(53.5)	112	(47.7)	195	(54.6)	134	(57.5)	0.086
Smoking (%Smoker)	118	(14.3)	36	(15.3)	46	(12.9)	36	(15.5)	0.596
IL6 (pg/mL)	2.05	(3.39)	2.09	(2.24)	1.90	(1.96)	2.23	(5.47)	0.441
CRP (ug/mL)	4.59	(7.39)	5.40	(10.73)	3.89	(4.45)	4.87	(6.83)	0.035
BMI (kg/m^2)	27.5	(4.0)	27.1	(4.2)	27.5	(4.2)	27.8	(3.6)	0.128
Years of Education (y)	5.58	(3.31)	5.53	(3.67)	5.45	(3.10)	5.85	(3.23)	0.311
MMSE	25.4	(3.4)	25.1	(3.8)	25.4	(3.3)	25.8	(3.0)	0.063
Total energy intake (kcal/day)	1942.7	(566.1)	1826.3	(582.1)	1917.9	(571.9)	2098.1	(505.7)	<0.001
Plasma α-tocopherol (μmol/L)	30.4	(8.3)	29.4	(8.3)	30.9	(8.3)	30.8	(8.2)	0.081
Plasma α-carotene (μmol/L)	0.06	(0.06)	0.05	(0.04)	0.06	(0.04)	0.07	(0.08)	0.144
Plasma β-carotene (μmol/L)	0.43	(0.26)	0.39	(0.24)	0.45	(0.28)	0.44	(0.25)	0.021
Plasma monosaturated fatty acid *	33.0	(3.7)	32.5	(3.8)	33.0	(3.7)	33.4	(3.8)	0.055
Frailty Index	0.13	(0.10)	0.16	(0.12)	0.13	(0.09)	0.11	(0.08)	<0.001

* p-values from one-way ANOVA or chi-square test.

3.2. Association of the Mediterranean-Type Diet with the Trajectory of FI

Participants were followed for a mean of 7.35 years (range from 1.9 to 10 years), and their FI increased an average of 0.014 units per year. Older baseline age; higher BMI; smokers; women; and higher plasma concentrations of CRP, MUFA, and α-carotene were associated with a higher FI across the whole follow-up period (Supplemental Table S3).

Conversely, higher β-carotene, vitamin E, and total energy intake were associated with a lower FI during the follow-up period. Compared to the low MTD-adherence group, the high adherence group had 0.03 units lower FI ($p < 0.0001$) and the medium adherence group had 0.013 units lower FI ($p = 0.0164$). The associations between adherence to the MTD and the FI remained significant after adjustment of covariates, and there was little change in the effect sizes (Supplemental Table S3). The high adherence group had 0.006 units slower progression of FI compared to the low adherence group (Table 2). No differences in the trajectory of the FI were observed for the medium adherence group (Table 2, Figure 2A).

Analyses of each MTD component show that alcohol consumption is associated with a lower FI throughout the follow-up period (Supplemental Table S4). There was signification interaction between the consumption of vegetables and fish with time indicating a slower trajectory of FI (Supplemental Table S4).

Table 2. Association of adherence to a Mediterranean-type diet at baseline with trajectories of the frailty index over 10 years.

	Model without Interaction			Model with Interaction		
All participants						
Adherence to MTD	**Beta**	**SE**	**p**	**Beta**	**SE**	**p**
Low	Reference			Reference		
Medium	−0.013	0.005	0.016	−0.010	0.006	0.099
High	−0.030	0.006	<0.001	−0.023	0.007	<0.001
Follow-up time	0.013	0.001	<0.001	0.016	0.002	<0.001
Low × Follow-up time				Reference		
Medium × Follow-up time				−0.003	0.002	0.249
High × Follow-up time				−0.006	0.002	0.021
Low frailty index at baseline						
Adherence to MTD	**Beta**	**SE**	**p**	**Beta**	**SE**	**p**
Low	Reference			Reference		
Medium	−0.001	0.004	0.820	0.002	0.005	0.612
High	−0.006	0.005	0.164	−0.003	0.005	0.574
Follow-up time	0.009	0.001	<0.001	0.012	0.002	<0.001
Low × Follow-up time				Reference		
Medium × Follow-up time				−0.004	0.002	0.040
High × Follow-up time				−0.005	0.002	0.030
High frailty index at baseline						
Adherence to MTD	**Beta**	**SE**	**p**	**Beta**	**SE**	**p**
Low	Reference			Reference		
Medium	−0.010	0.009	0.248	−0.010	0.010	0.295
High	−0.021	0.011	0.057	−0.016	0.012	0.186
Follow-up time	0.017	0.001	<0.001	0.018	0.003	<0.001
Low × Follow-up time				Reference		
Medium × Follow-up time				0.000	0.004	0.959
High × Follow-up time				−0.004	0.004	0.363

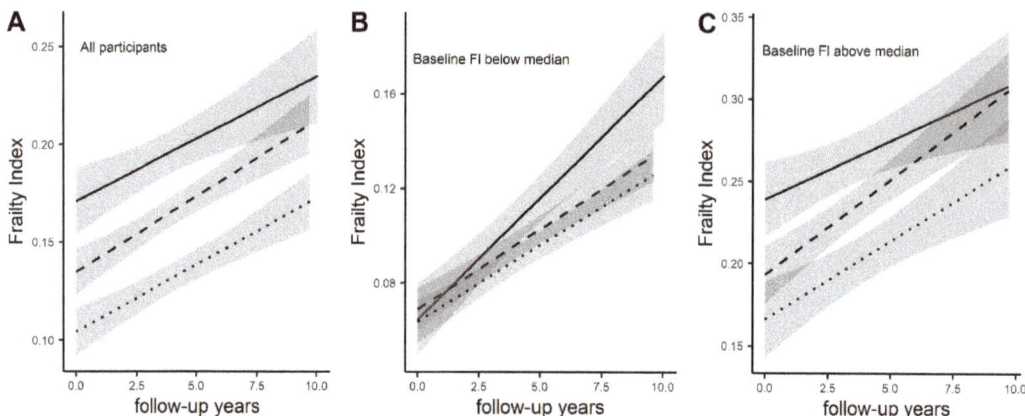

Figure 2. Association of MTD with trajectories of the Mediterranean-type diet (MTD). The associations of the MTD and the trajectory of frailty index (FI) were tested using a linear mixed model in all participants (**A**), participants with baseline FI below (**B**) or above (**C**) the median value of 0.103. The trajectories are stratified by low (solid line), medium (dashed line), or high (dotted line) adherence to a MTD. The trajectory of FI differed by MTD in subjects with low FI at baseline where the low adherence group had a faster progression of FI over time compared with the medium and high adherence groups.

3.3. Association of the Mediterranean-Type Diet with the Trajectory of FI by Baseline FI

We tested whether the association of the MTD with the FI differed by baseline FI values. In participants with a low FI (below the median value), there were significant differences in the slope of FI incline over time (Table 2). Compared to the low adherence to MTD group, both the medium and high adherence group had 0.004 and 0.005 unit/year slower progression in FI, respectively (Table 2, Figure 2B). In participants with a high FI (above the median value), there were no differences in the trajectory of FI increase and those in the higher MTD-adherence group maintained a lower FI throughout the follow-up period (Figure 2C).

4. Discussion

In this study, we report that adherence to the MTD is associated with a better FI over a 10 year follow-up period. We observed that the effect of the MTD on trajectories of FI depended on the participant's FI status at baseline. Overall, adherence to the MTD is protective against the progression of the FI, however, in participants that have a low FI at baseline low adherence to a MTD displayed faster worsening of the FI. This suggests that, for people who are more robust from the standpoint of the FI, promoting greater adherence to the MTD may be more beneficial in preventing health decline. All associations observed were independent of other risk factors, including inflammation, smoking status, years of education, and plasma nutrient biomarkers (vitamin E, carotenoids, and MUFA) at baseline.

There have been many studies that have examined the relationship between adherence to the MTD and the frailty phenotype. While the frailty phenotype and FI are correlated traits and often discussed interchangeably, the two traits are in fact complementary and independent constructs [25,26]. While the variables included in the FI are not predefined, the frailty phenotype is a construct from five defined criteria: unintentional weight loss, low grip strength, low energy, low walking speed, and low physical activity [27]. Frailty is considered when three or more of these conditions are met. Unlike the FI that is a continuous variable, the frailty phenotype is a categorical variable. There have been many studies that have shown the protective effect of adherence to a MTD on the incidence of frailty defined using the frailty phenotype [28–30]. A meta-analysis of four representative longitudinal studies of a MTD and the frailty phenotype showed that, over an average follow-up period of 3.9 years, medium and high adherence to a MTD was associated with

40% and 60% lower odds of developing frailty, respectively [31]. These studies reflect the overwhelming support for using a MTD in the prevention of frailty. The relative ease of operationalizing the frailty phenotype using the five set criteria perhaps explains why the number of studies examining the frailty phenotype with a MTD outweighs studies examining the FI. However, it is important to understand the effect the MTD exhibits on both frailty constructs since the specific variables required to ascertain the frailty phenotype are not available in many studies.

The associations of a MTD and three frailty constructs, including the frailty phenotype, the 61-variable FI, and the Tilburg Frailty Indicator, were investigated in 1740 subjects over 65 years of age in the Hellenic Longitudinal Investigation of Aging and Diet (HELIAD) study [30]. Higher adherence to the MTD was associated with a 4% decrease in the odds of frailty based on the 61-variable FI. There was also a trend for lower odds of frailty based on frailty phenotype, but the association was not significant. Interestingly, in this population the prevalence of frailty based on the three definitions differed considerably (4%–frailty phenotype, 18.7%–61-variable FI, and 25.4%–Tilburg Frailty Indicator) confirming the notion that these frailty constructs are different. The results from the InCHIANTI study are consistent with this prior report. Moreover we show that adherence to a MTD has the beneficial effect of maintaining a lower FI over a 10 year follow-up period. Moreover, our study indicates that low adherence to a MTD may accelerate the increase in the FI over time in those who have a low FI at baseline. The longitudinal effect of diet on the FI has been shown in another study, where the association of dietary patterns with changes in the FI over time was examined in 2632 individuals from the Rotterdam study [32]. Adherence to the Dutch national dietary guidelines was found to be associated with a lower FI both at baseline and over a 4 year follow-up period. Using principal component analysis, three dietary patterns were developed, including a "Traditional" pattern, characterized by higher intake of legumes, eggs, and savory snacks; a "Carnivore" pattern, with higher intake of meat and poultry; and a "Health Conscious" pattern, with higher intake of whole grain products, vegetables, and fruit. Interestingly, none of these patterns were associated with the FI at baseline but the "Traditional" pattern was associated with less frailty over time. This study, along with our study, suggests that following a higher quality diet can have long-lasting effects on the FI.

Adherence to a MTD is thought to promote health through various mechanisms. A MTD emphasizes the consumption of nutrient-rich foods, and as such, adherence to a MTD is associated with better nutrient status, including plasma levels of carotenoids and fatty acids [33–35]. Following a MTD is associated with a favorable chronic disease risk profile such as reduced blood cholesterol, lower inflammation, and increased antioxidant capacity [33,36–38]. Thus, adherence to a MTD most likely confers protection from the FI through these multiple mechanisms. In our study, the association of a MTD with the FI was independent of several of these factors, including nutrient status (carotenoids, vitamin E, and MUFA) and inflammation (CRP and IL-6), suggesting that the beneficial effects of a MTD cannot be fully explained by these factors.

This study has several strengths. First, this study was conducted in a well-characterized study that included repeated measures of the FI over a 10 year period, thereby allowing us to evaluate the long-term effect of the baseline diet. The study has comprehensive data on each participant, enabling us to adjust for several variables that may be important confounders or covariates in the relationship between the MTD and the FI. The study has several limitations. While the InCHIANTI study's data are rich, there likely are confounding factors that were not measured in our study. The MTD score was measured by self-report using a FFQ that is known to introduce some measurement error [39].

5. Conclusions

In conclusion, this study provides evidence that following a MTD has protective association with the FI. In particular, adherence to a MTD may be particularly important in older individuals who have low FI or are robust to maintain their health status. As the aging population grows worldwide, ensuring the health of this subgroup is of utmost importance. Our data suggest that promoting adherence to a MTD could be an effective strategy to reduce the burden of health deficits in older individuals.

Supplementary Materials: The following are available online at https://www.mdpi.com/article/10.3390/nu13041129/s1, Table S1. Comparison of demographic and clinical characteristics of InCHIANTI participants with and without follow up data; Table S2. Association of adherence to components Mediterranean-type diet with frailty index at baseline visit; Table S3. Association of adherence to Mediterranean-type diet at baseline with trajectories of frailty index over 10 years; Table S4. Association of components of Mediterranean-type diet at baseline with trajectories of frailty index over 10 years.

Author Contributions: Conceptualization, T.T. and L.F.; methodology, T.T., Y.J., S.A.T.; formal analysis, T.T.; resources, L.F., S.B.; data curation, S.B., Y.J.; writing—original draft preparation, T.T.; writing—review and editing, T.T., S.A.T., Y.J., S.B., L.F.; visualization, T.T.; supervision, L.F.; funding acquisition, L.F., S.B. All authors have read and agreed to the published version of the manuscript.

Funding: The InCHIANTI study baseline (1998–2000) was supported as a "targeted project" (ICS110.1/RF97.71) by the Italian Ministry of Health and in part by the U.S. National Institute on Aging (Contracts: 263 MD 9164 and 263 MD 821336); the InCHIANTI Follow-up 1 (2001–2003) was funded by the U.S. National Institute on Aging (Contracts: N.1-AG-1-1 and N.1-AG-1-2111); the InCHIANTI Follow-ups 2 and 3 studies (2004–2010) were financed by the U.S. National Institute on Aging (Contract: N01-AG-5-0002). This research was supported by the Intramural Research Program of the NIH, National Institute on Aging.

Institutional Review Board Statement: The study protocol was approved by the Italian National Institute of Research and Care of Aging Institutional Review and Medstar Research Institute (Baltimore, MD, USA).

Informed Consent Statement: Informed consent was obtained from all subjects involved in the study.

Data Availability Statement: InCHIANTI data is available through submission of research proposal at inchiantistudy.net.

Conflicts of Interest: The authors declare no conflict of interest.

References

1. Rockwood, K.; Mitnitski, A. Frailty in Relation to the Accumulation of Deficits. *J. Gerontol. Ser. A Boil. Sci. Med. Sci.* **2007**, *62*, 722–727. [CrossRef] [PubMed]
2. Mitnitski, A.B.; Mogilner, A.J.; Rockwood, K. Accumulation of Deficits as a Proxy Measure of Aging. *Sci. World J.* **2001**, *1*, 323–336. [CrossRef]
3. Hoogendijk, E.O.; Stenholm, S.; Ferrucci, L.; Bandinelli, S.; Inzitari, M.; Cesari, M. Operationalization of a frailty index among older adults in the InCHIANTI study: Predictive ability for all-cause and cardiovascular disease mortality. *Aging Clin. Exp. Res.* **2020**, *32*, 1025–1034. [CrossRef] [PubMed]
4. Brown, J.D.; Alipour-Haris, G.; Pahor, M.; Manini, T.M. Association between a Deficit Accumulation Frailty Index and Mobility Outcomes in Older Adults: Secondary Analysis of the Lifestyle Interventions and Independence for Elders (LIFE) Study. *J. Clin. Med.* **2020**, *9*, 3757. [CrossRef]
5. Fan, J.; Yu, C.; Guo, Y.; Bian, Z.; Sun, Z.; Yang, L.; Chen, Y.; Du, H.; Li, Z.; Lei, Y.; et al. Frailty index and all-cause and cause-specific mortality in Chinese adults: A prospective cohort study. *Lancet Public Health* **2020**, *5*, e650–e660. [CrossRef]
6. Kojima, G.; Iliffe, S.; Walters, K. Frailty index as a predictor of mortality: A systematic review and meta-analysis. *Age Ageing* **2018**, *47*, 193–200. [CrossRef] [PubMed]
7. Tanaka, T.; Talegawkar, S.A.; Jin, Y.; Colpo, M.; Ferrucci, L.; Bandinelli, S. Adherence to a Mediterranean Diet Protects from Cognitive Decline in the Invecchiare in Chianti Study of Aging. *Nutrients* **2018**, *10*, 2007. [CrossRef]
8. Milaneschi, Y.; Bandinelli, S.; Corsi, A.M.; Lauretani, F.; Paolisso, G.; Dominguez, L.J.; Semba, R.D.; Tanaka, T.; Abbatecola, A.M.; Talegawkar, S.A.; et al. Mediterranean diet and mobility decline in older persons. *Exp. Gerontol.* **2011**, *46*, 303–308. [CrossRef]
9. Agarwal, P.; Wang, Y.; Buchman, A.S.; Bennett, D.A.; Morris, M.C. Dietary Patterns and Self-reported Incident Disability in Older Adults. *J. Gerontol. Ser. A Boil. Sci. Med. Sci.* **2019**, *74*, 1331–1337. [CrossRef]
10. Kyprianidou, M.; Panagiotakos, D.; Faka, A.; Kambanaros, M.; Makris, K.C.; Christophi, C.A. Adherence to the Mediterranean diet in Cyprus and its relationship to multi-morbidity: An epidemiological study. *Public Health Nutr.* **2020**, *10*, 1–10. [CrossRef]
11. Eleftheriou, D.; Benetou, V.; Trichopoulou, A.; La Vecchia, C.; Bamia, C. Mediterranean diet and its components in relation to all-cause mortality: Meta-analysis. *Br. J. Nutr.* **2018**, *120*, 1081–1097. [CrossRef]

12. Talegawkar, S.A.; Bandinelli, S.; Bandeen-Roche, K.; Chen, P.; Milaneschi, Y.; Tanaka, T.; Semba, R.D.; Guralnik, J.M.; Ferrucci, L. A Higher Adherence to a Mediterranean-Style Diet Is Inversely Associated with the Development of Frailty in Community-Dwelling Elderly Men and Women. *J. Nutr.* **2012**, *142*, 2161–2166. [CrossRef] [PubMed]
13. Ferrucci, L.; Bandinelli, S.; Benvenuti, E.; Di Iorio, A.; Macchi, C.; Harris, T.B.; Guralnik, J.M. Subsystems Contributing to the Decline in Ability to Walk: Bridging the Gap Between Epidemiology and Geriatric Practice in the InCHIANTI Study. *J. Am. Geriatr. Soc.* **2000**, *48*, 1618–1625. [CrossRef] [PubMed]
14. Bartali, B.; Turrini, A.; Salvini, S.; Lauretani, F.; Russo, C.R.; Corsi, A.M.; Bandinelli, S.; D'Amicis, A.; Palli, D.; Guralnik, J.M.; et al. Dietary intake estimated using different methods in two Italian older populations. *Arch. Gerontol. Geriatr.* **2004**, *38*, 51–60. [CrossRef]
15. Trichopoulou, A.; Costacou, T.; Bamia, C.; Trichopoulos, D. Adherence to a Mediterranean Diet and Survival in a Greek Population. *N. Engl. J. Med.* **2003**, *348*, 2599–2608. [CrossRef] [PubMed]
16. Fabbri, E.; An, Y.; Zoli, M.; Simonsick, E.M.; Guralnik, J.M.; Bandinelli, S.; Boyd, C.M.; Ferrucci, L. Aging and the Burden of Multimorbidity: Associations With Inflammatory and Anabolic Hormonal Biomarkers. *J. Gerontol. Ser. A Boil. Sci. Med. Sci.* **2015**, *70*, 63–70. [CrossRef] [PubMed]
17. Katz, S.A.; Ford, A.B.; Moskowitz, R.W.; Jackson, B.A.; Jaffe, M.W. Studies of Illness in the Aged. The Index of Adl: A Standardized Measure of Biological and Psychosocial Function. *JAMA* **1963**, *185*, 914–919. [CrossRef]
18. Lawton, M.P.; Brody, E.M. Assessment of Older People: Self-Maintaining and Instrumental Activities of Daily Living. *Gerontology* **1969**, *9*, 179–186. [CrossRef]
19. Beekman, A.T.F.; Deeg, D.J.H.; Van Limbeek, J.; Braam, A.W.; De Vries, M.Z.; Van Tilburg, W. Criterion validity of the Center for Epidemiologic Studies Depression scale (CES-D): Results from a community-based sample of older subjects in The Netherlands. *Psychol. Med.* **1997**, *27*, 231–235. [CrossRef]
20. Folstein, M.F.; Folstein, S.E.; McHugh, P.R. "Mini-mental state". A practical method for grading the cognitive state of patients for the clinician. *J. Psychiatr. Res.* **1975**, *12*, 189–198. [CrossRef]
21. Wareham, N.J.; Jakes, R.W.; Rennie, K.L.; Mitchell, J.; Hennings, S.; Day, N.E. Validity and repeatability of the EPIC-Norfolk Physical Activity Questionnaire. *Int. J. Epidemiol.* **2002**, *31*, 168–174. [CrossRef]
22. Ferrucci, L.; Cherubini, A.; Bandinelli, S.; Bartali, B.; Corsi, A.; Lauretani, F.; Martin, A.; Andres-Lacueva, C.; Senin, U.; Guralnik, J.M. Relationship of Plasma Polyunsaturated Fatty Acids to Circulating Inflammatory Markers. *J. Clin. Endocrinol. Metab.* **2006**, *91*, 439–446. [CrossRef] [PubMed]
23. Dorgan, J.F.; Boakye, N.E.; Fears, T.R.; Schleicher, R.L.; Helsel, W.; Anderson, C.; Robinson, J.; Guin, J.D.; Lessin, S.; Ratnasinghe, L.D.; et al. Serum carotenoids and alpha-tocopherol and risk of nonmelanoma skin cancer. *Cancer Epidemiol. Biomark. Prev.* **2004**, *13*, 1276–1282.
24. Sowell, A.L.; Huff, D.L.; Yeager, P.R.; Caudill, S.P.; Gunter, E.W. Retinol, alpha-tocopherol, lutein/zeaxanthin, beta-cryptoxanthin, lycopene, alpha-carotene, trans-beta-carotene, and four retinyl esters in serum determined simultaneously by reversed-phase HPLC with multiwavelength detection. *Clin. Chem.* **1994**, *40*, 411–416. [CrossRef]
25. Malmstrom, T.K.; Miller, D.K.; Morley, J.E. A Comparison of Four Frailty Models. *J. Am. Geriatr. Soc.* **2014**, *62*, 721–726. [CrossRef]
26. Cesari, M.; Gambassi, G.; van Kan, G.A.; Vellas, B. The frailty phenotype and the frailty index: Different instruments for different purposes. *Age Ageing* **2014**, *43*, 10–12. [CrossRef]
27. Fried, L.P.; Tangen, C.M.; Walston, J.; Newman, A.B.; Hirsch, C.; Gottdiener, J.; Seeman, T.; Tracy, R.; Kop, W.J.; Burke, G.; et al. Frailty in Older Adults: Evidence for a Phenotype. *J. Gerontol. Ser. A Biol. Sci. Med. Sci.* **2001**, *56*, M146–M156. [CrossRef] [PubMed]
28. Alaghehband, F.R.; Erkkilä, A.T.; Rikkonen, T.; Sirola, J.; Kröger, H.; Isanejad, M. Association of Baltic Sea and Mediterranean diets with frailty phenotype in older women, Kuopio OSTPRE-FPS study. *Eur. J. Nutr.* **2021**, *60*, 821–831. [CrossRef]
29. Kwan, R.Y.; Cheung, D.S.; Lo, S.K.; Ho, L.Y.; Katigbak, C.; Chao, Y.-Y.; Liu, J.Y. Frailty and its association with the Mediterranean diet, life-space, and social participation in community-dwelling older people. *Geriatr. Nurs.* **2019**, *40*, 320–326. [CrossRef]
30. Ntanasi, E.; Yannakoulia, M.; Kosmidis, M.-H.; Anastasiou, C.A.; Dardiotis, E.; Hadjigeorgiou, G.; Sakka, P.; Scarmeas, N. Adherence to Mediterranean Diet and Frailty. *J. Am. Med. Dir. Assoc.* **2018**, *19*, 315–322.e2. [CrossRef]
31. Kojima, G.; Avgerinou, C.; Iliffe, S.; Walters, K. Adherence to Mediterranean Diet Reduces Incident Frailty Risk: Systematic Review and Meta-Analysis. *J. Am. Geriatr. Soc.* **2018**, *66*, 783–788. [CrossRef] [PubMed]
32. De Haas, S.C.M.; De Jonge, E.A.L.; Voortman, T.; Graaff, J.S.-D.; Franco, O.H.; Ikram, M.A.; Rivadeneira, F.; Jong, J.C.K.-D.; Schoufour, J.D. Dietary patterns and changes in frailty status: The Rotterdam study. *Eur. J. Nutr.* **2017**, *57*, 2365–2375. [CrossRef]
33. Bach-Faig, A.; Geleva, D.; Carrasco, J.; Ribas-Barba, L.; Serra-Majem, L. Evaluating associations between Mediterranean diet adherence indexes and biomarkers of diet and disease. *Public Health Nutr.* **2006**, *9*, 1110–1117. [CrossRef]
34. Panagiotakos, D.; Kalogeropoulos, N.; Pitsavos, C.; Roussinou, G.; Palliou, K.; Chrysohoou, C.; Stefanadis, C. Validation of the MedDietScore via the determination of plasma fatty acids. *Int. J. Food Sci. Nutr.* **2009**, *60* (Suppl. 5), 168–180. [CrossRef]
35. Féart, C.; Torrès, M.J.M.; Samieri, C.; Jutand, M.-A.; Peuchant, E.; Simopoulos, A.P.; Barberger-Gateau, P. Adherence to a Mediterranean diet and plasma fatty acids: Data from the Bordeaux sample of the Three-City study. *Br. J. Nutr.* **2011**, *106*, 149–158. [CrossRef]

36. Razquin, C.; Martinez, J.A.; Martinez-Gonzalez, M.A.; Mitjavila, M.T.; Estruch, R.; Marti, A. A 3 years follow-up of a Mediterranean diet rich in virgin olive oil is associated with high plasma antioxidant capacity and reduced body weight gain. *Eur. J. Clin. Nutr.* **2009**, *63*, 1387–1393. [CrossRef] [PubMed]
37. Calder, P.C.; Ahluwalia, N.; Brouns, F.; Buetler, T.; Clement, K.; Cunningham, K.; Esposito, K.; Jö Nsson, L.S.; Kolb, H.; Lansink, M.; et al. Dietary factors and low-grade inflammation in relation to overweight and obesity commissioned by the ILSI Europe Metabolic Syndrome and Diabetes Task Force. *Br. J. Nutr.* **2011**, *106*, S1–S78. [CrossRef]
38. Fitó, M.; Guxens, M.; Corella, D.; Sáez, G.; Estruch, R.; De La Torre, R.; Francés, F.; Cabezas, C.; López-Sabater, M.D.C.; Marrugat, J.; et al. Effect of a Traditional Mediterranean Diet on Lipoprotein Oxidation: A randomized controlled trial. *Arch. Intern. Med.* **2007**, *167*, 1195–1203. [CrossRef]
39. Kipnis, V.; Subar, A.F.; Midthune, D.; Freedman, L.S.; Ballard-Barbash, R.; Troiano, R.P.; Bingham, S.; Schoeller, D.A.; Schatzkin, A.; Carroll, R.J. Structure of Dietary Measurement Error: Results of the OPEN Biomarker Study. *Am. J. Epidemiol.* **2003**, *158*, 14–21, discussion 22–16. [CrossRef]

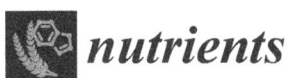

Article

Functional Frailty, Dietary Intake, and Risk of Malnutrition. Are Nutrients Involved in Muscle Synthesis the Key for Frailty Prevention?

Ana Moradell [1,2,3,4], Ángel Iván Fernández-García [1,2,3,4], David Navarrete-Villanueva [1,2,3,5], Lucía Sagarra-Romero [6], Eva Gesteiro [3,7], Jorge Pérez-Gómez [8], Irene Rodríguez-Gómez [9,10], Ignacio Ara [9,10], Jose A. Casajús [1,2,3,5,11], Germán Vicente-Rodríguez [1,2,3,4,11] and Alba Gómez-Cabello [1,2,3,4,11,12,*]

- [1] GENUD (Growth, Exercise, NUtrition and Development) Research Group, Universidad de Zaragoza, 50009 Zaragoza, Spain; amoradell@unizar.es (A.M.); angelivanfg@unizar.es (Á.I.F.-G.); dnavarrete@unizar.es (D.N.-V.); joseant@unizar.es (J.A.C.); gervicen@unizar.es (G.V.-R.)
- [2] Agrifood Research and Technology Centre of Aragón -IA2-, CITA-Universidad de Zaragoza, 50009 Zaragoza, Spain
- [3] Exercise and Health in Special Population Spanish Research Net (EXERNET), 50009 Zaragoza, Spain; eva.gesteiro@upm.es
- [4] Faculty of Health and Sport Science (FCSD), Department of Physiatry and Nursing, University of Zaragoza, Ronda Misericordia 5, 22001 Huesca, Spain
- [5] Department of Physiatry and Nursing, Faculty of Health, University of Zaragoza, 50009 Zaragoza, Spain
- [6] Faculty of Health Sciences, San Jorge University, Villanueva de Gállego, 50830 Zaragoza, Spain; lsagarra@usj.es
- [7] ImFINE Research Group, Department of Health and Human Performance, Faculty of Physical Activity and Sport Sciences-INEF, Polytechnic University of Madrid, 28040 Madrid, Spain
- [8] HEME (Health, Economy, Motricity and Education) Research Group, Faculty of Sport Science, University of Extremadura, 10003 Cáceres, Spain; jorgepg100@unex.es
- [9] GENUD Toledo Research Group, University of Castilla-La Mancha, 45071 Toledo, Spain; irene.rodriguez@uclm.es (I.R.-G.); ignacio.ara@uclm.es (I.A.)
- [10] Biomedical Research Networking Center on Frailty and Healthy Aging (CIBERFES), 28029 Madrid, Spain
- [11] Centro de Investigación Biomédica en Red de Fisiopatología de la Obesidad y Nutrición (CIBERObn), 28029 Madrid, Spain
- [12] Centro Universitario de la Defensa, 50090 Zaragoza, Spain
- * Correspondence: agomez@unizar.es; Tel.: +34-876-553-756

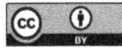

Abstract: Frailty is a reversible condition, which is strongly related to physical function and nutritional status. Different scales are used to screened older adults and their risk of being frail, however, Short Physical Performance Battery (SPPB) may be more adequate than others to measure physical function in exercise interventions and has been less studied. Thus, the main aims of our study were: (1) to describe differences in nutritional intakes by SPPB groups (robust, pre-frail and frail); (2) to study the relationship between being at risk of malnourishment and frailty; and (3) to describe differences in nutrient intake between those at risk of malnourishment and those without risk in the no-frail individuals. One hundred one participants (80.4 ± 6.0 year old) were included in this cross-sectional study. A validated semi-quantitative food frequency questionnaire was used to determine food intake and Mini Nutritional Assessment to determine malnutrition. Results revealed differences for the intake of carbohydrates, n-3 fatty acids (n3), and saturated fatty acids for frail, pre-frail, and robust individuals and differences in vitamin D intake between frail and robust (all $p < 0.05$). Those at risk of malnutrition were approximately 8 times more likely to be frail than those with no risk. Significant differences in nutrient intake were found between those at risk of malnourishment and those without risk, specifically in: protein, PUFA n-3, retinol, ascorbic acid, niacin equivalents, folic acid, magnesium, and potassium, respectively. Moreover, differences in alcohol were also observed showing higher intake for those at risk of malnourishment (all $p < 0.05$). In conclusion, nutrients related to muscle metabolism showed to have different intakes across SPPB physical function groups. The intake of these specific nutrients related with risk of malnourishment need to be promoted in order to prevent frailty.

Keywords: performance; frailty; nutritional status; vitamin D; protein

1. Introduction

Frailty is characterized by a loss of strength, endurance, and physical ability and cognitive function, which results in an increased risk of vulnerability to disease, dependence, and death [1,2]. Previously to this state and subsequently to a physiological decline, a pre-frail stage identifies a subset of high risk and potentially reversible condition before onset of established frailty [2]. Evidence shows that those in an intermediate stage between robust and frailty, namely, pre-frail, present an increased risk of becoming frail within just 3 years [3].

The most common method to assess frailty and pre-frailty stages is the Fried Phenotype [3]; however, the Short Physical Performance Battery (SPPB) is also frequently used [4] as a screening tool. Although the Fried phenotype has been widely used as a frailty scale, its applicability in the routine clinical practice is questionable because of the complexity of some measurements such as a handgrip dynamometer. Pre-disability condition of frailty can indeed be captured using the SPPB as a comprehensive measure of physical functioning impairment [5]. Even this first scale is the most widely cited [6], both have been widely used across the literature. However, components of the assessments differ, which may have implications on the feasibility of incorporating these assessments into clinical practice. For example, Pritchart et al. found different results when both scales were used to determine pre-frail and frail stages [7], and Lim et al. have recently suggested not overlapping the scales [8]. Nevertheless, the use of SPPB is increasing as it evaluates not only physical function but also physical performance through a mobility domain that could be of a higher interest in rehabilitation, physical exercise, and physical activity-related interventions.

Variety of health conditions contribute to the development of frailty, including environmental factors such as physical activity [9] or poor nutrition [10,11]. In addition, diseases as sarcopenia, defined as a generalized skeletal muscle mass disorder, often overlap with frailty and led to this detriment [12]. However, it implies not only muscle in limbs but also those involve in chewing and swallowing [13], which affects negatively food consumption. Optimal nutritional intake could delay frailty by avoiding chronic diseases such as cardiovascular diseases, obesity, and diabetes [14], increasing muscle mass and physical function, and even improving immune system [15]. In this regard, multiple studies have associated frailty, assessed by Fried phenotype, with different nutritional parameters such as low energy and low protein intake, vitamin B12 and vitamin D deficiency, or a higher risk of malnourishment [10,16]. However, to the best of our knowledge, a few studies differ between nutritional intake in these three-frailty stages determined by Fried [17–19], while no studies have been published reporting neither these dietary intake differences in frailty stages assessed by SPPB. This relationship could be interesting to design and implement more accurate strategies involving exercise and nutritional supplementation. There are existing exercise interventions including older adults and considering frail Fried phenotypes, which combine nutritional supplements and exercise in order to improve functional capacity [15,16,20]; they considered each nutrient's attributed effect without considering differences in dietary intakes between SPPB stages and taking these results into account could improve their outcomes. Thus, it should be of high importance to investigate which nutrients differ in frailty stages in order to design appropriate interventions according to the stage of frailty.

In light of the above, authors from the present study hypothesize to find deficiencies and lower intakes in nutrients that are strongly related to skeletal muscle synthesis in those people classified as frail or even in pre-frail compared with robust (according to SPPB). We also hypothesize that being at risk of malnutrition increases the likelihood of being frail.

Thus main purposes of this study were: (1) to investigate the differences in dietary intake between the different stages measured by SPPB (robust, frail, and pre-frail); (2) to describe the proportion of frail, pre-frail, and robust who meet the EFSA dietary references values in older adults; (3) to study the relationship between the risk of malnourishment and the development of functional frailty (measured by SPPB); and (4) to assesses possible key nutrients associated to possible development of frailty when there is a risk of malnutrition.

2. Materials and Methods

2.1. Study Design and Participants

This cross-sectional study was carried out in the framework of the EXERNET Elder 3.0 project. Participant recruitment was done in three health care centers and three nursing homes from the city of Zaragoza, Spain during 2018. Briefly, this study aims to implement a 6-month multicomponent exercise program in frail and pre-frail older adults in order to improve physical function and physical performance. Data for this report correspond to the evaluation previous to the intervention phase. This report also includes robust individuals who came to the recruitment phase. Inclusion criteria for the study were: (1) to be older than 65 years old, (2) not suffering from dementia and/or cancer, and (3) not being invalid (<4 points scored by SPPB). Participants with missing information of the food frequency questionnaire or mini nutritional assessment score were also excluded for the present study.

All methodology was described carefully elsewhere [21]. Information about functional capacity and other health/lifestyle outcomes such as daily walking and sitting hours, smoking, cognitive status (measured by Mini Mental State Examination [22]), or sleeping hours were collected through a structured questionnaire. The dietary information (food frequency questionnaire) was obtained once, in a separated day [23].

2.2. Ethics Statement

Oral and written information and possible benefits and risks derived from participation in this study were given to participants during the first day of attendance. Afterwards, from all the included participants, a written informed consent was obtained. National and European legislation related to data protection was followed rigorously.

The study was performed according to the Helsinki Declaration of 1961 revised in Fortaleza (2013) and the current legislation of human clinical research of Spain (Law 14/2007). The Hospital Universitario Fundación de Alcorcón (16/50) approved the study protocol.

2.3. Short Physical Performance Battery

The Short Physical Performance Battery (SPPB) was performed in order to evaluate the physical performance and functional status of the participants. Three tests composed the SPPB; balance (to stand up for 10 s with feet positioned in three ways: together side-by-side, semi-tandem, and tandem positions), usual gait speed (time to complete 4 m walking), and lower limb strength (time to rise 5 times from a chair) [24].

The total battery score from 0 to 12 points. Four functional stages were created in order to classify participants: dependent (<4 points), frail (4–6 points), pre-frail (7–9 points), and robust (>9 points) [4].

2.4. Anthropometrics and Body Composition Measurements

A portable stadiometer of 2.10 m (SECA, Hamburg, Germany) was used to measure height. To measure body weight (kg) and to estimate body total fat mass (TFM), percentage of body fat (FM%), and fat free mass (FFM), a portable bioelectrical impedance analyzer (BIA) (TANITA BC 418-MA Tanita Corp., Tokyo, Japan) was used. To standardize and avoid bias in the process, all participants had to come to the research center early in the morning with fasting. They were also advised to empty their bladder before the measurements. Older individuals had to remove shoes and heavy clothes. Body mass index (BMI) was calculated dividing weight (in kg) by the height in meters squared (($BMI = weight/height^2$; kg/m^2).

Mid-arm (relaxed) and calf circumferences were evaluated according to the International Society for the Advancement of Kinanthropometry (ISAK) protocol. A Rosscraft Anthrotape (Rosscraft Innovations Inc, Vancouver, BC, Canada) was used for this purpose.

2.5. Mediterranean Diet Adherence

The 14-point Mediterranean Diet Adherence questionnaire consist of 12 questions about food intake and 2 questions about food habits considered as characteristic from the Mediterranean diet. The result allows knowing the adherence to this diet [25]. Maximal score possibly obtain is 14, as each item point 0 or 1 depending on if the habit asked is complying each item. Results from the Mediterranean Diet Adherence were categorized as low adherence (<9 points) and high adherence (≥9 points).

2.6. Mini Nutritional Assessment

The Mini Nutritional Assessment (MNA) consists of 18-items 15 questions about diet, self-perception of nutritional and health state, and functional or independence and three anthropometric parameters (BMI, calf circumference and mid-arm circumference). All the items were specific for geriatric assessment. The final score classifies the participant as; well-nourished (>23.5 points), at risk of malnourishment (17–23.5 points), or malnourished (<17 points) [26,27].

2.7. Food Frequency Questionnaire

To assess dietary intake, a semiquantitative food frequency questionnaire, previously validated in Spain was used [23,28]. Information collected was relative to the last year. Moreover, 137 items accompanied by their typical portion size was complete. Participants selected the frequency of consumption between nine options ranging from never/almost never to six or more times per day. To obtain the daily intake, the portion size was multiplied by the frequency of consumption. Spanish food composition tables and other sources of information [29,30] were used to estimated nutrient intake. Data extracted from this questionnaire were total mean energy intake (kcal/day), macronutrients (protein, fat, and carbohydrates in g/day and % kcal of the total macronutrient energy distribution), alcohol (g and % kcal of the total macronutrient energy distribution), types of fatty acids (g/day), types of polyunsaturated fatty acids (PUFA) (n-3 and n-6) (g/day), vitamins and minerals (mg or ug/day as corresponding to the nutrient referred). Moreover, for each food item, we estimated the average amount of food consumed in grams and grouped them according to their nutrient contribution.

Dietary Reference Values were used in the study according to EFSA recommendations (2017) for adults [31].

2.8. Statistical Analysis

Calculations were performed using The Statistical Package for the Social Sciences (SPSS) v. 20.0 for Windows (SPSS, Inc., Chicago, IL, USA). Normality of the data was ensuring for the variables in three SPPB groups (robust, pre-frail, and frail). Differences between descriptive characteristics were assessed by analysis of variance (ANOVA) of one factor for continuous variables and chi-squared test for categorical variables. An additional ANOVA analysis was performed to describe differences between food group consumption. Groups according to dietary recommendations were created in order to describe how much people meet recommendations in each group and to show differences between SPPB groups by a chi-squared test. Moreover, an analysis of covariance (ANCOVA) adjusted by energy intake was performed to study differences in nutrient intake between the three groups. Further analyses were used to show differences in frail and pre-frail compared with robust as the reference group.

Additionally, a binary logistic regression analysis was used to study if being at risk of malnutrition was a predictor of being frailty. For this analysis, a non-frailty group was created including robust and pre-frail participants together and separated from frail, as a different group to compare them. The reason for this grouping was to increase the number of subjects and thus, the power of the analyses when comparing against frailty. Finally, differences in nutrient intake between those at risk of malnutrition and those with no risk in non-frail group were investigated by another ANOVA in order to elucidate possible key nutrients, which could influence frailty development in those no-frail, between those at risk of malnutrition, and those without risk. Statistical significance for all the analyses was set at $p < 0.05$.

3. Results

A total of 101 participants (78 females) with a mean age of 80.4 years met the inclusion criteria and were included in this report. Descriptive characteristics and differences between robust, pre-frail, and frail participants are shown in Table 1. Statistical differences between groups were observed for age, weight, and MNA.

Table 1. Descriptive characteristics of the participants of the study.

	Whole Sample (n = 101)	Robust (n = 13)	Pre-Frail (n = 68)	Frail (n = 20)	p Value
Sex					0.317
Males	23 (22.8)	1 (7.7)	18 (26.5)	4 (20.0)	
Females	78 (77.2)	12 (92.3)	50 (73.5)	16 (80.0)	
Age (years)	80.4 ± 6.0	77.3 ± 5.4	80.0 ± 5.8	83.0 ± 5.7	0.005
BMI (kg/m^2)	29.4 ± 5.4	27.2 ± 3.0	29.9 ± 5.0	29.4 ± 7.1	0.262
Weight (kg)	72.3 ± 14.2	66.0 ± 7.0	74.8 ± 13.7	69.2 ± 16.5	0.038
BF%	37.4 ± 6.9	37.6 ± 4.9	37.9 ± 7.1	36.2 ± 7.4	0.569
FFM (kg)	44.7 ± 8.7	41.0 ± 3.5	46.2 ± 9.3	43.1 ± 8.4	0.061
MNA	23.1 ± 3.1	24.6 ± 1.9	23.6 ± 3.0	21.2 ± 2.8	<0.001
Risk of malnutrition	42 (41.6)	3 (23.0)	23 (33.8)	16 (80.0)	<0.001
No risk of malnutrition	59 (58.4)	10 (77.0)	45 (66.2)	4 (20.0)	
ADM	7.6 ± 0.95	8.3 ± 2.4	7.5 ± 1.2	7.5 ± 2.7	0.363
Low ADM	78 (77.2)	7 (53.8)	54 (79.4)	17 (85.0)	
High ADM	23 (22.8)	6 (46.2)	14 (20.6)	3 (15.0)	
Smoking	3 (3.0)	0 (0.0)	3 (4.4)	0 (.055)	0.643
MMSE	26.6 ± 2.8	27.0 ± 3.0	26.8 ± 2.6	25.5 ± 2.8	0.134

BMI: body mass index, BF%: body fat percentage, FFM: fat free mass, SPPB: short physical performance battery, MNA: mini nutritional assessment, ADM: Adherence to Mediterranean Diet, MMSE: Mini mental state examination. n and (%) for categorical variables, mean and standard deviation for continuous variables. All statistical significance was set in $p < 0.05$.

Table 2 describes the intake of food group's consumption for each SPPB group. Differences were only observed for cheese between pre-frail and robust ($p < 0.05$).

Table 2. Differences of food group intakes between robust, pre-frail, and frail older adults.

	Robust (n = 13)	Pre-Frail (n = 68)	Frail (n = 20)	p Value
Yogurt (g/day)	71.2 ± 64.0	77.6 ± 62.0	88.2 ± 90.5	0.735
Milk (g/day)	190.0 ± 180.7	228.3 ± 167.5	300.0 ± 184.2	0.120
Cheese (g/day)	61.3 ± 41.1	27.0 ± 24.4 *	37.2 ± 44.1 *	0.002
Eggs (g/day)	27.4 ± 13.5	25.5 ± 12.8	25.1 ± 15.9	0.882
Red meat (g/day)	62.8 ± 51.0	57.7 ± 39.6	49.64 ± 6	0.614
White meat (g/day)	81.2 ± 71.7	64.6 ± 32.4	61.3 ± 41.1	0.331
Lean meat products (g/day)	32.6 ± 23	23.8 ± 20.9	19.1 ± 16.2	0.161
Fat meat products (g/day)	14.3 ± 19.5	11.4 ± 11.7	13.2 ± 12.6	0.671
White fish (g/day)	51.0 ± 30.1	45.5 ± 29.0	45.0 ± 30.5	0.809
Oily fish (g/day)	36.2 ± 41.1	25.2 ± 25.7	15.8 ± 17.5	0.079
Seafood (g/day)	25.3 ± 29.4	22.9 ± 28.6	30.4 ± 35.9	0.490
Vegetables (g/day)	463.9 ± 237.2	444.6 ± 218.1	391.34 ± 221.6	0.511
Fruit (g/day)	481.9 ± 222.0	454.4 ± 236.0	517.5 ± 637.6	0.753
Nuts (g/day)	42.1 ±43.30	33.6 ± 56.7	36.76 ± 58.7	0.871
Legumes (g/day)	22.8 ± 12.9	22.3 ± 13.5	28.6 ± 19.8	0.195
Cereals and potatoes (g/day)	169.9 ± 95.7	210 ± 106.6	200.5 ± 81.0	0.402
Olive oil (g/day)	32.9 ± 21.1	31.4 ± 21.6	31.1 ± 18.1	0.964
Fats and other oils (g/day)	4.5 ± 5.5	5.0 ± 6.7	3.86 ± 5.4	0.728
Fruit juices and beverages (g/day)	84.5 ± 91.9	67.3 ± 97.4	90.8 ± 127.3	0.964
Coffee and tea (g/day)	73.3 ± 52.1	57.6 ± 44.2	48.4 ± 58.5	0.331
Savory snacks (g/day)	48.3 ± 58.3	52.8 ± 71.1	92.3 ± 96.6	0.076
Sweet snacks (g/day)	92.1 ± 74.3	100.1 ± 75.6	107.6 ± 62.9	0.817
Alcoholic consumers	(n = 10)	(n = 54)	(n = 15)	
Beer (g/day)	65.7 ± 101.9	77.5 ± 169.0	13.8 ± 36.4	0.337
Wine (g/day)	48.8 ± 45.72	68.4 ± 76.8	66.6 ± 68.1	0.732

* differences between pre-frail and robust groups. p value stablished at <0.05. Beer and wine intake differences were calculated with alcohol consumers.

Percentages of the sample covering the Spanish DRI for vitamins and minerals in each SPPB group are shown in Table 3.

Table 3. Adequate intake or population reference intake and percentage of the sample covering recommendation from EFSA (European Food Safety Authority) of vitamins and minerals by Short Physical Performance Battery (SPPB) groups.

Nutrient Intake	AI or PRI (M/F)	Robust (%)	Pre-Frail (%)	Frail (%)	p value
Retinol equivalents (ug/day)	750/650	100	97.1	95.0	0.710
Vitamin D (µg/day)	15	15.4	0.0	0.0	0.001
Vitamin E (mg/day)	13/11	53.8	47.1	40	0.730
Ascorbic acid (C) (mg/day)	110/95	100.0	100.0	100.0	NC
Thiamine (B1) (mg/day)	1/0.8	100.0	100.0	100.0	NC
Riboflavin (B2) (mg/day)	1.6	100.0	77.9	70.0	0.105
Niacin equivalents (B3) (mg/day)	15.4/12.5	100.0	100.0	100.0	NC
Pyridoxin (B6) (mg/day)	1.7/1.6	100.0	94,1	90.0	0.494
Folic acid (B9) (µg/day)	330	92.3	85.3	72.0	0.373
Cobalamin (B12) (ug/day)	4	100.0	95.6	70.0	0.001
Calcium (mg/day)	950	76.9	60.3	76.9	0.427
Iron (mg/day)	11	100.0	100.0	100.0	NC
Magnesium (mg/day)	300	100.0	91.2	90.0	0.519
Potassium (mg/day)	3500	100.0	92.6	90.0	0.528
Iodine (µg/day)	150	84.6	80.9	85.0	0.887
Selenium (µg/day)	70	92.3	83.8	92.3	0.417
Zinc (mg/day)	16.3/12.7	69.2	38.2	35.0	0.092
Phosphorus (mg/day)	550	100.0	100.0	100	NC

AI: adequate intake represented in ordinary type; PRI: Population Recommended Intake, presented in bold type; dietary recommended intakes; M/F: values of reference for males and females; SPPB short physical performance battery; NC: not calculated.

Differences in percentage of people who cover these recommendations were found for vitamin D and B12. Concretely, for vitamin D, a high proportion of robust people met the recommendations (15.4%), while anyone in the other group reach the reference values. For B12, the whole sample of robust met the recommendations (100.0%), followed by pre-frail (95,6%) and frail (70%).

Differences between the amount of nutrients consumed, adjusted by energy intake are presented in Table 4.

Table 4. Differences between SPPB groups in nutrients adjusted by energy intake.

Nutrient intake	Robust (n = 13)	Pre-Frail (n = 68)	Frail (n = 20)	p Value
	Mean (SD)	Mean (SD)	Mean (SD)	
Carbohydrates (g/day)	234.3 ± 12.8 [a]	261.1 ± 5.6	279.1 ± 10.3	0.027
Protein (g/day)	112.7 ± 4.6 [a]	101.6 ± 2.0 [b]	99.2 ± 3.7	0.062
Total fat (g/day)	114.9 ± 5.0	106.3 ± 2.2	101.9 ± 4.0	0.130
Alcohol (g/day)	4.1 ± 2.5	6.1 ± 1.1	2.9 ± 2.0	0.319
n-3 (g/day)	3.2 ± 0.3 [a]	2.8 ± 0.1	2.0 ± 0.2	0.018
n-6 (g/day)	14.2 ± 1.6	15.5 ± 0.7	13.3 ± 1.3	0.277
MUFA (g/day)	51.5 ± 3.5	48.8 ± 1.5	46.9 ± 2.8	0.591
PUFA (g/day)	18.0 ± 1.9	19.0 ± 0.8	16.2 ± 1.5	0.254
SFA (g/day)	36.1 ± 2.0 [a]	30.0 ± 0.9 [b]	29.6 ± 1.6	0.018
Retinol equivalents (µg/day)	1737.9 ± 189.3	1612.1 ± 82.6	1470.0 ± 152.2	0.530
Vitamin D (µg/day)	7.8 ± 1.0 [a]	6.0 ± 0.4	4.6 ± 0.8	0.054
Vitamin E (mg/day)	10.9 ± 0.8	11.5 ± 0.3	11.6 ± 0.6	0.745
Ascorbic acid (mg/day)	306.3 ± 32.7	273.0 ± 14.3	237.0 ± 26.3	0.246
Thiamine (B1) (mg/day)	2.8 ± 0.3	2.6 ± 0.1	2.6 ± 0.2	0.801
Riboflavin (B2) (mg/day)	2.4 ± 0.2	2.2 ± 0.7	2.1 ± 0.1	0.460
Niacin equivalents (B3) (mg/day)	48.5 ± 2.5	43.0 ± 1.1	41.1 ± 2.0	0.063
Pyridoxin (B6) (mg/day)	2.8 ± 0.2	2.6 ± 0.6	2.4 ± 0.1	0.076
Folic acid (B9) (µg/day)	461.1 ± 33.8	450.4 ± 14.7	405.1 ± 27.2	0.294
Cobalamin (B12) (ug/day)	11.2 ± 1.3	9.8 ± 0.6	8.9 ± 1.0	0.346
Calcium (mg/day)	1299.7 ± 98.2	1127.5 ± 42.8	1145.4 ± 78.9	0.278
Iron (mg/day)	18.1 ± 1.0	17.8 ± 0.4	17.75 ± 0.8	0.956
Sodium (mg/day)	2710.1 ± 157.6	2451.3 ± 68.7	2632.1 ± 126.7	0.204
Magnesium (mg/day)	446.3 ± 13.3	428.7 ± 10.2	427.8 ± 18.7	0.777
Potassium (mg/day)	5158.5 ± 288.8	5043.7 ± 126.0	4622.2 ± 32.2	0.227
Iodine (ug/day)	280.7 ± 44.2	312.7 ± 19.3	349.2 ± 35.6	0.467
Selenium (µg/day)	112.5 ± 6.9	103.1 ± 3.0	102.3 ± 5.6	0.431
Zinc (mg/day)	14.0 ± 0.6	13.0 ± 0.3	13.2 ± 0.5	0.389
Phosphorus (mg/day)	2152.1 ± 108.7	1886.7 ± 47.4	1914.4 ± 87.4	0.086

Omega n-3, n-6: alpha linoleic fatty acid, MUFA: monounsaturated fatty acid, PUFA: polyunsaturated fatty acid, SFA: saturated fatty acid, SPPB short physical performance battery. [a] statistical difference between robust and frail groups [b] statistical differences between frail and pre-frail groups. All statistical significance was stablished at $p < 0.05$.

Globally, differences were observed between groups for carbohydrates, n3 fatty acids, and saturated fatty acids (SFA) (all $p < 0.05$). Specifically, differences were observed between robust and frail for carbohydrates (234.3 ± 12.8 vs. 279.1 ± 10.3 g/day), protein (112.6 ± 4.6 vs. 99.2 ± 3.7 g/day), n3 (3.2 ± 0.3 vs. 2.0 ± 0.2 g/day), SFA (36.1 ± 2.0 vs. 29.6 ± 1.6 g/day), and vitamin D (7.8 ± 1.0 vs. 4.6 ± 0.8 µg/day) (all $p <0.05$). In addition, differences were observed between pre-frail and frail, specifically for protein (101.6 ± 2.0 vs. 99.2 ± 3.7 g/day) and SFA (30.0 ± 0.9 vs. 29.6 ± 1.6 g/day) (both $p < 0.05$). No statistically significant differences were found between robust and pre-frail for any nutrient.

Moreover, Figures 1–4 show differences in dietary intakes between groups when referenced versus the robust group. Data about graphs is describe detailed in a supplementary file (Table S1). Figure 1 shows differences in macronutrient intake; frail presented a higher intake of carbohydrates (β = 44.9 ± 16.41) when compared to robust and a lower consumption of protein (β = −13.4 ± 6.0) and total fat (β = −13.0 ± 6.4), while pre-frail group only showed differences in protein (β = −11.0 ± 5.1) when compared to robust (all $p < 0.05$).

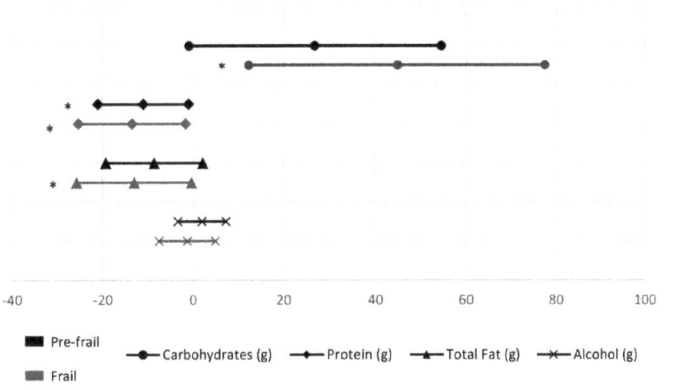

Figure 1. Macronutrient and alcohol intake in pre-frail and frail groups compared with robust (reference group). * Statistically significant differences (p value < 0.05).

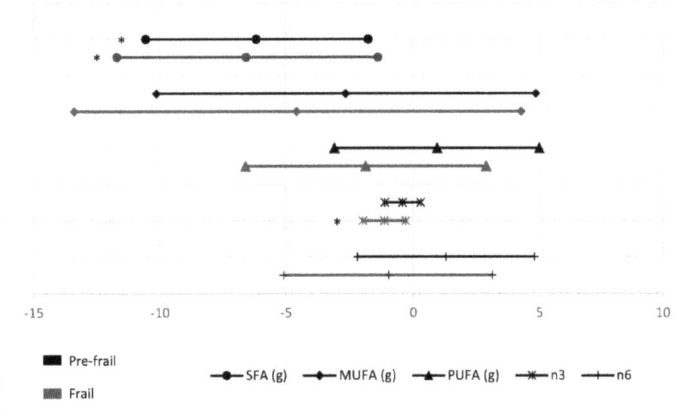

Figure 2. Fat type intake in pre-frail and frail groups compared with robust (reference group). * Statistically significant differences (p value < 0.05).

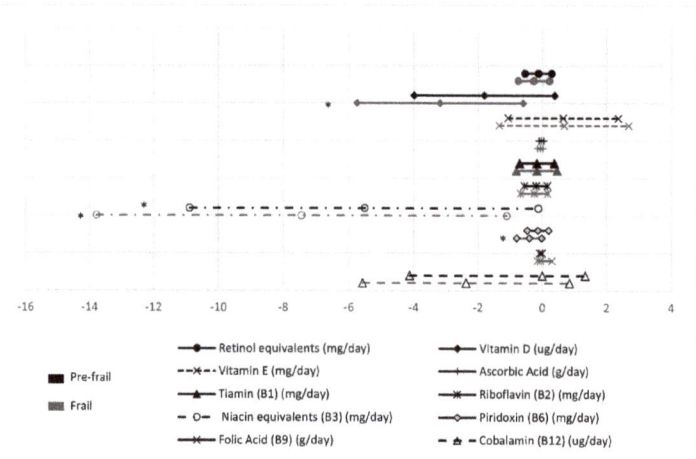

Figure 3. Vitamin intake in pre-frail and frail groups compared with robust (reference group). * Statistically significant differences (p value < 0.05).

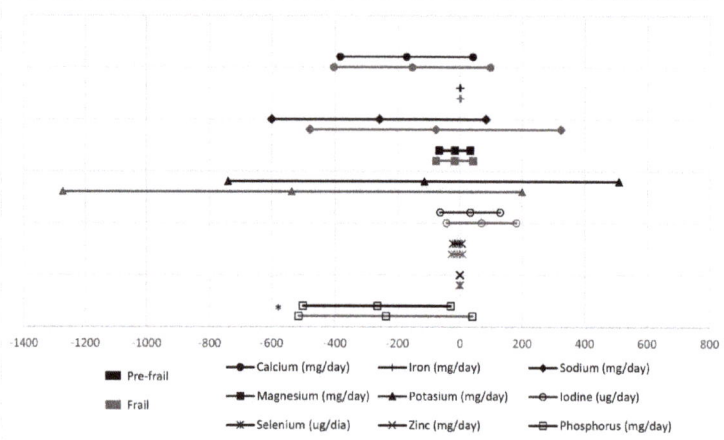

Figure 4. Mineral intake in pre-frail and frail groups compared with robust (reference group). * Statistically significant differences (p value < 0.05).

Data illustrating fat-type consumption are presented in Figure 2.

A lower consumption of SFA was observed in frail and pre-frail ($\beta = -6.6 \pm 2.6$ and $\beta = -6.2 \pm 2.2$, respectively) when considering robust as reference, and only frail presented a smaller intake of PUFA n-3 ($\beta = -1.1 \pm 0.4$) (all $p < 0.05$).

Regarding vitamins (Figure 3), frail group showed smaller intake for niacin equivalents ($\beta = -7.4 \pm 3.2$) and for pyridoxin ($\beta = -0.4 \pm 0.2$), while pre-frail only showed smaller intake for niacin equivalents ($\beta = -5.5 \pm 2.7$) when robust was taken as the reference (all $p < 0.05$; Figure 3).

For minerals (Figure 4), only pre-frail showed smaller intakes of phosphorus ($\beta = -265.5 \pm 118.7$) when compared with the reference group of robust ($p < 0.05$).

In addition, the binary logistic regression analysis was performed to predict the probability of being frail when there is a risk of malnourishment (adjusted by sex and age) and showed that those who were at risk of malnourishment were approximately 8 times more likely of being frail in comparison to those who are not at risk of malnourishment ($\beta = 7.7; p < 0.05$).

Finally, differences in nutritional intake of non-frail comparing those at risk of malnutrition and those without risk are presented in Table 5.

Table 5. Differences in nutrients intake between malnutrition groups in non-frail participants.

Nutrient Intake	At Risk of Malnutrition ($n = 26$)	No Risk of Malnutrition ($n = 55$)	p Value
	Mean (SD)	Mean (SD)	
Energy (kcal)	2485.3 ± 619.0	2444.5 ± 557.0	0.767
Carbohydrates (%)	42.3 ± 7.7	42.2 ± 7.2	0.959
Protein (%)	15.9 ± 3.3	17.6 ± 2.5	0.013
Total fat (%)	39.2 ± 7.0	39.1 ± 6.9	0.939
Alcohol (g)	2.6 ± 3.6	1.1 ± 1.9	0.020
n-3 (mg/day)	2.3 ± 1.0	3.2 ± 1.7	0.016
n-6 (mg/day)	15.3 ± 7.8	15.4 ± 7.7	0.924
MUFA (%)	18.4 ± 4.8	17.7 ± 4.7	0.559
PUFA (%)	6.3 ± 2.0	7.0 ± 2.7	0.258
SFA (%)	11.3 ± 2.7	11.2 ± 3.0	0.846
Retinol equivalents (ug/day)	1386.1 ± 552.8	1751.1 ± 722.4	0.025
Vitamin D (μg/day)	5.8 ± 3.3	6.5 ± 4.1	0.478
Vitamin E (mg/day)	11.1 ± 3.4	11.6 ± 3.2	0.505
Ascorbic acid (C) (mg/day)	238.2 ± 107.9	297.3 ± 128.4	0.041
Thiamine (B1) (mg/day)	2.5 ± 1.0	2.7 ± 0.9	0.290
Riboflavin (B2) (mg/day)	2.1 ± 0.6	2.7 ± 0.9	0.095
Niacin equivalents (B3) (mg/day)	40.4 ± 10.5	45.6 ± 10.5	0.040
Pyridoxin (B6) (mg/day)	2.4 ± 0.6	2.8 ± 0.6	0.003
Folic acid (B9) (μg/day)	403.9 ± 90.5	475.0 ± 131.3	0.014
Cobalamin (B12) (μg/day)	8.8 ± 3.8	10.7 ± 4.9	0.096
Calcium (mg/day)	1067.6 ± 325.5	1200.3 ± 402.8	0.146
Iron (mg/day)	16.5 ± 3.8	18.5 ± 4.6	0.055
Sodium (mg/day)	2487.9 ± 688.7	2506.5 ± 907.0	0.931
Magnesium (mg/day)	392.2 ± 83.9	451.3 ± 111.6	0.019
Potassium (mg/day)	4591.9 ± 829.8	5293.8 ± 1302.0	0.014
Iodine (μg/day)	272.2 ± 155.1	325.1 ± 161.1	0.167
Selenium (ug/day)	95.1 ± 32.9	109.4 ± 31.4	0.061
Zinc (mg/day)	12.3 ± 3.5	13.6 ± 3.3	0.090
Phosphorus (mg/day)	1795.1 ± 440.6	1997.7 ± 513.5	0.087

Omega n-3: alpha linolenic fatty acid, n-6: alpha linoleic fatty acid, MUFA: monounsaturated fatty acids, PUFA: polyunsaturated fatty acids, SFA: saturated fatty acids. %: percentage of total energy intake. Statistical significance stablished at $p < 0.05$.

Those non-frail participants at risk of malnourishment showed significant lower intake for protein (15.9 ± 3.3 vs. 17.6 ± 2.5% from the total energy intake), PUFA n-3 (2.3 ± 1.0 vs. 3.2 ± 1.7 g/day), retinol (1386.1 ± 552.8 vs. 1751.1 ± 722.4 μg/day), ascorbic acid (238.2 ± 107.9 vs. 297.3 ± 128.4 mg/day), niacin equivalents (40.4 ± 10.5 vs. 45.6 ± 10.5 mg/day), folic acid (403.9 ± 90.5 vs. 475.0 ± 131.3 μg/day), magnesium (392.2 ± 83.9 vs. 451.3 ± 111.6 mg/day), and potassium (4591.9 ± 829.8 vs. 5293.8 ± 1302.0 mg/day) (all $p < 0.05$). Moreover, those at risk of malnutrition also had a higher alcohol intake compared to the well-nourished (2.6 ± 3.6 vs. 1.1 ± 1.9 g, $p < 0.05$).

4. Discussion

The main findings of this study are: (1) some differences exist in the nutritional intake (carbohydrates, protein, vitamin D, PUFA n-3, and SFA) between robust, pre-frail, and frail older people but not for food groups; (2) vitamin D recommendations were met in higher proportions in robust group, while none of the pre-frail and pre-frail participants reached recommendations; (3) those older adults at risk of malnutrition were 7.7 times more likely to being frail compared to those without risk of malnutrition, (4) differences in intakes of protein, alcohol, PUFA n-3, retinol equivalents, ascorbic acid, niacin, pyridoxin, folic acid, magnesium, and phosphorus were observed between those non-frails at risk of malnourishment suggesting their important role in frailty prevention.

Nutrient deficiencies, nutrient intake, and diet quality have been widely studied in frail people determined by Fried phenotype [10,32]. Nevertheless, although SPPB has emerged as a tool for the screening of frailty in recent years, no comparable studies using this instrument have been found in the literature and, consequently, results found in this report have been compared with other studies using Fried phenotype.

Regarding differences in groups created with SPPB, frail, and pre-frail older adults showed lower consumption of protein, vitamin D, and PUFA n-3. These nutrients related to frailty have an important role in muscle mass synthesis during aging, sarcopenia, and inflammation [33,34]. Larger sample sizes found similar results regarding protein and vitamin D, however, in contrast to our results [35,36], no differences have been observed between frail and no-frail in other Spanish populations for PUFA n-3 [37]. However, it should be considered the ratio of PUFA n-3:n-6 as their assimilation depends on each other. In our study, not only frail groups presented lower consumption but also these ratios seemed to be unbalanced for those groups. Moreover, other differences such as higher intakes in carbohydrates and lower in SFA in the frail group also were found. Nevertheless, higher intakes of protein could be compensated by lower intakes of carbohydrates in robust, and the higher consumption of SFA in the robust group could be related to the quality of that protein source. If protein is obtained mainly from meat, it would lead to an increased consumption of SFA.

In addition to differences in nutrient intakes between frail, pre-frail, and robust individuals, most of our population did not meet the vitamin D recommended intakes (only 15% of the robust). This result and all the initials suggested the prioritization for the role of nutrition in frailty development, specially, when physical function is measured, or it is attempting to improve it. Thus, future exercise strategies with the main aim of improve physical function should consider all these nutrients.

Muscle mass and strength reduction due to aging may lead to muscle weakness and/or an impairment in physical function as well as physical activity, which may result in the reduction in total energy expenditure and also energy requirements [38]. Collectively, those factors could lead to complicate decrease in appetite, which is strongly related with risk of malnourishment [38]. Prior studies reveal that nutritional status could be helpful to screen frailty previously to the assessment by Fried [39]. Similarly, our study reveals that those at risk of malnutrition are approximately 8 times more likely to be frail than those without risk. Nutritional status and frailty have been also associated with quality of life [40,41]. Consequently, our results highlight even more the importance of ensure an adequate nutritional intake in this population.

Additionally, some nutrients' levels need to be remarkable for the prevention of frailty when nutritional status is considered. Differences were observed between those at risk and those without risk of being malnourished in the non-frail group. We observed higher intakes of protein, PUFA n-3, retinol equivalents, ascorbic acid, niacin, pyridoxin, folic acid, magnesium, and phosphorus in those without risk of malnourishment, while higher intakes of alcohol were observed in those at risk. Once more, PUFA n-3 and protein intake show their importance in these physiological statuses. Meanwhile, other nutrients such as vitamin A and ascorbic acid appear related to the risk of malnourishment and have been previously suggested to mediate in frailty due to their antioxidant effect, which may facilitate muscle mass synthesis [42]. Likewise, the importance of B group vitamins for their role in blood cell formation, macronutrient metabolism, and cognitive function, among others, has been also widely studied. Despite pyridoxin and vitamin B12 have been more associated in literature with frailty [43], folic acid and niacin seem also to be relevant in our sample. Furthermore, minerals such as magnesium and potassium, which appear to be significant in our sample, have been also associated with frailty and sarcopenia [44,45].

Globally, our results led us to focus not only on nutrients related to muscle mass synthesis but also on protein intake when approaching the dietary side of frailty. Moreover, future interventions using supplements, as those developed during last years with PUFA n-3 [46], vitamin D [47], or protein [48] and which have been demonstrated to be effectiveness to prevent frailty, should consider differently frailty stages. Interestingly, recent studies have reported different responses to protein intake between those stages [49], supporting our recommendation.

Limitations of this study should be highlighted. The present study has a cross-sectional design, reflecting associations but not revealing causality. Further research including larger sample sizes is required to verify these results in representative populations. Comparable groups with equal number of participants from both sexes need also to be performed. Although food frequency questionnaire is a validated method, this population could be over or underestimating their intakes as it is shown in the table of food group intake. Moreover, it could be also influenced by a possible cognitive impairment, however, no participants with these problems were included in this study as shown in the cognitive assessment. Some strengths like harmonized assessments and well instructed researchers should be considered as well as the novelty and practical potential of the topic. Finally, other variables such as quality of diet and nutrient food sources should be taken into account for future analyses.

5. Conclusions

In summary, our results showed lower intakes of protein, PUFA n-3, and vitamin D in frail group, while revealing higher intakes of carbohydrates. Moreover, those at risk of malnutrition have almost 8 times more probabilities to develop frailty. To prevent frailty, higher intakes in protein, PUFA n-3, retinol, ascorbic acid, folic acid, pyridoxin, niacin, magnesium, and potassium should be promoted in those at risk of malnutrition. Thus, it is an important role of nutritionists and dietitians to ensure healthy and specific diets in age populations and to stablish nutritional guidelines according to their functional capacity.

Supplementary Materials: The following are available online at https://www.mdpi.com/article/10.3390/nu13041231/s1, Table S1: Data about graphs; an analysis of covariance (ANCOVA) considering robust as reference group.

Author Contributions: Conceptualization, A.M., J.A.C., G.V.-R., and A.G.-C.; data curation, A.M.; formal analysis, A.M. and A.G.-C.; funding acquisition, I.A., J.A.C., and G.V.-R.; investigation, A.M., Á.I.F.-G., D.N.-V., L.S.-R., I.R.-G., and A.G.-C.; methodology, A.M., L.S.-R., J.A.C., and G.V.-R.; project administration, J.A.C., G.V.-R., and A.G.-C.; resources, Á.I.F.-G., D.N.-V., L.S.-R., and A.G.-C.; supervision, J.A.C., G.V.-R., and A.G.-C.; validation, E.G., J.P.-G., and I.A.; visualization, E.G., J.P.-G., I.R.-G., and I.A.; writing—original draft, A.M. and A.G.-C.; writing—review and editing, Á.I.F.-G., D.N.-V., E.G., J.P.-G., I.R.-G., I.A., J.A.C., and G.V.-R. All authors have read and agreed to the published version of the manuscript.

Funding: This study was funded by "Ministerio de Economía, Industria y Competitividad" (DEP2016-78309-R) and "Centro Universitario de la Defensa de Zaragoza" (UZCUD2017-BIO-01), Biomedical Research Networking Centre on Frailty and Healthy Aging (CIBERFES) and FEDER funds from the European Union (CB16/10/00477).

Institutional Review Board Statement: The study was conducted according to the guidelines of the Declaration of Helsinki, and approved by the Ethics Committee of Hospital Universitario de Alcorcón (protocol code: 16/50, date: 30/06/16).

Informed Consent Statement: Informed consent was obtained from all subjects involved in the study.

Data Availability Statement: The data are not publicly available due to privacy.

Acknowledgments: The authors are grateful to all the collaborators, nursing homes, health centers, council social services, and participants whose cooperation and dedication made this study possible. A.M.F. received a PhD grant from "Gobierno de Aragón" (2016-2021). D.N.V. received a grant from "Gobierno de Aragón" (DGAIIU/1/20). A.F.G. received a grant from the Spanish Government (BES-2017-081402). I.R-G. received a postdoctoral contract from the Government of Castilla-La Mancha (2019/9601).

Conflicts of Interest: The authors declare no conflict of interest. The funders had no role in the design of the study; in the collection, analyses, or interpretation of data; in the writing of the manuscript; or in the decision to publish the results.

References

1. Klein, B.E.; Klein, R.; Knudtson, M.D.; Lee, K.E. Frailty, morbidity and survival. *Arch. Gerontol. Geriatr.* **2005**, *41*, 141–149. [CrossRef] [PubMed]
2. Xue, Q.-L. The Frailty Syndrome: Definition and Natural History. *Clin. Geriatr. Med.* **2011**, *27*, 1–15. [CrossRef]
3. Fried, L.P.; Tangen, C.M.; Walston, J.D.; Newman, A.B.; Hirsch, C.; Gottdiener, J.S.; E Seeman, T.; Tracy, R.P.; Kop, W.J.; Burke, G.L.; et al. Frailty in Older Adults: Evidence for a Phenotype. *J. Gerontol. Ser. A Boil. Sci. Med. Sci.* **2001**, *56*, M146–M157. [CrossRef]
4. Treacy, D.; Hassett, L. The Short Physical Performance Battery. *J. Physiother.* **2018**, *64*, 61. [CrossRef] [PubMed]
5. Ramírez-Vélez, R.; De Asteasu, M.L.S.; Morley, J.E.; Cano-Gutierrez, C.A.; Izquierdo, M. Performance of the Short Physical Performance Battery in Identifying the Frailty Phenotype and Predicting Geriatric Syndromes in Community-Dwelling Elderly. *J. Nutr. Health Aging* **2021**, *25*, 209–217. [CrossRef]
6. Buta, B.J.; Walston, J.D.; Godino, J.G.; Park, M.; Kalyani, R.R.; Xue, Q.-L.; Bandeen-Roche, K.; Varadhan, R. Frailty assessment instruments: Systematic characterization of the uses and contexts of highly-cited instruments. *Ageing Res. Rev.* **2016**, *26*, 53–61. [CrossRef]
7. Pritchard, J.M.; Kennedy, C.C.; Karampatos, S.; Ioannidis, G.; Misiaszek, B.; Marr, S.; Patterson, C.; Woo, T.; Papaioannou, A. Measuring frailty in clinical practice: A comparison of physical frailty assessment methods in a geriatric out-patient clinic. *BMC Geriatr.* **2017**, *17*, 264. [CrossRef] [PubMed]
8. Lim, Y.J.; Ng, Y.S.; Sultana, R.; Tay, E.L.; Mah, S.M.; Chan, C.H.N.; Latib, A.B.; Abu-Bakar, H.M.; Ho, J.C.Y.; Kwek, T.H.H.; et al. Frailty Assessment in Community-Dwelling Older Adults: A Comparison of 3 Diagnostic Instruments. *J. Nutr. Health Aging* **2020**, *24*, 582–590. [CrossRef]
9. De Labra, C.; Guimaraes-Pinheiro, C.; Maseda, A.; Lorenzo, T.; Millán-Calenti, J.C. Effects of physical exercise interventions in frail older adults: A systematic review of randomized controlled trials. *BMC Geriatr.* **2015**, *15*, 154. [CrossRef]
10. Lorenzo-López, L.; Maseda, A.; De Labra, C.; Regueiro-Folgueira, L.; Rodríguez-Villamil, J.L.; Millán-Calenti, J.C. Nutritional determinants of frailty in older adults: A systematic review. *BMC Geriatr.* **2017**, *17*, 108. [CrossRef]
11. Cruz-Jentoft, A.J.; Kiesswetter, E.; Drey, M.; Sieber, C.C. Nutrition, frailty, and sarcopenia. *Aging Clin. Exp. Res.* **2017**, *29*, 43–48. [CrossRef]
12. Cruz-Jentoft, A.J.; Bahat, G.; Bauer, J.; Boirie, Y.; Bruyère, O.; Cederholm, T.; Cooper, C.; Landi, F.; Rolland, Y.; Sayer, A.A.; et al. Sarcopenia: Revised European consensus on definition and diagnosis. *Age Ageing* **2019**, *48*, 16–31. [CrossRef]
13. Azzolino, D.; Passarelli, P.C.; De Angelis, P.; Piccirillo, G.B.; D'Addona, A.; Cesari, M. Poor Oral Health as a Determinant of Malnutrition and Sarcopenia. *Nutrients* **2019**, *11*, 2898. [CrossRef]
14. Starr, K.N.P.; McDonald, S.R.; Bales, C.W. Obesity and Physical Frailty in Older Adults: A Scoping Review of Lifestyle Intervention Trials. *J. Am. Med. Dir. Assoc.* **2014**, *15*, 240–250. [CrossRef]
15. Kelaiditi, E.; van Kan, G.A.; Cesari, M. Frailty: Role of nutrition and exercise. *Curr. Opin. Clin. Nutr. Metab. Care* **2014**, *17*, 32–39. [CrossRef]
16. O'Connell, M.L.; Coppinger, T.; McCarthy, A.L. The role of nutrition and physical activity in frailty: A review. *Clin. Nutr. ESPEN* **2020**, *35*, 1–11. [CrossRef]
17. Coelho-Júnior, H.J.; Calvani, R.; Picca, A.; Gonçalves, I.O.; Landi, F.; Bernabei, R.; Cesari, M.; Uchida, M.C.; Marzetti, E. Protein-Related Dietary Parameters and Frailty Status in Older Community-Dwellers across Different Frailty Instruments. *Nutrients* **2020**, *12*, 508. [CrossRef]
18. Bollwein, J.; Diekmann, R.; Kaiser, M.J.; Bauer, J.M.; Uter, W.; Sieber, C.C.; Volkert, D. Distribution but not amount of protein intake is associated with frailty: A cross-sectional investigation in the region of Nürnberg. *Nutr. J.* **2013**, *12*, 109. [CrossRef]
19. Das, A.; Cumming, R.G.; Naganathan, V.; Blyth, F.; Ribeiro, R.V.; Le Couteur, D.G.; Handelsman, D.J.; Waite, L.M.; Simpson, S.J.; Hirani, V. Prospective Associations Between Dietary Antioxidant Intake and Frailty in Older Australian Men: The Concord Health and Ageing in Men Project. *J. Gerontol. Ser. A Boil. Sci. Med. Sci.* **2019**, *75*, 348–356. [CrossRef]
20. Morante, J.J.H.; Martínez, C.G.; Morillas-Ruiz, J.M. Dietary Factors Associated with Frailty in Old Adults: A Review of Nutritional Interventions to Prevent Frailty Development. *Nutrients* **2019**, *11*, 102. [CrossRef]
21. Fernández-García, Á.I.; Gómez-Cabello, A.; Moradell, A.; Navarrete-Villanueva, D.; Pérez-Gómez, J.; Ara, I.; Pedrero-Chamizo, R.; Subías-Perié, J.; Muniz-Pardos, B.; Casajús, J.A.; et al. How to Improve the Functional Capacity of Frail and Pre-Frail Elderly People? Health, Nutritional Status and Exercise Intervention. The EXERNET-Elder 3.0 Project. *Sustainability* **2020**, *12*, 6246. [CrossRef]
22. Folstein, M.F.; Folstein, S.E.; McHugh, P.R. "Mini-mental state": A practical method for grading the cognitive state of patients for the clinician. *J. Psychiatr. Res.* **1975**, *12*, 189–198. [CrossRef]
23. Fernandez-Ballart, J.D.; Pinol, J.L.; Zazpe, I.; Corella, D.; Carrasco, P.; Toledo, E.; Perez-Bauer, M.; Martinez-Gonzalez, M.; Salas-Salvado, J.; Martin-Moreno, J. Relative validity of a semi-quantitative food-frequency questionnaire in an elderly Mediterranean population of Spain. *Br. J. Nutr.* **2010**, *103*, 1808–1816. [CrossRef]

24. Guralnik, J.M.; Simonsick, E.M.; Ferrucci, L.; Glynn, R.J.; Berkman, L.F.; Blazer, D.G.; Scherr, P.A.; Wallace, R.B. A Short Physical Performance Battery Assessing Lower Extremity Function: Association With Self-Reported Disability and Prediction of Mortality and Nursing Home Admission. *J. Gerontol.* **1994**, *49*, M85–M94. [CrossRef]
25. Trichopoulou, A.; A Martínez-González, M.; Tong, T.Y.; Forouhi, N.G.; Khandelwal, S.; Prabhakaran, D.; Mozaffarian, D.; De Lorgeril, M. Definitions and potential health benefits of the Mediterranean diet: Views from experts around the world. *BMC Med.* **2014**, *12*, 112. [CrossRef]
26. Vellas, B.; Guigoz, Y.; Garry, P.J.; Nourhashemi, F.; Bennahum, D.; Lauque, S.; Albarede, J.L. The Mini Nutritional Assessment (MNA) and its use in grading the nutritional state of elderly patients. *Nutrition* **1999**, *15*, 116–122. [CrossRef]
27. Bauer, J.M.; Kaiser, M.J.; Anthony, P.; Guigoz, Y.; Sieber, C.C. The Mini Nutritional Assessment®—Its History, Today's Practice, and Future Perspectives. *Nutr. Clin. Pr.* **2008**, *23*, 388–396. [CrossRef]
28. Martin-Moreno, J.M.; Boyle, P.; Gorgojo, L.; Maisonneuve, P.; Fernandez-Rodriguez, J.C.; Salvini, S.; Willett, W.C. Development and validation of a food frequency questionnaire in Spain. *Int. J. Epidemiol.* **1993**, *22*, 512–519. [CrossRef] [PubMed]
29. Moreiras, O.; Carbajal, A.; Cabrera, L.C.C. *Tablas de Composición de los Alimentos. GUÍA de Prácticas*; Ed.Pirámide: Madrid, Spain, 2015.
30. Mataix, J. *Tabla de Composición de Alimentos*, 5th ed.; Universidad de Granada: Granada, Spain, 2009.
31. EFSA. *Dietary Reference Values for Nutrients Summary Report*; Wiley Online Library: Hoboken, NJ, USA, 2017.
32. Michel, J.P.; Cruz-Jentoft, A.J.; Cederholm, T. Frailty, Exercise and Nutrition. *Clin. Geriatr. Med.* **2015**, *31*, 375–387. [CrossRef] [PubMed]
33. Dupont, J.; Dedeyne, L.; Dalle, S.; Koppo, K.; Gielen, E. The role of omega-3 in the prevention and treatment of sarcopenia. *Aging Clin. Exp. Res.* **2019**, *31*, 825–836. [CrossRef] [PubMed]
34. Gray, S.R.; Mittendorfer, B. Fish oil-derived n-3 polyunsaturated fatty acids for the prevention and treatment of sarcopenia. *Curr. Opin. Clin. Nutr. Metab. Care* **2018**, *21*, 104–109. [CrossRef]
35. Balboa-Castillo, T.; A Struijk, E.; Lopez-Garcia, E.; Banegas, J.R.; Rodríguez-Artalejo, F.; Guallar-Castillon, P. Low vitamin intake is associated with risk of frailty in older adults. *Age Ageing* **2018**, *47*, 872–879. [CrossRef]
36. Schoufour, J.D.; Franco, O.H.; Jong, J.C.K.-D.; Trajanoska, K.; Stricker, B.; Brusselle, G.; Rivadeneira, F.; LaHousse, L.; Voortman, T. The association between dietary protein intake, energy intake and physical frailty: Results from the Rotterdam Study. *Br. J. Nutr.* **2019**, *121*, 393–401. [CrossRef]
37. Sandoval-Insausti, H.; Pérez-Tasigchana, R.F.; López-García, E.; García-Esquinas, E.; Rodríguez-Artalejo, F.; Guallar-Castillón, P. Macronutrients Intake and Incident Frailty in Older Adults: A Prospective Cohort Study. *J. Gerontol. Ser. A Boil. Sci. Med. Sci.* **2016**, *71*, 1329–1334. [CrossRef]
38. Morley, J.E.; Vellas, B.; Van Kan, G.A.; Anker, S.D.; Bauer, J.M.; Bernabei, R.; Cesari, M.; Chumlea, W.; Doehner, W.; Evans, J.; et al. Frailty Consensus: A Call to Action. *J. Am. Med. Dir. Assoc.* **2013**, *14*, 392–397. [CrossRef]
39. Soysal, P.; Veronese, N.; Arik, F.; Kalan, U.; Smith, L.; Isik, A.T. Mini Nutritional Assessment Scale-Short Form can be useful for frailty screening in older adults. *Clin. Interv. Aging* **2019**, *14*, 693–699. [CrossRef]
40. Salminen, K.S.; Suominen, M.H.; Kautiainen, H.; Pitkälä, K.H. Associations Between Nutritional Status, Frailty and Health-Related Quality of Life Among Older Long-Term Care Residents in Helsinki. *J. Nutr. Health Aging* **2020**, *24*, 319–324. [CrossRef]
41. Rizzoli, R.; Reginster, J.-Y.; Arnal, J.-F.; Bautmans, I.; Beaudart, C.; Bischoff-Ferrari, H.; Biver, E.; Boonen, S.; Brandi, M.-L.; Chines, A.; et al. Quality of Life in Sarcopenia and Frailty. *Calcif. Tissue Int.* **2013**, *93*, 101–120. [CrossRef]
42. Welch, A.A.; Jennings, A.; Kelaiditi, E.; Skinner, J.; Steves, C.J. Cross-Sectional Associations Between Dietary Antioxidant Vitamins C, E and Carotenoid Intakes and Sarcopenic Indices in Women Aged 18–79 Years. *Calcif. Tissue Int.* **2020**, *106*, 331–342. [CrossRef]
43. Behrouzi, P.; Grootswagers, P.; Keizer, P.L.C.; Smeets, E.T.H.C.; Feskens, E.J.M.; De Groot, L.C.P.G.M.; A Van Eeuwijk, F. Dietary Intakes of Vegetable Protein, Folate, and Vitamins B-6 and B-12 Are Partially Correlated with Physical Functioning of Dutch Older Adults Using Copula Graphical Models. *J. Nutr.* **2020**, *150*, 634–643. [CrossRef]
44. Van Dronkelaar, C.; Van Velzen, A.; Abdelrazek, M.; Van Der Steen, A.; Weijs, P.J.; Tieland, M. Minerals and Sarcopenia; The Role of Calcium, Iron, Magnesium, Phosphorus, Potassium, Selenium, Sodium, and Zinc on Muscle Mass, Muscle Strength, and Physical Performance in Older Adults: A Systematic Review. *J. Am. Med. Dir. Assoc.* **2018**, *19*, 6–11.e3. [CrossRef]
45. Arnaud, M.J. Update on the assessment of magnesium status. *Br. J. Nutr.* **2008**, *99*, S24–S36. [CrossRef]
46. Stocks, J.; Valdes, A.M. Effect of dietary omega-3 fatty acid supplementation on frailty-related phenotypes in older adults: A systematic review and meta-analysis protocol. *BMJ Open* **2018**, *8*, e021344. [CrossRef]
47. De Koning, E.J.; Van Schoor, N.M.; Penninx, B.W.; Elders, P.J.; Heijboer, A.C.; Smit, J.H.; Bet, P.M.; Van Tulder, M.W.; Heijer, M.D.; Van Marwijk, H.W.; et al. Vitamin D supplementation to prevent depression and poor physical function in older adults: Study protocol of the D-Vitaal study, a randomized placebo-controlled clinical trial. *BMC Geriatr.* **2015**, *15*, 151. [CrossRef]
48. Oktaviana, J.; Zanker, J.; Vogrin, S.; Duque, G. The effect of protein supplements on functional frailty in older persons: A systematic review and meta-analysis. *Arch. Gerontol. Geriatr.* **2020**, *86*, 103938. [CrossRef]
49. Buhl, S.F.; Beck, A.M.; Christensen, B.; Caserotti, P. Effects of high-protein diet combined with exercise to counteract frailty in pre-frail and frail community-dwelling older adults: Study protocol for a three-arm randomized controlled trial. *Trials* **2020**, *21*, 637. [CrossRef]

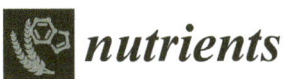

Article

Dietary Annatto-Extracted Tocotrienol Reduces Inflammation and Oxidative Stress, and Improves Macronutrient Metabolism in Obese Mice: A Metabolic Profiling Study

Chwan-Li Shen [1,2,3,*], Sivapriya Ramamoorthy [4], Gurvinder Kaur [2,5], Jannette M. Dufour [2,6], Rui Wang [1], Huanbiao Mo [7] and Bruce A. Watkins [8,*]

1. Department of Pathology, Texas Tech University Health Sciences Center, Lubbock, TX 79430, USA; rui.wang@ttuhsc.edu
2. Center of Excellence for Integrative Health, Texas Tech University Health Sciences Center, Lubbock, TX 79430, USA; Gurvinder.Kaur@ttuhsc.edu (G.K.); Jannette.Dufour@ttuhsc.edu (J.M.D.)
3. Center of Excellence for Translational Neuroscience and Therapeutics, Texas Tech University Health Sciences Center, Lubbock, TX 79430, USA
4. Metabolon, Inc., Morrisville, NC 27560, USA; SRamamoorthy@metabolon.com
5. Department of Medical Education, Texas Tech University Health Sciences Center, Lubbock, TX 79430, USA
6. Department of Cell Biology and Biochemistry, Texas Tech University Health Sciences Center, Lubbock, TX 79430, USA
7. Department of Nutrition, Georgia State University, Atlanta, GA 30303, USA; hmo@gsu.edu
8. Department of Nutrition, University of California at Davis, Davis, CA 95616, USA
* Correspondence: leslie.shen@ttuhsc.edu (C.-L.S.); bawatkins@ucdavis.edu (B.A.W.); Tel.: +1-(806)-743-2815 (C.-L.S.)

Citation: Shen, C.-L.; Ramamoorthy, S.; Kaur, G.; Dufour, J.M.; Wang, R.; Mo, H.; Watkins, B.A. Dietary Annatto-Extracted Tocotrienol Reduces Inflammation and Oxidative Stress, and Improves Macronutrient Metabolism in Obese Mice: A Metabolic Profiling Study. *Nutrients* **2021**, *13*, 1267. https://doi.org/10.3390/nu13041267

Academic Editor: Cristian Del Bo

Received: 22 February 2021
Accepted: 10 April 2021
Published: 13 April 2021

Publisher's Note: MDPI stays neutral with regard to jurisdictional claims in published maps and institutional affiliations.

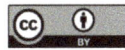

Copyright: © 2021 by the authors. Licensee MDPI, Basel, Switzerland. This article is an open access article distributed under the terms and conditions of the Creative Commons Attribution (CC BY) license (https://creativecommons.org/licenses/by/4.0/).

Abstract: Obesity and its related complications are a world-wide health problem. Dietary tocotrienols (TT) have been shown to improve obesity-associated metabolic disorders, such as hypercholesterolemia, hyperglycemia, and gut dysbiosis. This study examined the hypothesis that the antioxidant capacity of TT alters metabolites of oxidative stress and improves systemic metabolism. C57BL/6J mice were fed either a high-fat diet (HFD control) or HFD supplemented with 800 mg annatto-extracted TT/kg (HFD+TT800) for 14 weeks. Sera from obese mice were examined by non-targeted metabolite analysis using UHPLC/MS. Compared to the HFD group, the HFD+TT800 group had higher levels of serum metabolites, essential amino acids (lysine and methionine), sphingomyelins, phosphatidylcholine, lysophospholipids, and vitamins (pantothenate, pyridoxamine, pyridoxal, and retinol). TT-treated mice had lowered levels of serum metabolites, dicarboxylic fatty acids, and inflammatory/oxidative stress markers (trimethylamine N-oxide, kynurenate, 12,13-DiHOME, and 13-HODE + 9-HODE) compared to the control. The results suggest that TT supplementation lowered inflammation and oxidative stress (oxidized glutathione and GSH/GSSH) and improved macronutrient metabolism (carbohydrates) in obese mice. Thus, TT actions on metabolites were beneficial in reducing obesity-associated hypercholesterolemia/hyperglycemia. The effects of a non-toxic dose of TT in mice support the potential for clinical applications in obesity and metabolic disease.

Keywords: vitamin E; tocotrienol; metabolites; obesity; mice; inflammation

1. Introduction

Obesity is characterized by an excessive amount of adipose tissue, which has been recognized as a major endocrine organ that releases a wide variety of signaling molecules (hormones, growth factors, cytokines and chemokines) [1,2]. These signaling molecules play central roles in the regulation of energy metabolism and homeostasis, inflammation, and immunity [1,2].

Obesity is accompanied by a state of chronic low-grade systemic inflammation that accelerates the development of insulin resistance in type 2 diabetes (T2DM) [3] and hyperlipidemia in fatty liver diseases and cardiovascular diseases [4]. Hyperglycemia and high intracellular glucose metabolism, a hallmark of T2DM, is associated with excessive mitochondrial reactive oxygen species (ROS) and oxidative stress [5], which can impair insulin signaling and lead to insulin resistance of skeletal muscle glucose transport [6]. Moreover, there is growing evidence that excess generation of ROS, largely due to hyperglycemia, causes oxidative stress in a variety of tissues [5].

Studies in cell cultures, animal models, and human participants have provided compelling evidence that vitamin E, mainly tocopherols, play a role in preventing T2DM due to their antioxidant and anti-inflammatory capacities [7]. Until recently, tocotrienols (TTs), vitamin E molecules that differ from tocopherols by possessing an unsaturated isoprenoid side chain, have been overlooked for their potential effects in preventing T2DM [8,9]. TTs are more lipophilic, making them more easily incorporated into the cell membrane [10] and more rapidly absorbed than tocopherols [11]. Among all eight vitamin E isomers, δ-TT is considered as the most potent antioxidant/anti-inflammatory agent [12]. δ-TT has also been shown to be more protective than α-tocopherol against chronic diseases, such as T2DM, obesity, metabolic syndrome, fatty liver diseases, and cardiovascular diseases [13].

Tocotrienols have received increased attention due to their ability to attenuate obesity-associated complications via various molecular/cellular mechanisms, such as induction of apoptosis in preadipocytes, inhibition of fat cell adipogenesis and differentiation, activation of energy sensing pathways, protection of cell membranes against oxidative damage, inhibition of lipid peroxidation, and suppression of inflammation [8,14]. In animal models of obesity and T2DM [8,9,15], the anti-proliferative, antioxidant and anti-inflammatory properties of TTs contributed to their effects on hypo-cholesterolemia [16] and improved glucose homeostasis [8,9]. TT supplementation improved lipid metabolism as shown in reduced adipocyte hypertrophy, serum free fatty acids, triglycerides, and cholesterol [8,17] and hepatic steatosis in obese mice with increased markers of fatty acid β-oxidation (i.e., carnitine palmitoyltransferase 1A, carnitine palmitoyltransferase 2, and Forkhead box A2) and reduced markers of fatty acid synthesis (e.g., fatty acid synthase, acetyl-co-carboxylase-1) in adipose tissue [8]. In addition, TT supplementation significantly improved glucose tolerance in obese mice, as shown by a decreased area under the curve of the glucose tolerance test [8,9], which in part is attributed to the suppression of tumor necrosis factor-α (TNF-α), interleukin-1 beta (IL-1β), and interleukin-6 (IL-6) in lipopolysaccharide-stimulated peritoneal macrophages of obese mice [18]. In humans, TT administration significantly reduced serum levels of total cholesterol, low density lipoproteins (LDL), and triglycerides [13].

The present study used global non-targeted metabolomics to determine the metabolic effects of TT supplementation in mice with high-fat-diet (HFD)-induced obesity. Our approach focused on six broad pathways involving the metabolism of lipids, amino acids, cofactors and vitamins, nucleotides, peptides, and xenobiotics. We hypothesized that a diet supplemented with TT would reduce lipid peroxidation and oxidative stress, and alter the metabolism of amino acids, fatty acids, phospholipids, and sphingolipids in obese mice in ways that would be beneficial on lipid metabolism and glucose homeostasis in obese mice.

2. Materials and Methods

2.1. Animals and Treatments

Twenty male C57BL/6J mice (5-week-old, Jackson Laboratory, Bar Harbor, ME, USA), housed in cages of four mice and maintained at a controlled temperature of 21 ± 2 °C with a 12 h light-dark cycle, were fed chow diet and distilled water at libitum for 5 days. After acclimation, mice were weighed and assigned to two groups: control group fed high-fat diet (HFD; 21%, 20%, and 58% of energy from protein, carbohydrates, and fat, respectively, Research Diets Inc., New Brunswick, NJ, USA) and the treatment group fed the HFD supplemented with annatto-extracted TT at 800 mg/kg diet (HFD+TT800). TT was extracted from annatto oil with 71.3% purity, containing 86.1% δ-TT and 13.9% γ-TT, free of tocopherol (American River Nutrition, LLC, Hadley, MA, USA). The remaining 30% components of TT are mainly fatty acids of annatto oil itself, with a very small amount of plant terpenes, sterols, and waxes.

TT was premixed with tocopherol-stripped soybean oil (Dytes Inc., Bethlehem, PA, USA) before being incorporated into the ingredients of the HFD. Both groups were given the diets for 14 weeks with free access to water and diet during the study period. Previous rodent studies showed the anti-inflammatory actions of δ-TT at 400 and 1600 mg/kg diet/ in obese mice [8]; the TT dose used in our current study, 800 mg/kg diet, is within this range. Table 1 lists the ingredient composition in g/kg of the two dietary groups. Body weight, food intake, and water consumption were recorded weekly. All conditions and handling of the mice were approved by the Texas Tech University Health Sciences Center Institutional Animal Care and Use Committee. All procedures and animal use were performed in accordance with the relevant guidelines and regulations.

Table 1. Ingredient composition of the experimental diets (g/kg).

Ingredient	HFD	HFD+TT800
Casein, 80 Mesh	267.1	267.1
L-Cystine	4	4
Maltodextrin 10	166.9	166.9
Sucrose	91.9	91.9
Cellulose, BW 200	66.8	66.8
Soybean oil [a]	33.38	33.38
Lard	327.2	327.2
Mineral mix [b], S10026B	13.4	13.4
Dicalcium phosphate	17.4	17.4
Calcium carbonate	7.3	7.3
Potassium citrate, 1 H_2O	22	22
Vitamin mix [c], V13401 (without E)	13.4	13.4
Vitamin E acetate (500 IU/gm)	0.1	0.1
Choline bitartrate	2.7	2.7
Tocotrienol [d]	0	0.56

HFD, high-fat diet control group; HFD+TT800, a high-fat diet supplemented with tocotrienol (TT800) at 800 mg/kg diet. [a] Soybean oil tocopherol stripped (catalog number: 404365, Dyets Inc., Bethlehem, PA, USA). [b] Mineral mix provides (g/kg diet): calcium phosphate, dibasic, 260; calcium carbonate, 110; potassium citrate,1H_2O, 330; sodium chloride, 51.8; magnesium oxide, 8.38; magnesium sulfate, 7H_2O, 51.52; chromium K sulfate, 12H_2O, 0.385; cupric carbonate, 0.21; sodium fluoride, 0.04; potassium iodate, 0.007; ferric citrate, 4.2; manganous carbonate, 2.45; ammonium molybdate, 4H_2O, 0.06, sodium selenite, 0.007, zinc carbonate, 1.12; sucrose, 179.821. [c] Vitamin mix provides (g/kg diet): vitamin A acetate (500,000 IU/g), 0.8; vitamin D3 (100,000 IU/g), 1.0; vitamin K1 (menadione sodium bisulfite, 62.5% menadione), 0.08; biotin (1%), 2.0; cyanocobalamin (B12) (0.1%), 1.0; folic acid, 0.2; nicotinic acid, 3.0; calcium pantothenate, 1.6; pyridoxine-HCl, 0.7; riboflavin, 0.6; thiamine HCl, 0.6; sucrose, 988.42. [d] Tocotrienols was an extract of annatto oil containing 86.1% δ-tocotrienol and 13.9% γ-tocotrienol (American River Nutrition, Hadley, MA, USA). High-performance liquid chromatography determined the purity content to be 71.3%.

2.2. Sample Collection

At the end of the experiment, mice were fasted for 4-h, anesthetized with isoflurane, and then euthanized. Blood was collected into microtainer blood collector tubes (BD Biosciences, San Jose, CA, USA) and then centrifuged at $1500\times g$ for 20 min to isolate serum. The serum samples were kept at $-80\,^\circ$C until further analyses.

2.3. Metabolomics Analyses of Serum

Sample preparation and non-targeted metabolomics analysis of serum samples were conducted at Metabolon, Inc. (Morrisville, NC, USA) as described in a previous study [19]. Briefly, individual samples were subjected to methanol extraction and then split into aliquots for analysis by ultrahigh performance liquid chromatography/mass spectrometry (UHPLC/MS). The global biochemical profiling analysis comprised of four unique arms consisting of reverse phase chromatography positive ionization methods optimized for hydrophilic (LC/MS Pos Polar) and hydrophobic compounds (LC/MS Pos Lipid), reverse phase chromatography with negative ionization conditions (LC/MS Neg), and a HILIC chromatography method coupled to negative ionization (LC/MS Polar) [20]. All of the methods alternated between full scan MS and data dependent multi-stage mass spectrometry (MSn) scans. The scan range varied slightly between methods but generally covered 70–1000 m/z.

Metabolites were identified by automated comparison of the ion features in the experimental samples to a reference library of standard chemical entries [21] that included retention time, molecular weight (m/z), preferred adducts, in-source fragments, and associated MS spectra and curated by visual inspection for quality control using software developed at Metabolon, Inc. (Morrisville, NC, USA).

2.4. Statistical Analyses

Principal components analysis (PCA) and hierarchical clustering were used for classification analysis. For the scaled intensity graphics, each biochemical in original scale (raw area count) was rescaled to set the median across all animals and time-points as equal to 1. To gain insight into individual metabolites that may be able to differentiate the groups, we also performed random forest analysis. This method attempts to bin individual samples in groups based on their metabolite similarities and differences. The method is unbiased since the prediction for each sample is based on trees built from a subset of samples that do not include that sample [22]. Random forest also defines which metabolites contribute most strongly to the group binning.

Two types of statistical analyses for metabolites were performed: (1) significance tests; and (2) classification analysis. Standard statistical analyses were performed in ArrayStudio on log-transformed data. For analyses not standard in ArrayStudio, the R program (http://cran.r-project.org/ (accessed on 27 October 2016)) was used. Following log transformation and imputation of missing values, if any, with the minimum observed value for each compound, Welch's two sample *t*-Test was used as significance test to identify biochemicals that differed significantly ($p < 0.05$) between experimental groups. An estimate of the false discovery rate (q-value) was calculated to take into account the multiple comparisons that normally occur in metabolomic-based studies.

3. Results

There were no differences in body weight, food intake, and water consumption between the HFD group and the HFD+TT800 group throughout the study period (data not shown).

3.1. Metabolite Summary and Significantly Altered Biochemicals

A comprehensive non-targeted mass spectrometry-based metabolomics profiling analysis was performed on sera from the HFD and HFD+TT800 mice after a 14-week feeding period. Overall, a total of 566 metabolites, or biochemicals, of known identity were detected and categorized into six broad categories including amino acids, cofactors and vitamins, lipids, nucleotides, peptides, and xenobiotics. Among these 566 compounds, 68 biochemicals were primarily responsible for the observed significant difference due to TT ($p \leq 0.05$) with 44 additional biochemicals showing a tendency of change due to TT ($0.05 < p < 0.1$). Among the 68 biochemicals ($p \leq 0.05$) with changes in concentration, 32 biochemicals edged higher whereas 36 others went lower. Similarly, among the 44 biochemicals ($0.05 < p < 0.1$), 18 biochemicals were higher whereas 26 others were lower.

The PCA analysis revealed adequate segregation of the HFD group from the HFD+TT800 group, suggesting distinct biochemical compositions (Figure 1a). About 30% of the samples from each group showed overlapping distribution, demonstrating similar biochemical composition between these groups. The observed variability in 30% of the samples from each group could be attributed to potential variances in sample collection that lead to global changes in the amount of metabolites in the samples.

Figure 1b presents a heatmap of hierarchical clustering of serum metabolites between the HFD and HFD+TT800 groups. Most of the HFD+TT800 biochemicals show a single branch of the dendrogram whereas the HFD samples segregate to a separate branch. The groups have eight distinguishable metabolic signatures/superpathways, including amino acids, carbohydrates, cofactors and vitamins, energy metabolites, lipids, nucleotides, peptides, and xenobiotics.

Figure 1c shows the biochemical importance plot based on the results of the random forest test. The 30 top ranking biochemical differences of importance to group classification separations are shown, indicating key differences in lipid metabolism and amino acid metabolism between the groups.

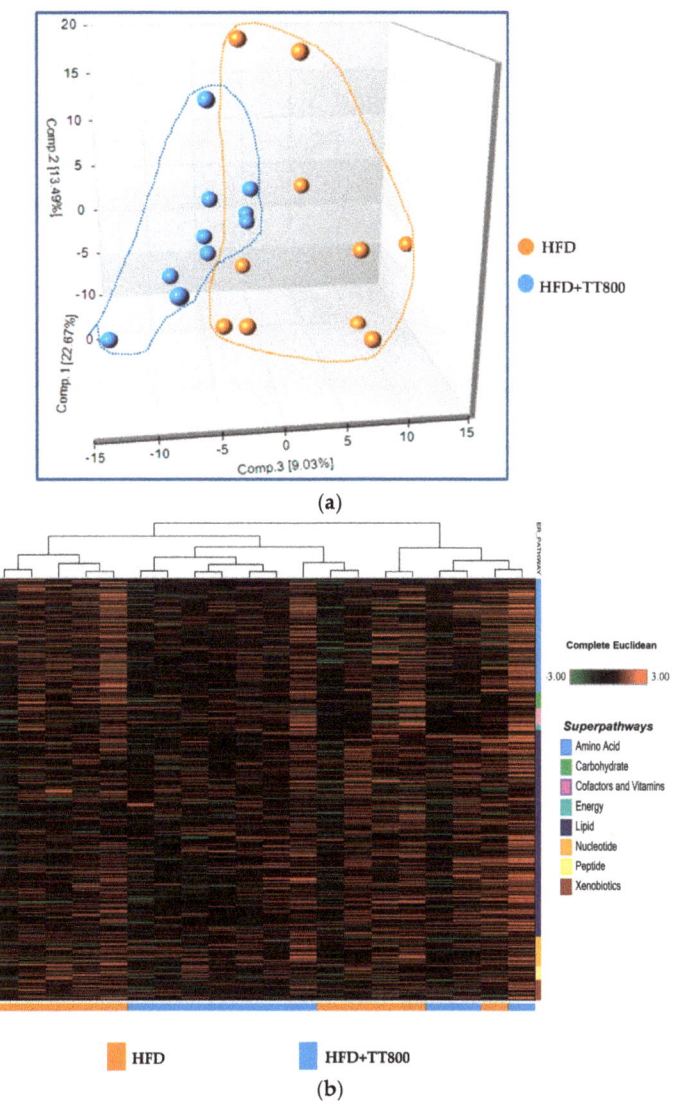

Figure 1. *Cont.*

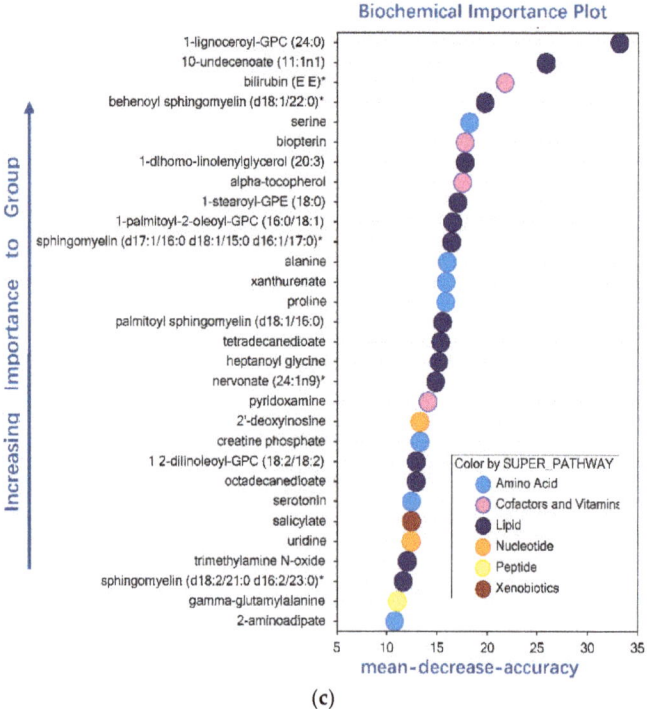

(c)

Figure 1. (**a**) Principal component analysis (PCA) showed differences in metabolites of serum samples in mice between the control HFD group and the treatment HFD+TT800 group. Each ball represents the cumulative metabolites from each mouse. The 10 orange balls are mice from the control HFD group and 10 blue balls are mice from the HFD+TT800 group. Metabolites associated with mice in the TT800 group are more tightly associated or closer together than those from mice in the control HFD group. TT supplementation appears to narrow the range of metabolite data in the mice fed the HFD. Each dietary group was comprised of $n = 10$ mice. (**b**) Differences in eight superpathways of serum metabolites between the control HFD group and the HFD+TT800 group. Heatmap of the hierarchical cluster analysis of serum metabolites by Student's *t*-test to distinguish the eight superpathways of metabolites between the control HFD group and the HFD+TT800 group. The eight superpathways include amino acids, carbohydrates, cofactors and vitamins, energy metabolites, lipids, nucleotides, peptides, and xenobiotics. Color in red indicates up-regulation and color in green indicates down-regulation (fold changes, $p < 0.05$). Each dietary group was comprised of $n = 10$ mice. (**c**) Biochemical importance plot based on random forest classification of the overall metabolomics profile for mouse serum samples. Random forest analysis distinguishes between the control HFD group subsets of superpathways and the treated HFD+TT800 group subsets of superpathways. Progression to TT800 supplementation was set as the response variable and all serum metabolites or biochemicals identified by the platform were set as predictors. The biochemicals are plotted according to the increasing importance to group separation to elucidate the metabolic fingerprint for TT800 supplementation as compared to the control HFD group. The figure presents the 30 top-ranked metabolites and their classification (indicated in the figure, lower right) based on their importance for the identification of the two treatment subsets. Light blue = amino acid, pink = cofactors and vitamins, dark blue = lipid, orange = nucleotide, light yellow = peptide, burgundy = xenobiotics. Each dietary group was comprised of $n = 10$ mice.

3.2. Effects of TT on Lipid Metabolism

The effects of TT supplementation on the serum level of fatty acid metabolites, presented as the ratio of (HFD+TT800)/HFD, are presented in Table 2. Relative to the HFD group, the HFD+TT800 group had lower serum levels of 13-methylmyristate (a branched chain fatty acid), two medium-chain fatty acids-pelargonate (C9:0) and 10-undecenoate (C11:1n1), and several fatty acid dicarboxylates, including azelate, sebacate, 1,11-undecanedicarboxylate, dodecanedioate, tetradecanedioate and octadecanedioate ($p \leq 0.05$). Other fatty acid dicarboxylates, including 2-hydroxyadipate, suberate, undecanedioate and hexadecanedioate, showed a trend of reduction ($0.05 < p < 0.1$). The HFD+TT800 group had lower levels of several fatty acid acyl glycine metabolites, including valerylglycine, hexanoylglycine, heptanoyl glycine, 3,4-methylene heptanoylglycine, and N-octanoylglycine, than the HFD group ($p \leq 0.05$). In addition, the HFD+TT800 group had altered fatty acid acyl carnitine metabolites—lower hexanoylcarnitine (C6) levels and higher lignoceroylcarnitine (C24) levels—and a higher level of serum carnitine ($p \leq 0.05$) (Table 3).

Table 2. Effects of TT supplementation on serum fatty acid metabolites in mice fed HFD compared to the HFD control group.

Sub Pathway	Metabolite Name	HFD+TT800/HFD
Fatty acid branched	13-methylmyristate	0.80
Medium chain fatty acid	heptanoate (C7:0)	1.13
	pelargonate (C9:0)	0.84
	10-undecenoate (C11:1n1)	0.69
Fatty acid monohydroxy	2-hydroxyoctanoate	0.84
	9-HODE + 13-HODE	0.71
	14-HDoHE/17-HDoHE	0.82
Fatty acid, dicarboxylate	2-hydroxyadipate	0.69
	suberate (octanedioate)	0.81
	azelate (nonanedioate)	0.79
	sebacate (decanedioate)	0.77
	Undecanedioate	0.81
	1,11-undecanedicarboxylate	0.75
	dodecanedioate	0.81
	tetradecanedioate	0.80
	hexadecanedioate	0.85
	Octadecanedioate	0.79
Eicosanoid	Thromboxane B2	0.45
	12-HHTE	0.72
	12-HHTrE	0.47
Endocannabinoid	oleoyl ethanolamide	1.07
	palmitoyl ethanolamide	1.09
	linoleoyl ethanolamide	1.11
Fatty acid acyl glycine	Valerylglycine	0.61
	Hexanoylglycine	0.51
	heptanoyl glycine	0.53
	3,4-methylene heptanoylglycine	0.63
	N-octanoylglycine	0.57
	N-palmitoylglycine	0.93
Fatty acid acyl carnitine	hexanoylcarnitine (C6)	0.71
	decanoylcarnitine (C10)	1.29
	lignoceroylcarnitine (C24)	1.18
Carnitine	Carnitine	1.22

Metabolite values are expressed as the ratio of HFD+TT800/HFD which is the fold change of the treated HFD+TT800 group compared to the HFD control group. A ratio greater than 1 indicates a value larger for the treated group (HFD+TT800) and less than 1 the value for HFD+TT800 group is lower compared to the HFD control group. Green indicates fold reduction and red is for fold increase by TT supplementation with $p \leq 0.05$ obtained from the Student's *t*-test. Yellow indicates fold reduction and pink is for fold increase by TT supplementation with $0.05 < p < 0.1$ that was obtained from the Student's *t*-test.

Table 3. Effects of TT supplementation on serum sphingolipid, phospholipid, and other lipid metabolites in mice fed HFD compared to the HFD control group.

Sub Pathway	Metabolite Name	HFD+TT800/HFD
Sphingolipid Metabolism	palmitoyl dihydrosphingomyelin (d18:0/16:0)	1.08
	palmitoyl sphingomyelin (d18:1/16:0)	0.31
	behenoyl sphingomyelin (d18:1/22:0)	1.32
	sphingomyelin (d17:1/16:0, d18:1/15:0, d16:1/17:0)	1.19
	sphingomyelin (d18:2/16:0, d18:1/16:1)	1.11
	sphingomyelin (d18:1/18:1, d18:2/18:0)	1.26
	sphingomyelin (d18:1/20:1, d18:2/20:0)	1.24
	sphingomyelin (d18:1/24:1, d18:2/24:0)	1.14
	sphingomyelin (d18:2/21:0, d16:2/23:0)	0.78
	sphingomyelin (d18:2/24:2)	1.21
	sphingomyelin (d18:1/22:2, d18:2/22:1, d16:1/24:2)	1.21
	sphingomyelin (d18:2/18:1)	1.24
	sphingomyelin (d18:1/19:0, d19:1/18:0)	0.72
Phospholipid Metabolism	glycerophosphorylcholine (GPC)	1.25
	glycerophosphoinositol (GPI)	1.20
	trimethylamine N-oxide (TMAO)	0.58
Phosphatidylcholine (PC)	1-palmitoyl-2-palmitoleoyl-GPC (16:0/16:1)	1.15
	1-palmitoyl-2-oleoyl-GPC (16:0/18:1)	1.12
	1,2-dilinoleoyl-GPC (18:2/18:2)	1.24
Lysophospholipid	1-lignoceroyl-GPC (24:0)	1.39
	1-stearoyl-GPE (18:0)	1.17
Plasmalogen	1-(1-enyl-palmitoyl)-2-palmitoyl-GPC (P-16:0/16:0)	1.23
	1-(1-enyl-palmitoyl)-2-linoleoyl-GPC (P-16:0/18:2)	1.17
Monoacylglycerol	1-dihomo-linolenylglycerol (20:3)	1.66
Diacylglycerol	palmitoyl-linoleoyl-glycerol (16:0/18:2)	0.40
Ceramides	glycosyl ceramide (d18:1/20:0, d16:1/22:0)	1.21
Mevalonate Metabolism	Mevalonate	0.84
Primary Bile Acid Metabolism	beta-muricholate	0.69

Metabolite values are expressed as the ratio of HFD+TT800/HFD which is the fold change of the treated HFD+TT800 group compared to the HFD control group. A ratio greater than 1 indicates a value larger for the treated group (HFD+TT800) and less than 1 the value for HFD+TT800 group is lower compared to the HFD control group. Green indicates fold reduction and red is for fold increase by TT supplementation with $p \leq 0.05$ obtained from the Student's t-test. Yellow indicates fold reduction and pink is for fold increase by TT supplementation with $0.05 < p < 0.1$ that was obtained from the Student's t-test.

Some oxylipins (bioactive lipids) were changed favorably in mice supplemented with TT, as shown by the (HFD+TT800)/HFD ratio (Table 2). In this case, 9-HODE and 13-HODE and 14 HDoHE/17-HDoHE were lower, suggesting lower acute pain and inflammation and auto-oxidation of DHA. Thromboxane B2, an inactive metabolite of thromboxane A2, was lower as well for the ratio values (ratio 0.45). Furthermore, 14 HDoHe/17-HDoHe showed a lower ratio (ratio 0.72), and this lipokine appears to lower circulating triglycerides. 12-HETE, which activates protein kinase C and mediates biological functions of growth factor cytokines was lower. Interestingly, the ratio for 12 HHTrE, a COX metabolite of arachidonate that may promote or limit inflammatory and promote allergic responses, was lower with TT supplementation. In contrast, the ratios for oleoyl ethanolamide, palmitoyl ethanolamide and linoleoyl ethanolamide in serum were not different between the groups.

The effects of TT supplementation on sphingolipids, phospholipids, and other lipid metabolites are shown in Table 3. The HFD+TT800 group showed significantly higher concentrations of intermediates of sphingolipid metabolism, such as palmitoyl dihydrosphingomyelin and behenoyl subgroups of shingomeylins, and a variety of sphingomyelin isomers. Regarding phospholipid metabolism, the HFD+TT800 group had (i) lower levels of trimethylamine N-oxide (TMAO), an intermediate of phospholipid metabolism ($p \leq 0.05$); and (ii) higher levels of glycerophosphorylcholine (GPC) and glycerophosphoinositol (GPI) ($0.05 < p < 0.1$).

TT supplementation resulted in higher levels of phosphatidylcholine intermediates (e.g., 1-palmitoyl-2-palmitoleoyl-GPC, 1-palmitoyl-2-oleoyl-GPC, and 1,2-dilinoleoyl-GPC, $p \leq 0.05$) and lysophospholipid intermediates (e.g., 1-lignoceroyl-GPC and 1-stearoyl-GPE, $p \leq 0.05$). TT supplementation also led to higher ratios for the levels of 1-(1-enyl-palmitoyl)-2-palmitoyl-GPC and 1-(1-enyl-palmitoyl)-2-linoleoyl-GPC (plasmalogen metabolites, 0.05 < p < 0.1), 1-dihmo-linolenyglycerol (a monoacylglycerol metabolite, $p \leq 0.05$), and glycosyl ceramide (a ceramides metabolite, 0.05 < p < 0.1). TT supplementation led to lower levels of palmitoyl-linoleoyl-glycerol (a metabolite of diacylglycerol, 0.05 < p < 0.1), mevalonate (an intermediate of mevalonate metabolism, $p \leq 0.05$), and beta-muricholate (a metabolite of bile acid metabolism, 0.05 < p < 0.1).

3.3. Effects of TT on Amino Acid Metabolism

Table 4 shows the effects of TT supplementation on serum amino acid metabolites in obese mice, again presented as ratios of (HFD+TT800)/HFD. Relative to the control HFD group, the HFD+TT800 group had higher levels of intermediates involved in amino acid metabolism, including serine (serine metabolism), alanine (alanine metabolism), pyroglutamine (glutamate metabolism), histidine and 1-methylhistamine (histidine metabolism), phenylpyruvate (phenylalanine metabolism), tyrosine and 2-hydroxyphenylacetate (tyrosine metabolism), serotonin and indoleacetate (tryptophan metabolism), 3-methylglutaconate and 3-methyl-2-oxobutyrate (leucine, isoleucine, and valine metabolism), S-methylcysteine (cysteine metabolism), 2-monomethylarginine (arginine metabolism), and creatine phosphate (creatine metabolism). The increases in two gluconeogenic amino acids, serine and alanine, could mean greater gluconeogenesis and improved glucose homeostasis to reduce obesity found in obese mice [15].

Table 4. Effects of TT supplementation on serum amino acid metabolites in mice fed HFD compared to the HFD control group.

Sub Pathway	Biochemical Name	HFD+TT800/HFD
Glycine, Serine, and Threonine Metabolism	N-acetylglycine	0.75
	Serine	1.13
Alanine and Aspartate Metabolism	Alanine	1.17
Glutamate Metabolism	Pyroglutamine	1.15
Histidine Metabolism	Histidine	1.06
	N-acetyl-3-methylhistidine	0.68
	Imidazole propionate	0.35
	1-Methylhistamine	1.28
Lysine Metabolism	N2-acetyllysine	0.76
	N2,N6-diacetyllysine	0.83
	N6,N6,N6-trimethyllysine	0.76
	2-Aminoadipate	0.84
Phenylalanine Metabolism	Phenylpyruvate	1.28
Tyrosine Metabolism	Tyrosine	1.12
	2-Hydroxyphenylacetate	1.29
Tryptophan Metabolism	Kynurenate	0.70
	Xanthurenate	0.43
	Serotonin	1.39
	Indoleacetate	1.31
Leucine, Isoleucine, and Valine Metabolism	3-Methylglutaconate	2.00
	Alpha-hydroxyisovalerate	0.88
	Ethylmalonate	0.84
	3-Methyl-2-oxobutyrate	1.35
Methionine, Cysteine, SAM, and Taurine Metabolism	S-methylcysteine	1.42
	N-acetyltaurine	0.77
Urea cycle, Arginine, and Proline Metabolism	2-Oxoarginine	0.81
	N-monomethylarginine	1.22
Creatine Metabolism	Creatine phosphate	1.86
Guanidino and Acetamido Metabolism	4-Guanidinobutanoate	0.80
Glutathione Metabolism	2-Hydroxybutyrate/2-Hydroxyisobutyrate	0.75

Metabolite values are expressed as the ratio of HFD+TT800/HFD which is the fold change of the treated HFD+TT800 group compared to the HFD control group. A ratio greater than 1 indicates a value larger for the treated group (HFD+TT800) and less than 1 the value for HFD+TT800 group is lower compared to the HFD control group. Green indicates fold reduction and red is for fold increase by TT supplementation with $p \leq 0.05$ that was obtained from the Student's t-test. Yellow indicates fold reduction and pink is for fold increase by TT supplementation with 0.05 < p < 0.1 that was obtained from the Student's t-test.

Furthermore, relative to the HFD group, the HFD+TT800 group had lower levels of intermediates of amino acid metabolism (Table 4), including N-acetylglycine (glycine metabolism), N-acetyl-3-methylhistidine and imidazole propionate (histidine metabolism), N2-acetyllysine, N2,N6-diacetyllysine, N6,N6,N6-trimethyllysine and 2-aminoadipate (lysine metabolism), kynurenate and xanthurenate (tryptophan metabolism), alpha-hydroxyisovalerate and ethylmalonate (leucine, isoleucine, and valine metabolism), N-acetyltaurine (taurine metabolism), 2-oxoarginine (arginine metabolism), 4-guanidinobutanoate (guanidine metabolism), and 2-hydroxybutyrate/2-hydroxyisobutyrate (glutathione metabolism).

3.4. Effects of TT on Carbohydrate Metabolism and Energy Cycle

Figure 2 shows the effects of TT supplementation on carbohydrate metabolism and TCA cycle in obese mice. Compared to the control HFD group, the HFD+TT800 group had lower levels of serum ribitol (pentose metabolism, Figure 2a), galactonate (galactose metabolism, Figure 2b), N-acetylneuraminate (amino sugar metabolism, Figure 2c), erythronate (amino sugar metabolism, Figure 2d), and citrate (TCA cycle, Figure 2e).

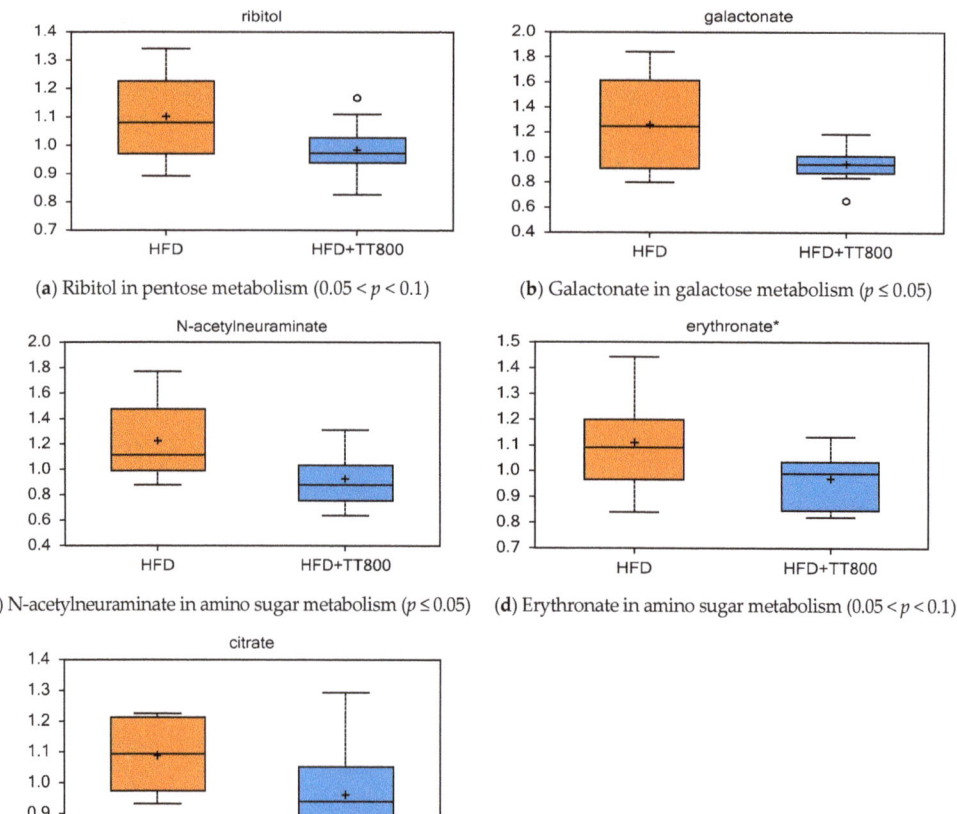

(a) Ribitol in pentose metabolism ($0.05 < p < 0.1$)

(b) Galactonate in galactose metabolism ($p \leq 0.05$)

(c) N-acetylneuraminate in amino sugar metabolism ($p \leq 0.05$)

(d) Erythronate in amino sugar metabolism ($0.05 < p < 0.1$)

(e) Citrate in TCA cycle ($0.05 < p < 0.1$)

Figure 2. Effect of TT supplementation on carbohydrate metabolism. Importance of compounds relative to flux through carbohydrate metabolism and biosynthetic pathways in mice given TT. A lower level of citrate (e) in mice given TT might indicate a higher flux of TCA to support better energy production and use, and lower macronutrient carbon to support fat deposition when a HFD is fed. Generally, figures (a–d) suggest lower formation of these anabolic pathway intermediates. Each dietary group was comprised of $n = 10$ mice.

3.5. Effect of TT on Cofactors and Vitamin Metabolism

The HFD+TT800 group had lower serum concentrations of threonate (ascorbate and aldarate metabolism, Figure 3a), glucuronate (vitamin B6 metabolism, Figure 3b), and biopterin (tetrahydrobiopterin metabolism, Figure 3c) than the HFD group (Figure 3). Furthermore, the HFD+TT800 group had higher concentrations of pantothenate (pantothenate and CoA metabolism, Figure 3d), bilirubin (hemoglobin and porphyrin metabolism, Figure 3e), retinol (vitamin A metabolism, Figure 3f), pyridoxamine (vitamin B6 metabolism, Figure 3g), and pyridoxal (vitamin B6 metabolism, Figure 3h).

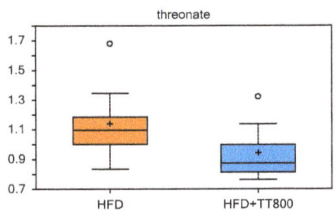

(**a**) Threonate in ascorbate and aldarate metabolism ($p \leq 0.05$)

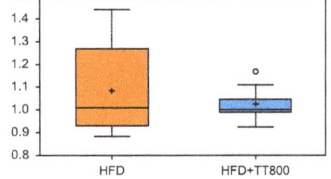

(**b**) Glucuronate in Vitamin B6 metabolism ($0.05 < p < 0.1$)

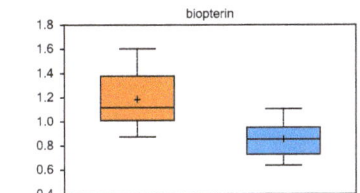

(**c**) Biopterin in tetrahydrobiopterin metabolism ($p \leq 0.05$)

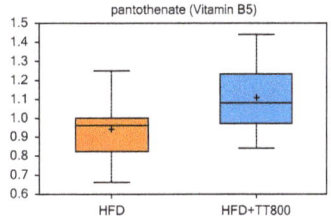

(**d**) Pantothenate (vitamin B5) in pantothenate and CoA metabolism ($0.05 < p < 0.1$)

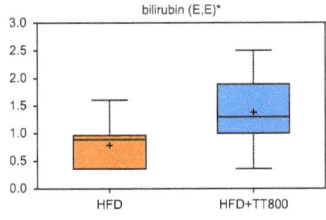

(**e**) Bilirubin (E,E) in hemoglobin and porphyrin metabolism ($p \leq 0.05$)

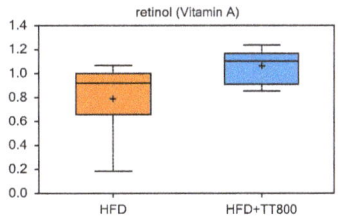

(**f**) Retinol in vitamin A metabolism ($0.05 < p < 0.1$)

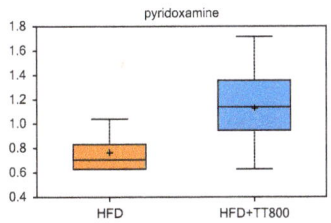

(**g**) Pyridoxamine in vitamin B6 metabolism ($p \leq 0.05$)

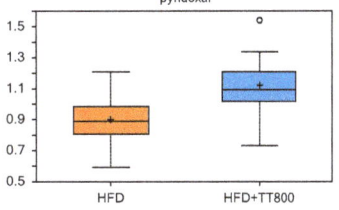

(**h**) Pyridoxal in vitamin B6 metabolism ($p \leq 0.05$)

Figure 3. Effect of TT supplementation on serum cofactor and vitamin metabolites. TT may conserve pantothenate and CoA use for oxidative and biosynthetic reactions in intermediary metabolism, and intermediates of retinoic acid metabolism in mice, in contrast to a HFD that leads to anabolic responses for fat deposition. TT supplementation appears to reduce levels of biopterin for amino acid metabolism in support of neurotransmitter formation. Each dietary group was comprised of $n = 10$ mice.

3.6. Effect of TT on Nucleotide Metabolism

Table 5 shows the HFD+TT800 group had lower levels of intermediates involved in purine metabolism including (i) xanthine/inosine-containing metabolites, such as hypoxanthine, xanthine, xanthosine, 2′-deoxyinosine and allantoin; and (ii) guanine-containing metabolites, such as 7-methylguanine. In addition, the HFD+TT800 group had higher levels of intermediates involved in purine metabolism including (i) adenine-containing metabolites, such as adenosine-3′,5′-cyclic monophosphate, (ii) orotate-containing metabolites, such as dihydroorotate, and (iii) uracil-containing metabolites, such as uracil.

Table 5. Effects of TT supplementation on serum nucleotide metabolites in mice fed HFD compared to the HFD control group.

Sub Pathway	Biochemical Name	HFD+TT800/HFD
Purine metabolism, xanthine/Inosine containing	Hypoxanthine	0.23
	Xanthine	0.41
	Xanthosine	0.53
	2′-Deoxyinosine	0.15
	Allantoin	0.85
Purine metabolism, Adenine containing	Adenosine-3′,5′-cyclic monophosphate (cAMP)	1.55
Purine metabolism, Guanine containing	7-Methylguanine	0.74
Purine Metabolism, Orotate containing	Dihydroorotate	1.55
Pyrimidine Metabolism, Uracil containing	Uridine	1.18

Metabolite values are expressed as the ratio of HFD+TT800/HFD which is the fold change of the treated HFD+TT800 group compared to the HFD control group. A ratio greater than 1 indicates a value larger for the treated group (HFD+TT800) and less than 1 the value for HFD+TT800 group is lower compared to the HFD control group. Green indicates fold reduction and red is for fold increase by TT supplementation with $p \leq 0.05$ that was obtained from the Student's t-test. Yellow indicates fold reduction and pink is for fold increase by TT supplementation with $0.05 < p < 0.1$ that was obtained from the Student's t-test.

3.7. Effect of TT on Xenobiotics Metabolism

Figure 4 illustrates that TT-supplementation decreased the levels of intermediates involved in (i) benzoate metabolism (e.g., 4-hydroxyhippurate, Figure 4a, $p \leq 0.05$; 4-methylcartechol sulfate, Figure 4b, $p \leq 0.05$; and o-cresol sulfate Figure 4c, $0.05 < p < 0.1$); and (ii) food component metabolism (glucoronate, Figure 4d, $p \leq 0.05$). TT supplementation may have reduced the amount of these compounds by changing gut microflora in mice. Annatto seed is a medium to high source of salicylates, consistent with the higher level of salicylates found in sera of mice given TT800 as shown in panel Figure 4e.

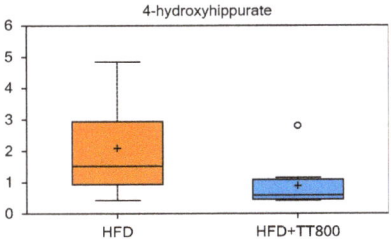
(a) 4-Hydroxyhippurate in benzoate metabolism ($p \leq 0.05$)

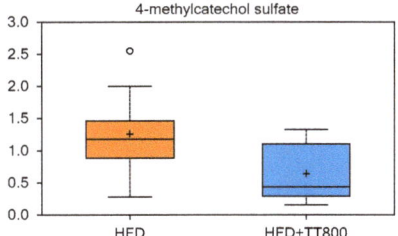
(b) 4-Methylcatechol sulfate in benzoate metabolism ($p \leq 0.05$)

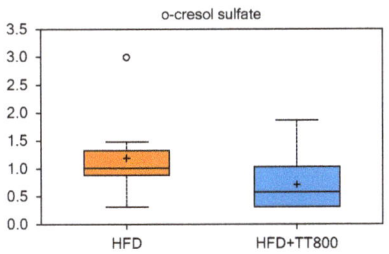
(c) O-cresol sulfate in benzoate metabolism ($0.05 < p < 0.1$)

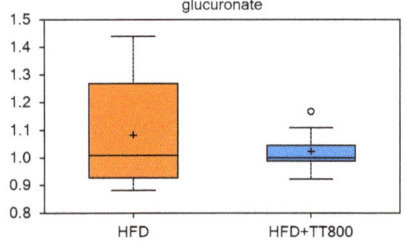
(d) Glucuronate in food component ($p \leq 0.05$)

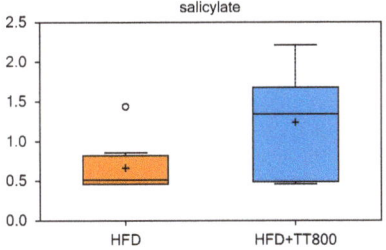
(e) Salicylate in drug metabolism ($p \leq 0.05$)

Figure 4. Effect of TT supplementation on serum xenobiotic metabolites. Supplementation with TT800 in mice fed a HFD may help reduce bacterial products of phenylalanine metabolism, and 4 hyrdoxyhippurate, as well as lower glucuranate. These compounds may be reduced with TT supplementation by changing gut microflora in mice. Each dietary group was comprised of n = 10 mice.

4. Discussion

The present study showed that 14 weeks of annatto-TT (90% δ-TT+10% γ-TT) supplementation significantly increased TT levels and reduced the intermediate metabolites of lipid peroxidation, dicarboxylic fatty acids (such as azelate, sebacate, 1,11-undecanedicarboxylate, dodecanedioate, tetradecanedioate and octadecanedioate) in mice fed a high fat diet. Dicarboxylic fatty acids are produced by fatty acid omega-oxidation, which can serve as a 'rescue pathway' when beta-oxidation is impaired or overwhelmed (e.g., at times of high energy demand) [23]. The decrease in dicarboxylates in the HFD+TT800 group may suggest reduced omega-oxidation in response to TT supplementation, perhaps reflecting a more efficient β-oxidation of fatty acids or an enhanced ability to handle the excess load of fatty acids imposed by HFD. Fang et al. reported TT-enriched palm oil enhanced the interaction between the purified ligand-binding domain of PPARα with the receptor-interacting motif of coactivator PPARγ coactivator-1α in a cell-free in vitro system [24]. We previously reported PPARα mRNA was significantly higher in animals fed with an HFD supplemented with TT400 in the diet, relative to those fed without TT400 supplementation [8]. Thus, in the present study, the observed decrease in intermediate metabolites of dicarboxylic fatty acids in the HFD+TT800 group confirms one of the molecular mechanisms for the anti-oxidation activity of TT. Specifically, in mice given TT compared to the control group, medium chain fatty acids and fatty acid metabolism (acyl glycine) decreased, however, carnitine metabolism and fatty acid acyl carnitine (medium and long-chain fatty acids) increased.

Some oxylipins were changed favorably in mice supplemented with TT, and the ratio values of HFD+TT800/HFD for 13-HODE and 9-HODE, 14 HDoHe/17-HDoHe, and thromboxane B2 were lower, suggesting actions of lower acute pain and inflammation and auto-oxidation of DHA. The amount for 14 HDoHe/17-HDoHe showed a lower ratio which may support lower circulating triglycerides as we previously reported in male mice given TT with a high fat diet compared mice not given TT [8]. Furthermore, the lower value for 12-HETE would suggest a reduced production of growth factor cytokines. The reduced arachidonic acid COX metabolite 12 HHTrE would lower inflammation in obese mice.

Sphingomyelins are a class of phospholipids that are found in animal cell membranes and form lipid microdomains with cholesterol [25]. The unique composition of sphingomyelins allows them to play important roles in both membrane stabilization and lipid signaling [25]. In addition to the role of sphingolipids as structural components of cell membranes, sphingolipids also function as intracellular and extracellular mediators that regulate cellular processes including cell survival, proliferation, apoptosis, differentiation, migration, and immune processes [26]. Emerging evidence suggests that biosynthesis or metabolism of sphingolipids is altered in obesity, diabetes, and cardiovascular diseases [25–27]. Our study demonstrated a substantial accumulation of several sphingomyelin components in the HFD+TT800 group. The increase in the sphingomyelin pool observed in the HFD+TT800 group may correlate with several factors including fatty acid availability, ceramide utilization, membrane turnover, and/or uptake. Evidence suggests that TT supplementation leads to intracellular accumulation of dihydroceramide and sphinganine, two key sphingolipid intermediates in the de novo synthesis of the sphingolipid pathway that contribute to TT-supplemented apoptosis of adipocytes [28]. In the present study, an increase in glycosyl ceramide and sphingomyelin intermediates by TT supplementation could indicate changes in the de novo synthesis of sphingolipids, and a role in the pro-death effect on adipocytes in prevention of obesity [28].

Mice given TT compared to the controls in our study showed higher levels of PC, an abundant phospholipid of mammalian cells and subcellular organelles. There was a higher amount of complex lipid composition supporting phospholipid metabolism (e.g., GPC, GPI), PC (e.g., 1-palmitoyl-2-oleoyl-GPC, 1-2-dilinoleoyl-GPC) and lysophospholipid (e.g., 1-lignoceroyl-GPC, 1-stearoyl-GPE) in the TT-supplemented obese mice compared to the controls. These differences likely suggest that TT could play a supporting role in regulating lipid, lipoprotein, and energy metabolism.

In our current study, TT-supplemented obese mice had significantly lower trimethylamine N-oxide (TMAO) in serum relative to the controls. TMAO has been shown in animal models to up-regulate macrophage receptors associated with atherosclerosis [29]. Elevated serum concentrations of TMAO have been linked to adverse cardiovascular outcomes in humans [29,30] and TMAO has been identified as a cardiovascular disease risk factor and biomarker in humans [31]. TMAO is also a product of phospholipid and carnitine metabolism by the intestinal microbiome. Li et al. reported the serum content of TMAO and inflammatory cytokines (i.e., interleukin-1, interleukin-2, and monocyte chemoattractantprotein-1) were significantly higher in the T2DM rats than those in the control [32]. Authors also reported that the gut microbiota of T2DM rats had decreased abundance of beneficial bacteria, such as *Allobaculum, Bifidobacterium, Eubacterium,* and *Anaerotruncus,* while those of opportunistic pathogens (e.g., *Enterococcus, Corynebacterium, Aerococcus,* and *Facklamia*) were increased, suggesting the role of TMAO in modification of gut microbiome during the development of T2DM [32]. In our previous study [15], we reported that dietary TT supplementation increased Bacteroidetes/Firmicutes ratio and the number of bacteria which belong to Clostridiales order, especially the Oscillospira genus (Firmicutes phylum) was decreased by two-fold in the feces of obese mice. The current finding that TT supplementation favors a beneficial gut microbiome [15] along with decreased serum TMAO in obese mice suggests a potential for TT to improve glucose homeostasis, which is consistent with our previous observation that TT supplementation improved glucose and insulin tolerance in HFD mice [8,9].

Dietary supplementation with TMAO decreased the expression of a number of bile acid transport genes in the liver (Cyp7a1 and Cyp27a1) adversely affecting cholesterol elimination [30] and blocking reverse cholesterol transport, providing another potential link between TMAO and vascular disease. Further, we previously reported that TT supplementation lowers triglyceride accumulation and inflammation in liver of obese mice [8]. Thus, the decreased serum TMAO level in the TT-treated obese mice compared to controls provides a supportive mechanism for the role of TT in promoting metabolically healthy obesity.

Lysophosphatidylcholine (LPC) is an important signaling molecule with diverse biological functions [33]. LPC is involved in inflammation [34] and insulin resistance in obesity [35] and can exert positive effects on glucose metabolism [36]. Barber et al. (2012) has demonstrated that exposing mice to chronic HFD markedly reduced plasma LPC (14:0, 15:0, 20:0, 20:1, 20:5, 16:1, and 18:1) along with an increase in fat mass and the development of glucose intolerance and hyperinsulinemia [37]. Such a reduction in LPC species observed in obese mice was also reported in plasma from obese animals [37] and obese T2DM individuals [38]. Yea et al. (2009) demonstrated that LPC activates adipocyte glucose uptake and lowers blood glucose levels in murine models of diabetes [36]. Our findings that TT increases LPC suggested reduced inflammation.

One of the earliest observed biological activities of TT is the ability to downregulate the mevalonate pathway via suppression of its rate-limiting enzyme, 3-hydroxy-3-methylglutaryl coenzyme A reductase (HMGCR) [38]. Among the TT isomers, delta- and gamma-TTs have been shown to be the most potent in suppressing HMGCR [39]. The TT appears to downregulate HMGCR at the transcriptional level by mimicking the action of its transcription factors or enhance the ubiquitination and degradation of HMGCR at the post-translational level [40]. The reduced serum level of mevalonate in TT-supplemented mice compared to controls is consistent with these previous findings.

The association of obesity, insulin resistance, and chronic oxidative stress/low-grade inflammation has been evident for more than a decade [41]. The pathways for ROS production and oxidative stress are upregulated in a coordinated way in HFD mice, along with hyperglycemia and insulin resistance [42]. Insulin metabolism has been linked to oxidized LDL [42]. For instance, Linna et al. has shown the highest HOMA-IR quartile consistently had the highest concentrations of oxidized-LDL and ratio of oxidized-LDL/HDL-cholesterol [42], suggesting a strong positive association between insulin resistance and damage caused by oxidized lipids in T2DM individuals. Bioactive oxidized linoleic acid metabolites, such as 9- and 13-hydroxyoctadecadienoic acid (9-HODE+13-HODE), have been linked to oxidative stress, inflammation and numerous pathological and physiological states [43]. In the present study, TT supplementation decreased the levels of 9-HODE and 13-HODE in serum of obese mice, indicating TT mitigated the potential of linoleic acid metabolites to oxidized products.

We previously reported TT supplementation improved glucose homeostasis (improved insulin resistance and decreased hyperglycemia) in obese mice via a reduction of inflammation and oxidative stress [8,15]. We showed that compared to the HFD group without TT, TT supplementation to an HFD lowered values of TNF-α, IL-6 and MCP-1 in adipose tissue [8,15]. Fang et al. also demonstrated the tocotrienol-rich fraction of palm oil improved whole body glucose utilization and insulin sensitivity of diabetic Db/Db mice by selectively regulating PPAR target genes [24] In the current study, the HFD +TT800 mice showed a relative decrease in some of the oxidative stress and stress response markers. As shown in Figure 5, the methionine/cysteine circuit is tightly linked to glutathione production to actively manage oxidative stress. Noticeable ($p > 0.1$) decreases in the ratios for oxidized glutathione (0.4056), cysteine-glutathione disulfide (0.7438), methionine sulfoxide (0.974), 5-oxoproline (0.949), and cystine (0.8775) were observed in TT-treated mice in relation to control mice. Reduction in these metabolites is reminiscent of an improved redox environment and might be an indication of lower oxidative insult by TT supplementation. In addition, lower activity of the γ-glutamyl cycle, which is important for recycling and regeneration of GSH, was noted in TT-treated mice, as evidenced by a decline in γ-glutamyl amino acids. Furthermore, compared to the HFD mice, the oxidative stress markers including oxidized lipids (12,13-DiHOME, 9-HODE + 13-HODE) and inflammatory molecule kynurenate were significantly reduced while an antioxidant marker threonate was significantly increased in the HFD +TT800 mice. Thus, the observed decrease in the levels of these oxidative stress markers provides added support for the notion that treatment with TT lowers HFD-induced oxidative stress.

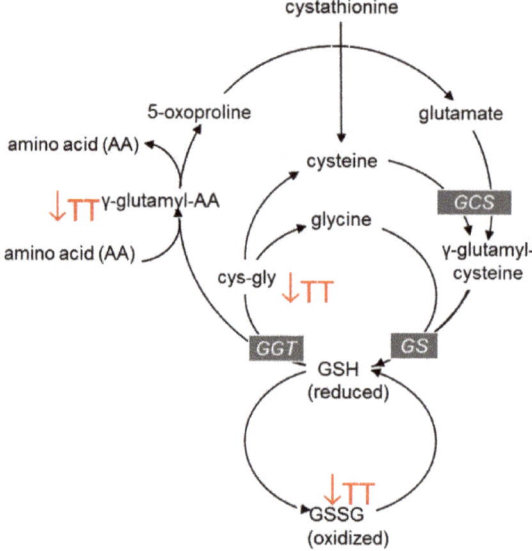

Figure 5. Effects of TT supplementation on the methionine-cysteine cycle and GSH/GSSH redox status. Supplementation of mice fed a HFD with TT alters the amounts of intermediates in amino acid metabolism and oxidized glutathione that reflect a lowered ratio of reduced glutathione/oxidized glutathione (GSH/GSSH), and thus, a lowered oxidative stress. TT, tocotrienol.

Xanthine oxidase (XO) oxidizes hypoxanthine to xanthine and uric acid, producing hydrogen peroxide. A large body of work has demonstrated that enhanced XO activity is considered a damage signal, contributing to a damage-associated molecular pattern [44]. Endothelial xanthine oxidoreductase (XOR) together with NADPH oxidase and nitric oxide (NO) synthase plays a physiological role in inflammatory signaling, the regulation of NO production and vascular function [44]. The role of XOR in adipogenesis is also connected with insulin resistance and obesity, two main features of T2DM [44]. In the present study, consistent with TT-mediated reduction in oxidative stress, we observed a significant decrease in purine breakdown products such as hypoxanthine, xanthine, xanthosine and allantoin in obese mice, suggesting TT reduced XO activity and ROS production and protected against HFD-induced oxidative stress. Collectively, these results point towards TT as a potent antioxidant against obesity-induced oxidative damage.

A noticeable increase in vitamin B metabolites including pyridoxamine and pyridoxal was displayed by mice supplemented with TT. Vitamin B6 is an essential cofactor in various transamination, decarboxylation, glycogen hydrolysis, and synthesis pathways involving carbohydrate, sphingolipid, amino acid, heme, and neurotransmitter metabolism.

Since the gut microbiota is associated with the biosynthesis of B vitamins, the observed fluctuation in vitamin B molecules in the HFD+TT800 animals could be linked to TT-mediated favorable alterations in microbiome composition [15]. A consequential increase in serotonin (a tryptophan-derived neurotransmitter that has roles in mediating behavior, mood, gut movement, growth, and learning) was noted in the TT-supplemented obese mice. Consistent with this finding, we also observed changes in the benzoate pathway intermediates (4-hydroxyhippurate and 4-methylcatechol sulfate), which are derived from microbiome metabolism of aromatic amino acids. Collectively, these changes are reflective of favorable gut microbial influences associated with TT supplementation [15].

5. Conclusions

This global metabolomic profiling study was conducted to gain an understanding of the changes in metabolites associated with TT supplementation in HFD-induced obesity in mice. Overall, the results from the serum profiling demonstrate alterations in biochemical pathways, including those of amino acids, lipid oxidation and peroxidation, oxidative stress, sphingolipids, and xanthine oxidase along with changes in serum metabolites that may be related to the intestinal microbiome. As a path forward, it is important to measure metabolic changes under TT treatment using a complex lipid platform which will shed light on the comprehensive changes in lipid metabolism with TT supplementation. Additionally, research on adipose tissue adipokines and composition of fatty acids in obesity should reveal the role of TT in inflammation and fatty acid metabolism in regard to oxylipins and endocannabinoids. Finally, the level of TT used is well within the safety range of TT [45], suggesting the potential of TT for clinical applications. It is not only the potent antioxidant capacity, but also the safety and efficacy of TT that enhances their clinical potential [45].

Author Contributions: Conceptualization, C.-L.S., S.R, and B.A.W.; methodology, C.-L.S., S.R, and B.A.W.; software, S.R.; validation, C.-L.S., S.R, and B.A.W.; writing—original draft preparation, C.-L.S., S.R, and B.A.W.; writing—review and editing, G.K., J.M.D., R.W., H.M., and B.A.W.; supervision, project administration, and funding acquisition, C.-L.S. All authors have read and agreed to the published version of the manuscript.

Funding: This research was funded by American River Nutrition, LLC, Hadley, MA and internal funding from Texas Tech University Health Sciences Center.

Institutional Review Board Statement: Texas Tech University Health Sciences Center IACUC# 15003.

Informed Consent Statement: Not applicable.

Data Availability Statement: Available upon request.

Acknowledgments: We thank Michael M. Tomison for animal care. We thank American River Nutrition, LLC, Hadley, MA for supplying the annatto-extracted tocotrienols and funding this animal study. J.M.D. and G.K. were supported in part by The Jasper L. and Jack Denton Wilson Foundation. We also thank Texas Tech University Health Sciences Center for providing funds for metabolomics analysis.

Conflicts of Interest: The authors declare that they have no competing interests. The contents of this manuscript are solely the responsibility of the authors and do not necessarily represent the official views of American River Nutrition. The American River Nutrition declares that they have no competing interests in the design of the study and collection, analysis, and interpretation of data and in writing the manuscript.

References

1. Kalupahana, N.S.; Moustaid-Moussa, N.; Claycombe, K.J. Immunity as a link between obesity and insulin resistance. *Mol. Asp. Med.* **2012**, *33*, 26–34. [CrossRef]
2. Malagón, M.M.; Díaz-Ruiz, A.; Guzmán-Ruiz, R.; Jiménez-Gómez, Y.; Moreno, N.R.; García-Navarro, S.; Vázquez-Martínez, R.; Peinado, J.R. Adipobiology for novel therapeutic approaches in metabolic syndrome. *Curr. Vasc. Pharmacol.* **2014**, *11*, 954–967. [CrossRef]

3. Xu, H.; Barnes, G.T.; Yang, Q.; Tan, G.; Yang, D.; Chou, C.J.; Sole, J.; Nichols, A.; Ross, J.S.; Tartaglia, L.A.; et al. Chronic inflammation in fat plays a crucial role in the development of obesity-related insulin resistance. *J. Clin. Investig.* **2003**, *112*, 1821–18930. [CrossRef]
4. Klop, B.; Elte, J.W.F.; Cabezas, M.C. Dyslipidemia in Obesity: Mechanisms and Potential Targets. *Nutrition* **2013**, *5*, 1218–1240. [CrossRef]
5. Rochette, L.; Zeller, M.; Cottin, Y.; Vergely, C. Diabetes, oxidative stress and therapeutic strategies. *Biochim. Biophys. Acta* **2014**, *1840*, 2709–2729. [CrossRef]
6. Henriksen, E.J. Dysregulation of glycogen synthase kinase-3 in skeletal muscle and the etiology of insulin resistance and type 2 diabetes. *Curr. Diabetes Rev.* **2010**, *6*, 285–293. [CrossRef]
7. Pazdro, R.; Burgess, J.R. The role of vitamin E and oxidative stress in diabetes complications. *Mech. Ageing Dev.* **2010**, *131*, 276–286. [CrossRef] [PubMed]
8. Allen, L.; Ramalingam, L.; Menikdiwela, K.; Scoggin, S.; Shen, C.; Tomison, M.D.; Kaur, G.; Dufour, J.M.; Chung, E.; Kalupahana, N.S.; et al. Effects of delta-tocotrienol on obesity-related adipocyte hypertrophy, inflammation and hepatic steatosis in high-fat-fed mice. *J. Nutr. Biochem.* **2017**, *48*, 128–137. [CrossRef]
9. Shen, C.L.; Kaur, G.; Wanders, D.; Sharma, S.; Tomison, M.D.; Ramalingam, L.; Chung, E.; Moustaid-Moussa, N.; Mo, H.; Dufour, J.M. Annatto-extracted tocotrienols improve glucose homeostasis and bone properties in high-fat diet-induced type 2 diabetic mice by decreasing the inflammatory response. *Sci. Rep.* **2018**, *8*, 11377. [CrossRef] [PubMed]
10. Yoshida, Y.; Niki, E.; Noguchi, N. Comparative study on the action of tocopherols and tocotrienols as antioxidant: Chemical and physical effects. *Chem. Phys. Lipids* **2003**, *123*, 63–75. [CrossRef]
11. Viola, V.; Pilolli, F.; Piroddi, M.; Pierpaoli, E.; Orlando, F.; Provinciali, M.; Betti, M.; Mazzini, F.; Galli, F. Why tocotrienols work better: Insights into the in vitro anti-cancer mechanism of vitamin E. *Genes Nutr.* **2011**, *7*, 29–41. [CrossRef] [PubMed]
12. Aggarwal, B.B.; Sundaram, C.; Prasad, S.; Kannappan, R. Tocotrienols, the vitamin E of the 21st century: Its potential against cancer and other chronic diseases. *Biochem. Pharmacol.* **2010**, *80*, 1613–1631. [CrossRef] [PubMed]
13. Ahsan, H.; Ahad, A.; Iqbal, J.; Siddiqui, A.W. Pharmacological potential of tocotrienols: A review. *Nutr. Metab.* **2014**, *11*, 52. [CrossRef] [PubMed]
14. Zhao, L.; Fang, X.; Marshall, M.R.; Chung, S. Regulation of Obesity and Metabolic Complications by Gamma and Delta Tocotrienols. *Molecules* **2016**, *21*, 344. [CrossRef]
15. Chung, E.; Elmassry, M.M.; Kottapalli, P.; Kottapalli, K.R.; Kaur, G.; Dufour, J.M.; Wright, K.; Ramalingam, L.; Moustaid-Moussa, N.; Wang, R.; et al. Metabolic benefits of annatto-extracted tocotrienol on glucose homeostasis, inflammation, and gut microbiome. *Nutr. Res.* **2020**, *77*, 97–107. [CrossRef]
16. Prasad, K. Tocotrienols and Cardiovascular Health. *Curr. Pharm. Des.* **2011**, *17*, 2147–2154. [CrossRef]
17. Zhao, L.; Kang, I.; Fang, X.; Wang, W.; Lee, M.A.; Hollins, R.R.; Marshall, M.R.; Chung, S. Gamma-tocotrienol attenuates high-fat diet-induced obesity and insulin resistance by inhibiting adipose inflammation and M1 macrophage recruitment. *Int. J. Obes.* **2015**, *39*, 438–446. [CrossRef]
18. Malavolta, M.; Pierpaoli, E.; Giacconi, R.; Basso, A.; Cardelli, M.; Piacenza, F.; Provinciali, M. Anti-inflammatory Activity of Tocotrienols in Age-related Pathologies: A SASPected Involvement of Cellular Senescence. *Biol. Proced. Online* **2018**, *20*, 22. [CrossRef]
19. Hatano, T.; Saiki, S.; Okuzumi, A.; Mohney, R.P.; Hattori, N. Identification of novel biomarkers for Parkinson's disease by metabolomic technologies. *J. Neurol. Neurosurg. Psychiatry* **2016**, *87*, 295–301. [CrossRef]
20. Evans, A.M.; Bridgewater, B.R.; Liu, Q.; Mitchell, M.W.; Robinson, R.J.; Dai, H.; Stewart, S.J.; DeHaven, C.D.; Miller, L.A.D. High resolution mass spectrometry improves data quantity and quality as compared to unit mass resolution mass spectrometry in high-throughput profiling metabolomics. *Metabolomics* **2014**, *4*, 132.
21. Dehaven, C.D.; Evans, A.M.; Dai, H.; Lawton, K.A. Organization of GC/MS and LC/MS metabolomics data into chemical libraries. *J. Cheminform.* **2010**, *2*, 9. [CrossRef]
22. Breiman, L. Random Forests. *Mach. Learn.* **2001**, *45*, 5–32. [CrossRef]
23. Ribel-Madsen, A.; Hellgren, L.I.; Brøns, C.; Ribel-Madsen, R.; Newgard, C.B.; Vaag, A.A. Plasma amino acid levels are elevated in young, healthy low birth weight men exposed to short-term high-fat overfeeding. *Physiol. Rep.* **2016**, *4*, e13044. [CrossRef]
24. Fang, F.; Kang, Z.; Wong, C. Vitamin E tocotrienols improve insulin sensitivity through activating peroxisome proliferator-activated receptors. *Mol. Nutr. Food Res.* **2010**, *54*, 345–352. [CrossRef]
25. Mitsutake, S.; Igarashi, Y. Sphingolipids in Lipid Microdomains and Obesity. *Vitam. Horm.* **2013**, *91*, 271–284.
26. Boini, K.M.; Xia, M.; Koka, S.; Gehr, T.W.B.; Li, P.-L. Sphingolipids in obesity and related complications. *Front. Biosci.* **2017**, *22*, 96–116.
27. Mitsutake, S.; Zama, K.; Yokota, H.; Yoshida, T.; Tanaka, M.; Mitsui, M.; Ikawa, M.; Okabe, M.; Tanaka, Y.; Yamashita, T.; et al. Dynamic modification of sphingomyelin in lipid microdomains controls development of obesity, fatty liver, and type 2 diabetes. *J. Biol. Chem.* **2011**, *286*, 28544–28555. [CrossRef]
28. Zhao, L.; Ha, J.-H.; Okla, M.; Chung, S. Activation of autophagy and AMPK by gamma-tocotrienol suppresses the adipogenesis in human adipose derived stem cells. *Mol. Nutr. Food Res.* **2013**, *58*, 569–579. [CrossRef] [PubMed]
29. Wang, Z.; Klipfell, E.; Bennett, B.J.; Koeth, A.R.; Levison, B.S.; Dugar, B.; Feldstein, A.E.; Britt, E.B.; Fu, X.; Chung, Y.-M.; et al. Gut flora metabolism of phosphatidylcholine promotes cardiovascular disease. *Nat. Cell Biol.* **2011**, *472*, 57–63. [CrossRef] [PubMed]

30. Koeth, R.A.; Wang, Z.; Levison, B.S.; Buffa, J.A.; Org, E.; Sheehy, B.T.; Britt, E.B.; Fu, X.; Wu, Y.; Li, L.; et al. Intestinal microbiota metabolism of l-carnitine, a nutrient in red meat, promotes atherosclerosis. *Nat. Med.* **2013**, *19*, 576–585. [CrossRef]
31. Bordoni, L.; Samulak, J.J.; Sawicka, A.K.; Pelikant-Malecka, I.; Radulska, A.; Lewicki, L.; Kalinowski, L.; Gabbianelli, R.; Olek, R.A. Trimethylamine N-oxide and the reverse cholesterol transport in cardiovascular disease: A cross-sectional study. *Sci. Rep.* **2020**, *10*, 18675. [CrossRef] [PubMed]
32. Li, H.; Qi, T.; Huang, Z.-S.; Ying, Y.; Zhang, Y.; Wang, B.; Ye, L.; Zhang, B.; Chen, D.-L.; Chen, J. Relationship between gut microbiota and type 2 diabetic erectile dysfunction in Sprague-Dawley rats. *Acta Acad. Med. Wuhan* **2017**, *37*, 523–530. [CrossRef]
33. Xu, Y. Sphingosylphosphorylcholine and lysophosphatidylcholine: G protein-coupled receptors and receptor-mediated signal transduction. *Biochim. Biophys. Acta* **2002**, *1582*, 81–88. [CrossRef]
34. Xing, F.; Liu, J.; Mo, Y.; Liu, Z.; Qin, Q.; Wang, J.; Fan, Z.; Long, Y.; Liu, N.; Zhao, K.; et al. Lysophosphatidylcholine up-regulates human endothelial nitric oxide synthase gene transactivity by c-Jun N-terminal kinase signalling pathway. *J. Cell. Mol. Med.* **2009**, *13*, 1136–1148. [CrossRef] [PubMed]
35. Han, M.S.; Lim, Y.-M.; Quan, W.; Kim, J.R.; Chung, K.W.; Kang, M.; Kim, S.; Park, S.Y.; Han, J.-S.; Park, S.-Y.; et al. Lysophosphatidylcholine as an effector of fatty acid-induced insulin resistance. *J. Lipid Res.* **2011**, *52*, 1234–1246. [CrossRef] [PubMed]
36. Yea, K.; Kim, J.; Yoon, J.H.; Kwon, T.; Kim, J.H.; Lee, B.D.; Lee, H.; Lee, S.J.; Kim, J.; Lee, T.G.; et al. Lysophosphatidylcholine activates adipocyte glucose uptake and lowers blood glucose levels in murine models of diabetes. *J. Biol. Chem.* **2009**, *284*, 33833–33840. [CrossRef]
37. Barber, M.N.; Risis, S.; Yang, C.; Meikle, P.J.; Staples, M.; Febbraio, M.A.; Bruce, C.R. Plasma Lysophosphatidylcholine Levels Are Reduced in Obesity and Type 2 Diabetes. *PLoS ONE* **2012**, *7*, e41456. [CrossRef]
38. Pearce, B.C.; Parker, R.A.; Deason, M.E.; Qureshi, A.A.; Wright, J.J.K. Hypocholesterolemic activity of synthetic and natural tocotrienols. *J. Med. Chem.* **1992**, *35*, 3595–3606. [CrossRef]
39. Mo, H.; Jeter, R.; Bachmann, A.; Yount, S.T.; Shen, C.-L.; Yeganehjoo, H. The Potential of Isoprenoids in Adjuvant Cancer Therapy to Reduce Adverse Effects of Statins. *Front. Pharmacol.* **2019**, *9*, 1515. [CrossRef]
40. Song, B.L.; DeBose-Boyd, R.A. Insig-dependent ubiquitination and degradation of 3-hydroxy-3-methylglutaryl coenzyme a reductase stimulated by delta- and gamma-tocotrienols. *J. Biol. Chem.* **2006**, *281*, 25054–25061. [CrossRef]
41. Zeyda, M.; Stulnig, T.M. Obesity, Inflammation, and Insulin Resistance—A Mini-Review. *Gerontology* **2009**, *55*, 379–386. [CrossRef]
42. Linna, M.S.; Ahotupa, M.; Kukkonen-Harjula, K.; Fogelholm, M.; Vasankari, T.J. Co-existence of insulin resistance and high concentrations of circulating oxidized LDL lipids. *Ann. Med.* **2015**, *47*, 394–398. [CrossRef]
43. Nieman, D.C.; Shanely, R.A.; Luo, B.; Meaney, M.P.; Dew, D.A.; Pappan, K.L. Metabolomics approach to assessing plasma 13- and 9-hydroxy-octadecadienoic acid and linoleic acid metabolite responses to 75-km cycling. *Am. J. Physiol. Integr. Comp. Physiol.* **2014**, *307*, R68–R74. [CrossRef]
44. Battelli, M.G.; Polito, L.; Bolognesi, A. Xanthine oxidoreductase in atherosclerosis pathogenesis: Not only oxidative stress. *Atherosclerosis* **2014**, *237*, 562–567. [CrossRef]
45. Ramanathan, N.; Tan, E.; Loh, L.J.; Soh, B.S.; Yap, W.N. Tocotrienol is a cardioprotective agent against ageing-associated cardiovascular disease and its associated morbidities. *Nutr. Metab.* **2018**, *15*, 6. [CrossRef]

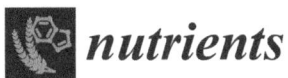

Article

Diet–Cognition Associations Differ in Mild Cognitive Impairment Subtypes

Qiumin Huang, Xiaofang Jia, Jiguo Zhang, Feifei Huang, Huijun Wang, Bing Zhang, Liusen Wang, Hongru Jiang and Zhihong Wang *

National Institute for Nutrition and Health, Chinese Center for Disease Control and Prevention, 29 Nanwei Road, Beijing 100050, China; qmhuangx@163.com (Q.H.); jiaxf@ninh.chinacdc.cn (X.J.); zhangjg@ninh.chinacdc.cn (J.Z.); fayekobe@163.com (F.H.); wanghj@ninh.chinacdc.cn (H.W.); zzhangb327@aliyun.com (B.Z.); wangls@ninh.chinacdc.cn (L.W.); jianghr@ninh.chinacdc.cn (H.J.)
* Correspondence: wangzh@ninh.chinacdc.cn; Tel.: +86-10-6623-7076

Citation: Huang, Q.; Jia, X.; Zhang, J.; Huang, F.; Wang, H.; Zhang, B.; Wang, L.; Jiang, H.; Wang, Z. Diet–Cognition Associations Differ in Mild Cognitive Impairment Subtypes. *Nutrients* **2021**, *13*, 1341. https://doi.org/10.3390/nu13041341

Academic Editors: Emiliana Giacomello and Luana Toniolo

Received: 22 March 2021
Accepted: 16 April 2021
Published: 17 April 2021

Publisher's Note: MDPI stays neutral with regard to jurisdictional claims in published maps and institutional affiliations.

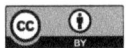

Copyright: © 2021 by the authors. Licensee MDPI, Basel, Switzerland. This article is an open access article distributed under the terms and conditions of the Creative Commons Attribution (CC BY) license (https://creativecommons.org/licenses/by/4.0/).

Abstract: Cognitive function is not generally associated with diet, and there is debate over that association. Moreover, little is known about such associations with the specific cognitive domains and subtypes of mild cognitive impairment (MCI). We analyzed data of 4309 Chinese adults aged 55 and over from the Community-based Cohort Study on Nervous System Diseases from 2018–2019. Dietary habits were assessed at inclusion using a validated semi-quantitative food frequency questionnaire. Cognitive function of the participants was measured by using the Montreal Cognitive Assessment. Analyses were performed using multiple logistic regression and quantile regression with adjustment for socio-demographic, lifestyle, and health-related factors. Compared with normal cognition participants, those with a worse cognition state were characterized as being an older age and lower economic level. After adjustment for potential factors, participants with higher consumption of rice, legumes, fresh vegetables, fresh fruit, pork, poultry, fish, and nuts tended to have higher scores of global cognitive function and domains, and to have lower odds of MCI, while those with higher consumption levels of wheat and eggs had worse cognition, compared with the corresponding bottom consumption level of each food. Participants with a medium consumption level of beef or mutton had 57% (OR: 1.57, 95%CI: 1.07–2.32) higher odds of aMCI-SD, whereas they had 50% (OR: 0.50, 95%CI: 0.34–0.73) lower odds of naMCI-MD. Similarly, the highest consumption level of dairy was positively associated with the odds of aMCI-SD (OR:1.51, 95%CI:1.00–2.29), but inversely linked to the odds of naMCI-SD (OR: 0.60, 95%CI: 0.38–0.93) and naMCI-MD (OR: 0.49, 95%CI: 0.29–0.82). Most diet global cognitive benefits were observed to be associated with the preexisting higher consumption of rice, legumes, fresh vegetables, fresh fruit, meat, and nuts. In addition, the heterogeneity of associations between the consumption of certain foods and MCI subtypes was observed among Chinese adults aged over 55 years. These cross-sectional observations require validation in prospective studies.

Keywords: diet; food consumption; cognition; cognitive domains; MCI subtypes; China

1. Introduction

Age-related diseases have gradually imposed a heavy burden on public health worldwide, of which dementia is a primary concern, particularly Alzheimer's disease (AD), with increases in the proportion of the aging population in both developed and developing countries [1]. In 2020, an estimated 5.8 million Americans age 65 and older were living with AD, and 9.8 million of the Chinese population aged 60 years or older are reported to have AD [2]. Mild cognitive impairment (MCI), an intermediate state between normal cognitive aging and AD, is a known early manifestation of AD and the annual conversion rate from MCI to AD may be 8.1% in a community setting [3], characterized as amnestic or non-amnestic deficit, therefore providing valuable information about the population at risk for developing AD [4]. To date, no effective cure is available to delay the progression of

AD [5], while nutrition plays an important role in the aging process of the brain [6]. Hence, it is critical to explore the evidence on the association between dietary factors and MCI risk in the elderly population to shift focus towards prevention methods of this pre-dementia phase of AD.

The links between diets and cognition have been of public interest. Special attention has been devoted to fresh vegetables and fruit because they are a good source of antioxidant nutrients, such as vitamin C, vitamin E, and carotenoids, as well as the consumption of fish and nuts due to their richness in unsaturated fatty acids that were proved to have anti-inflammatory benefits [7,8]. The effect of the consumption of these vegetables and fruits on cognition function have been summarized in a systematic review of nine cohort studies, indicating that high consumption of vegetables was associated with slower rates of cognitive decline in older age, but not fruit consumption [9]. Yet, there are abundant studies on analytically combined fruit and vegetable consumption showing that fruit and vegetable intakes [10–12] and, in addition, berry intake [13], have been associated with better cognitive outcomes. Moreover, intervention studies have also shown positive findings in relation to fruit and cognition. For example, in studies in which grape, blueberry, orange, or cherry juice was consumed daily by participants for a period of 8–16 weeks, positive findings in respect to cognition were reported [14]. The increased consumption of fish or nuts was observed to reduce the risk of MCI [7,15,16], benefiting cognitive abilities. Few studies have examined the effect of staple foods [17] or meat [18] that are generally considered to have negative effects on health because of their high contents of carbohydrate or saturated fat. Most previous studies, however, tended to focus on the outcome of MCI, without data specifically on subtypes of MCI, including single domain/multidomain amnestic and non-amnestic subtypes [19], which feature as deficits of distinct cognitive domains related to unequal brain function and have varied prevalence. Moreover, some Chinese studies suggested the above foods may have a beneficial effect on cognitive abilities [20–22], but were mainly based on a limited number of respondents recruited in a localized region and there were inconsistent results [21,23]. Therefore, the present study aims to examine the association of diet, covering various foods, with the odds of MCI and its subtypes using a sample of Chinese people aged 55 years and older from the Community-based Cohort Study on Nervous System Diseases (CCSNSD), as well as with a focus on various cognitive domains.

2. Materials and Methods

2.1. Study Population

Data in the present study were derived from the baseline of the CCSNSD, an ongoing and longitudinal study established from 2018–2019 by the National Institute for Nutrition and Health, Chinese Center for Disease Control and Prevention, which focused on the potential factors associated with risks of three nervous diseases, including epilepsy for subjects aged >1 year, and AD and Parkinson's disease for the population aged ≥55 years old. Participants without such diseases were enrolled using a multistage stratified random sampling approach in Hebei, Zhejiang, Shaanxi, and Hunan provinces, respectively. Two cities and two counties were randomly selected in each province. Urban and suburban neighborhoods within the cities and townships and villages within the counties were selected randomly. In each community, all members meeting the inclusion and exclusion criteria of any of three nervous diseases in a randomly selected household were interviewed. The protocol of this study was reviewed and approved by the Institutional Review Board of the National Institute for Nutrition and Health (No. 2017020, 6 November 2017). Additionally, written informed consent was obtained for each participant before the survey.

The present study targeted subjects recruited in the cohort of AD. The samples eligible for inclusion were (1) 55 years old and older, (2) resident population living in the sampled community, (3) absence of clinically diagnosed AD, and (4) free of comorbid conditions that could affect assessment, such as congenital or acquired mental retardation, MCI, and visual/hearing abnormalities, even with correction. Subjects with completed data of sociodemographic characteristics, disease history, cognitive examination, food frequency questionnaire (FFQ), psychological evaluation, and survey of basic abilities of daily living were selected to participate in the present study. We excluded subjects because of their inability to perform basic activities of daily living involving eating, dressing, bathing, toileting, grooming, transferring to bed or chair, walking across a room, and urinary or fecal continence. Finally, a total of 4309 participants were involved in the analysis.

2.2. Assessment of Food Consumption

Dietary consumptions were assessed by a validated semi-quantitative FFQ covering 81 food items categorized as 13 major food groups and items in this study: rice, wheat, tubers, legumes, fresh vegetables, fresh fruit, pork, poultry, fish, beef or mutton, eggs, dairy, and nuts (Table S1). Participants were asked about the frequency of habitual consumption of each item during the last 12 months and chose among five categories of frequency (daily, weekly, monthly, annually, or never) and the amount consumed during the previous 12 months. For each item, if the participant was a non-consumer, then his/her consumption was set to zero grams daily or weekly. For consumers, their consumption of each food group or item was calculated by its reported average consumption frequency and quantity. Finally, the consumptions of rice, wheat, tubers, legumes, fresh vegetables, fresh fruit, pork, beef or mutton, dairy, and eggs were converted to daily grams, respectively, which were categorized into four levels by quartiles. The consumptions of fish, poultry, or nuts were grouped into four levels to reflect non-consumers for more than 25% of participants whose consumption of these three foods was zero, and tertiles of weekly consumption among corresponding consumers.

2.3. Assessment of Cognitive Function

The cognitive function of participants was evaluated using the Montreal Cognitive Assessment (MoCA). The MoCA included 52 items, of which scores of 32 items were calculated for the total MoCA scores ranging from 0 to 30 points which were positively associated with global cognitive function [24]. The criteria for MCI were according to Chinese MoCA norms [25]: total MoCA score ≤13 for illiterate individuals, ≤19 for individuals with 1 to 6 years of education, and ≤24 for those with 7 or more years of education.

The memory index score (MIS), executive index score (EIS), visuospatial index score (VIS), language index score (LIS), attention index score (AIS), and orientation index score (OIS) were applied to evaluate the cognitive domain function of memory, execution, visuospatial, language, attention, and orientation, respectively, and calculated based on the MoCA cognitive domain index score [24]. Participants who scored less than 1.5 SD below the age- and education-adjusted mean value in each cognitive domain were considered as being impaired in that cognitive domain [4]. Participants screened as having MCI and characterized by different cognitive domain deficits were categorized into 4 groups [26,27]: amnestic MCI single domain (aMCI-SD): only memory impairment; non-amnestic MCI single domain (naMCI-SD): a deficit in one cognitive domain other than memory; amnestic MCI multiple domains (aMCI-MD): memory impairment plus one other impaired domain; non-amnestic MCI multiple domains (naMCI-MD): deficits in at least 2 domains other than memory.

2.4. Assessment of Covariates

Interviewers with a degree in medicine or public health were required, and received two rounds of training conducted by national experts and provincial professionals, respectively. Then, those who passed a qualification test were appointed to use questionnaires to collect information on sociodemographic and health-related factors, including age, education (illiterate, ≤primary school, and ≥secondary school), resident area (rural, urban), current employment (no, yes), smoking (never, ever/current), alcohol intake (never, ever/current), monthly household income per capita (<1000, 1000–3999, ≥4000 (RMB)), physical activity, sleep duration, medical history, and medication use. Physical activity was assessed from four aspects: occupational, household chore, leisure time, and transportation activities. The intensity of total physical activity was assessed using metabolic equivalent of task (MET) hours per week based on the American College of Sports Medicine Association's recommended standard [28], by tertiles (low, medium, and high), in the analysis. According to the National Sleep Foundation's recommendations of sleep duration [29], the recommendation for the sleep duration of participants aged 55 to 64 years is 7–9 h, and for those aged ≥65 years it is 7–8 h. The individual total energy intake was summed up from all items in the FFQ linked to the China Food Composition Table [30].

Trained health workers measured individual waist circumference midway between the lowest rib and the iliac crest with a tape measure. Central obesity is defined as a waist circumference of ≥90 cm for men and ≥85 cm for women according to the criteria of weight for adults in China [31]. We used the Chinese body mass index (BMI) cutoff of 28 kg per square meter (kg/m^2) to determine obesity [31]. Participants with a history of diet-related chronic diseases were defined as having hospital diagnosis of hypertension, diabetes, stroke, or myocardial infarction by professional doctors or receiving treatment for these diseases.

2.5. Statistical Analysis

Data were expressed as mean (SD) and n (%) for continuous variables and categorical variables, respectively. Differences in the prevalence of MCI and its subtypes of participants by different consumption levels of each food subgroup were analyzed by using a chi-square test. Differences in the distribution of global cognitive function score and cognitive domain subscores by different consumption levels of each food subgroup were examined using a Kruskal–Wallis H test. A series of multiple logistic regression models were conducted to assess the odds ratio (OR) and 95% confidence interval (CI) by levels of dietary consumption of each food item by adjusting for potential confounders, including demographics, socioeconomic status, lifestyle, energy intake, diet-related disease history, obesity, and central obesity. Quantile regression models were used to assess associations of food consumption with global cognitive score and cognitive domain subscores by adjusting for potential confounders.

We conducted all statistical analyses using SAS version 9.4 (SAS Institute, Inc., Cary, NC, USA) and Stata version 12.0 (StataCorp., College Station, TX, USA). All statistical tests were two-tailed and considered significant at $p < 0.05$.

3. Results

3.1. Characteristics of Study Population

Among the 4309 participants included in the study, the mean age was 68.4 years (range 55 to 86), of which 80.1% were 55~74 years old; 54.6% were women, 49.4% were from urban areas, 76.4% had a monthly household income per capita of more than RMB 1000, 85.8% of the subjects had a primary or above education level, and less than 40% of participants had histories of diet-related chronic diseases (Table S2). Overall, participants tended to consume rice, wheat, fresh vegetables, and pork, and close to 25% of them reported to not consume beef or mutton, poultry, fish, eggs, dairy, or nuts (Table 1).

Table 1. Food consumption levels of Chinese adults aged 55 years and above in four provinces in CCSNSD 2018–2019 [a].

Foods	Q1/T0	Q2/T1	Q3/T2	Q4/T3
Rice (g/day)	10.0 (3.3, 21.4)	74.6 (45.7, 100.0)	180.0 (150.0, 200.0)	300.0 (300.0, 450.0)
Wheat (g/day)	7.1 (0.0, 14.3)	50.0 (40.0, 60.0)	100.0 (100.0, 120.0)	300.0 (200.0, 360.0)
Tubers (g/day)	0.0 (0.0, 3.9)	13.1 (9.3, 15.0)	28.6 (24.8, 35.0)	67.1 (51.4, 100.0)
Legumes (g/day)	3.3 (0.0, 7.1)	20.0 (14.3, 25.4)	44.2 (37.1, 57.1)	113.1 (85.7, 158.9)
Fresh vegetables (g/day)	47.4 (30.0, 63.6)	117.0 (98.4, 140.0)	228.0 (195.6, 259.9)	408.2 (342.5, 530.2)
Fresh fruit (g/day)	6.7 (0.0, 11.4)	27.1 (21.5, 33.2)	57.5 (48.7, 70.8)	144.3 (107.1, 205.7)
Pork (g/day)	2.7 (0.0, 5.0)	14.3 (11.5, 17.9)	32.9 (28.6, 42.9)	100.0 (71.4, 161.0)
Beef or mutton (g/day)	0.0 (0.0, 0.0)	0.5 (0.3, 0.7)	2.5 (1.6, 3.3)	10.0 (8.0, 16.7)
Poultry (g/week)	0.0 (0.0, 0.0)	18.4 (11.7, 23.3)	50.0 (46.7, 70.0)	150.0 (100.0, 220.0)
Fish (g/week)	0.0 (0.0, 0.0)	23.3 (11.7, 28.0)	80.0 (51.5, 100.0)	300.0 (200.0, 432.0)
Eggs (g/day)	6.3 (0.0, 8.7)	20.0 (15.4, 21.7)	42.9 (32.0, 50.0)	60.5 (60.0, 81.8)
Dairy (g/day)	0.0 (0.0, 0.0)	21.4 (8.6, 31.2)	80.0 (57.5, 100.0)	206.3 (163.8, 257.1)
Nuts (g/week)	0.0 (0.0, 0.0)	5.8 (2.9, 9.6)	23.3 (18.7, 42.0)	140.0 (93.3, 210.0)

[a]: expressed as median (P25, p75). Q1–Q4 are consumption levels of foods (except dairy and nuts) grouped by quartile consumption; T0 = non-consumer group for dairy and nuts, T1–T3 are consumption levels of dairy and nuts grouped by the tertile consumption of consumers.

3.2. Cognitive Function by Demographics and Health-Related Factors

Six hundred and five participants were found to have MCI, resulting in a prevalence of 42.6%. The prevalence of each subtype of MCI was less than 10%, of which the highest one was 8.2%, observed in the group with aMCI-MD. Compared to normal cognition participants, those with MCI or its subtypes tended to be older, have a lower monthly income, live in a rural area, and have other health-related problems (Table S2).

The average score of global cognitive function among participants was 21.53, and each cognitive domain score was more than half of the total score of the corresponding subdomain. The scores of global cognitive function and cognitive domains were strongly significantly different by age group, education level, residential area, monthly income, and health-related factors. Generally, the older population, women, and those with a lower education level and a worse economic or health state had lower scores of global cognitive function and cognitive domains, compared to those of their counterparts (Table S3).

3.3. Association of Food Consumptions with MCI and Its Subtypes

The prevalence of MCI and its subtypes in the bottom quartile consumption level of rice was significantly higher than that of other rice consumption levels, while among all wheat consumption levels, the highest prevalence of MCI, naMCI-SD, aMCI-MD, and naMCI-MD was observed in its top quartile consumption level. The prevalence of MCI in the highest consumption level of legumes, fresh vegetables, pork, poultry, beef of mutton, fish, or nuts was obviously lower as compared with that of other consumption levels of the corresponding food. Moreover, participants with one of the MCI subtypes tended to cluster in the lower consumption levels of fresh vegetables and fish, and those with aMCI-MD and naMCI-MD consumed less of legumes, pork, and nuts (Table 2).

Table 2. Prevalence of MCI and its subtypes of participants according to consumption levels of food subgroups [a].

Foods	MCI		p Value	MCI Subtypes				p Value
	Yes	No		aMCI-SD	naMCI-SD	aMCI-MD	naMCI-MD	
Rice			<0.001					0.005
Q1	586 (51.0)	564 (49.0)		73 (6.3)	90 (7.8)	127 (11.0)	91 (7.9)	
Q2	504 (44.8)	620 (55.2)		53 (4.7)	76 (6.8)	75 (6.7)	54 (4.8)	
Q3	374 (36.3)	657 (63.7)		37 (3.6)	65 (6.3)	61 (5.9)	75 (7.3)	
Q4	370 (36.9)	634 (63.1)		42 (4.2)	66 (6.6)	92 (9.2)	39 (3.9)	

Table 2. Cont.

Foods	MCI		p Value	MCI Subtypes				p Value
	Yes	No		aMCI-SD	naMCI-SD	aMCI-MD	naMCI-MD	
Wheat			<0.001					0.045
Q1	330 (31.6)	713 (68.4)		32 (3.1)	55 (5.3)	78 (7.5)	59 (5.7)	
Q2	479 (44.4)	600 (55.6)		47 (4.4)	72 (6.7)	75 (7.0)	49 (4.5)	
Q3	495 (44.9)	607 (55.1)		72 (6.5)	68 (6.2)	85 (7.7)	64 (5.8)	
Q4	530 (48.8)	555 (51.2)		54 (5.0)	102 (9.4)	117 (10.8)	87 (8.0)	
Tubers			0.698					<0.001
Q1	444 (42.0)	613 (58.0)		33 (3.1)	74 (7.0)	95 (9.0)	101 (9.6)	
Q2	455 (41.6)	638 (58.4)		60 (5.5)	76 (7.0)	93 (8.5)	54 (4.9)	
Q3	473 (44.0)	602 (56.0)		54 (5.0)	72 (6.7)	87 (8.1)	52 (4.8)	
Q4	462 (42.6)	622 (57.4)		58 (5.4)	75 (6.9)	80 (7.4)	52 (4.8)	
Legumes			<0.001					<0.001
Q1	533 (50.1)	531 (49.9)		47 (4.4)	86 (8.1)	149 (14.0)	105 (9.9)	
Q2	468 (42.8)	625 (57.2)		63 (5.8)	78 (7.1)	104 (9.5)	63 (5.8)	
Q3	438 (40.7)	637 (59.3)		41 (3.8)	74 (6.9)	59 (5.5)	55 (5.1)	
Q4	395 (36.7)	682 (63.3)		54 (5.0)	59 (5.5)	43 (4.0)	36 (3.3)	
Fresh vegetables			<0.001					0.007
Q1	504 (46.8)	573 (53.2)		68 (6.3)	82 (7.6)	121 (11.2)	75 (7.0)	
Q2	513 (47.6)	564 (52.4)		53 (4.9)	73 (6.8)	119 (11.0)	74 (6.9)	
Q3	448 (41.6)	629 (58.4)		46 (4.3)	72 (6.7)	69 (6.4)	69 (6.4)	
Q4	369 (34.2)	709 (65.8)		38 (3.5)	70 (6.5)	46 (4.3)	41 (3.8)	
Fresh fruit			<0.001					0.004
Q1	536 (49.8)	540 (50.2)		45 (4.2)	99 (9.2)	133 (12.4)	96 (8.9)	
Q2	492 (45.8)	582 (54.2)		62 (5.8)	69 (6.4)	95 (8.8)	62 (5.8)	
Q3	384 (35.4)	700 (64.6)		41 (3.8)	59 (5.4)	54 (5.0)	57 (5.3)	
Q4	422 (39.3)	653 (60.7)		57 (5.3)	70 (6.5)	73 (6.8)	44 (4.1)	
Pork			<0.001					0.009
Q1	546 (50.3)	540 (49.7)		76 (7.0)	83 (7.6)	118 (10.9)	69 (6.4)	
Q2	482 (45.1)	586 (54.9)		51 (4.8)	86 (8.1)	75 (7.0)	78 (7.3)	
Q3	404 (37.6)	671 (62.4)		35 (3.3)	59 (5.5)	99 (9.2)	58 (5.4)	
Q4	402 (37.2)	678 (62.8)		43 (4.0)	69 (6.4)	63 (5.8)	54 (5.0)	
Beef or mutton			<0.001					<0.001
Q1	758 (46.5)	872 (53.5)		59 (3.6)	123 (7.5)	173 (10.6)	141 (8.7)	
Q2	243 (46.6)	278 (53.4)		37 (7.1)	29 (5.6)	68 (13.1)	26 (5.0)	
Q3	442 (40.9)	640 (59.1)		72 (6.7)	66 (6.1)	71 (6.6)	44 (4.1)	
Q4	391 (36.3)	685 (63.7)		37 (3.4)	79 (7.3)	43 (4.0)	48 (4.5)	
Poultry			<0.001					0.063
Q1	534 (49.4)	548 (50.6)		53 (4.9)	83 (7.7)	114 (10.5)	85 (7.9)	
Q2	503 (46.9)	570 (53.1)		74 (6.9)	80 (7.5)	114 (10.6)	67 (6.2)	
Q3	420 (40.4)	620 (59.6)		42 (4.0)	79 (7.6)	65 (6.3)	50 (4.8)	
Q4	377 (33.8)	737 (66.2)		36 (3.2)	55 (4.9)	62 (5.6)	57 (5.1)	
Fish			<0.001					<0.001
Q1	522 (48.5)	555 (51.5)		42 (3.9)	100 (9.3)	107 (9.9)	79 (7.3)	
Q2	527 (49.6)	535 (50.4)		78 (7.3)	62 (5.8)	126 (11.9)	52 (4.9)	
Q3	416 (38.7)	658 (61.3)		45 (4.2)	74 (6.9)	67 (6.2)	50 (4.7)	
Q4	369 (33.7)	727 (66.3)		40 (3.6)	61 (5.6)	55 (5.0)	78 (7.1)	
Eggs			0.007					0.018
Q1	415 (38.5)	664 (61.5)		44 (4.1)	56 (5.2)	102 (9.5)	64 (5.9)	
Q2	480 (43.3)	629 (56.7)		48 (4.3)	99 (8.9)	79 (7.1)	58 (5.2)	
Q3	447 (42.7)	599 (57.3)		50 (4.8)	69 (6.6)	76 (7.3)	66 (6.3)	
Q4	492 (45.8)	583 (54.2)		63 (5.9)	73 (6.8)	98 (9.1)	71 (6.6)	
Dairy			0.242					<0.001
T0	1049 (43.2)	1378 (56.8)		99 (4.1)	172 (7.1)	223 (9.2)	187 (7.7)	
T1	289 (44.2)	365 (55.8)		38 (5.8)	54 (8.3)	63 (9.6)	27 (4.1)	
T2	236 (39.2)	366 (60.8)		21 (3.5)	43 (7.1)	31 (5.1)	26 (4.3)	
T3	260 (41.5)	366 (58.5)		47 (7.5)	28 (4.5)	38 (6.1)	19 (3.0)	

Table 2. Cont.

Foods	MCI		p Value	MCI Subtypes				p Value
	Yes	No		aMCI-SD	naMCI-SD	aMCI-MD	naMCI-MD	
Nuts			<0.001					<0.001
T0	874 (46.8)	993 (53.2)		54 (2.9)	151 (8.1)	166 (8.9)	140 (7.5)	
T1	376 (46.2)	438 (53.8)		72 (8.8)	34 (4.2)	96 (11.8)	48 (5.9)	
T2	317 (38.8)	501 (61.2)		44 (5.4)	59 (7.2)	51 (6.2)	45 (5.5)	
T3	267 (33.0)	543 (67.0)		35 (4.3)	53 (6.5)	42 (5.2)	26 (3.2)	

[a]: expressed as the number of subjects for each category (%). Q1–Q4 are consumption levels of foods (except dairy and nuts) grouped by their quartile consumption; T0 = non-consumer group for dairy and nuts, T1–T3 are consumption levels of dairy and nuts grouped by the tertile consumption of consumers. p value < 0.05 was considered to be statistically significant, examined by chi-square test.

Table 3 shows the odds ratio (95% CI) between the consumption level of food items and MCI and its subtypes in Chinese people aged above 55 years old. After adjusting for potential factors, participants in the top quartile level of rice, legumes, fresh vegetables, fresh fruit, pork, beef or mutton, poultry, fish, and nuts had lower ORs of MCI, whereas those with the highest consumption level of wheat and egg had higher ORs of MCI in comparison to their bottom level ($p < 0.05$). In addition, compared to the first quartile of consumption, participants in the second quartile level of beef or mutton, poultry, and fish had 89% (OR = 1.89, 95%CI: 1.18~3.02), 64% (OR = 1.64, 95%CI: 1.10~2.45), and 82% (OR = 1.82, 95%CI: 1.19~2.78) higher odds of aMCI-SD, respectively, while those in higher consumption levels of these foods were inversely associated with ORs of other subtypes of MCI. As compared with non-consumers, dairy or nut consumers had higher odds of aMCI-SD and aMCI-MD and, inversely, those with higher consumption of these foods were associated with decreased odds of naMCI-SD and naMCI-MD.

Table 3. Associations of food consumption with MCI and its subtypes using multiple logistic regression model [a].

Foods	MCI	MCI Subtypes			
		aMCI-SD	naMCI-SD	aMCI-MD	naMCI-MD
Rice					
Q2	0.87 (0.73, 1.05)	0.69 (0.45, 1.06)	0.90 (0.62, 1.29)	0.93 (0.66, 1.31)	0.86 (0.58, 1.27)
Q3	0.65 (0.54, 0.78) [†]	0.47 (0.30, 0.75) [†]	0.69 (0.48, 1.00)	0.70 (0.49, 1.01)	1.05 (0.73, 1.50)
Q4	0.83 (0.68, 1.00) [†]	0.69 (0.45, 1.08)	0.94 (0.65, 1.37)	1.25 (0.90, 1.76)	0.74 (0.48, 1.15)
Wheat					
Q2	1.52 (1.26, 1.83) [†]	1.35 (0.83, 2.19)	1.46 (0.99, 2.15)	1.09 (0.76, 1.57)	0.88 (0.58, 1.34)
Q3	1.43 (1.18, 1.73) [†]	1.84 (1.16, 2.91) [†]	1.15 (0.78, 1.72)	1.25 (0.87, 1.80)	1.08 (0.72, 1.62)
Q4	1.52 (1.25, 1.85) [†]	1.41 (0.86, 2.32)	1.89 (1.29, 2.77) [†]	1.06 (0.75, 1.51)	1.19 (0.79, 1.77)
Tubers					
Q2	0.93 (0.77, 1.12)	1.61 (1.02, 2.55) [†]	0.99 (0.69, 1.41)	0.99 (0.71, 1.38)	0.56 (0.39, 0.81) [†]
Q3	1.02 (0.85, 1.22)	1.42 (0.89, 2.26)	0.96 (0.67, 1.38)	0.98 (0.70, 1.38)	0.53 (0.36, 0.77) [†]
Q4	1.03 (0.85, 1.23)	1.57 (0.99, 2.52)	1.12 (0.78, 1.62)	0.79 (0.56, 1.12)	0.52 (0.36, 0.77) [†]
Legumes					
Q2	0.72 (0.60, 0.86) [†]	0.91 (0.60, 1.38)	0.71 (0.50, 1.01)	0.71 (0.53, 0.96) [†]	0.59 (0.41, 0.84) [†]
Q3	0.68 (0.57, 0.82) [†]	0.63 (0.39, 0.99) [†]	0.71 (0.50, 1.02)	0.49 (0.34, 0.69) [†]	0.61 (0.42, 0.88) [†]
Q4	0.57 (0.48, 0.69) [†]	0.75 (0.48, 1.17)	0.55 (0.38, 0.80) [†]	0.35 (0.24, 0.51) [†]	0.37 (0.25, 0.57) [†]
Fresh vegetables					
Q2	1.03 (0.86, 1.23)	0.72 (0.48, 1.08)	0.94 (0.66, 1.34)	1.06 (0.78, 1.43)	1.13 (0.79, 1.62)
Q3	0.88 (0.73, 1.06)	0.60 (0.39, 0.91) [†]	0.96 (0.67, 1.37)	0.69 (0.49, 0.97) [†]	1.10 (0.76, 1.59)
Q4	0.66 (0.54, 0.80) [†]	0.39 (0.25, 0.62) [†]	0.83 (0.58, 1.20)	0.46 (0.31, 0.67) [†]	0.69 (0.45, 1.06)
Fresh fruit					
Q2	0.93 (0.77, 1.11)	1.58 (1.02, 2.45) [†]	0.72 (0.51, 1.02)	0.89 (0.65, 1.23)	0.73 (0.51, 1.05)
Q3	0.56 (0.47, 0.68) [†]	0.77 (0.48, 1.25)	0.51 (0.35, 0.73) [†]	0.49 (0.34, 0.70) [†]	0.64 (0.44, 0.92) [†]
Q4	0.71 (0.58, 0.85) [†]	1.14 (0.72, 1.81)	0.64 (0.45, 0.92) [†]	0.88 (0.62, 1.24)	0.62 (0.41, 0.93) [†]

Table 3. Cont.

Foods	MCI	MCI Subtypes			
		aMCI-SD	naMCI-SD	aMCI-MD	naMCI-MD
Pork					
Q2	0.83 (0.70, 1.00) †	0.61 (0.41, 0.91) †	1.03 (0.73, 1.45)	0.68 (0.49, 0.96) †	1.16 (0.80, 1.67)
Q3	0.68 (0.56, 0.82) †	0.39 (0.25, 0.61) †	0.73 (0.50, 1.06)	0.93 (0.67, 1.29)	0.92 (0.62, 1.36)
Q4	0.74 (0.61, 0.89) †	0.48 (0.32, 0.74) †	0.93 (0.64, 1.35)	0.68 (0.48, 0.98) †	1.02 (0.68, 1.54)
Beef or mutton					
Q2	0.99 (0.81, 1.23)	1.89 (1.18, 3.02) †	0.79 (0.50, 1.24)	1.18 (0.84, 1.65)	0.56 (0.35, 0.89) †
Q3	0.80 (0.67, 0.94) †	1.57 (1.07, 2.32) †	0.75 (0.53, 1.05)	0.74 (0.54, 1.02)	0.50 (0.34, 0.73) †
Q4	0.74 (0.62, 0.88) †	0.79 (0.50, 1.25)	0.99 (0.71, 1.37)	0.54 (0.37, 0.79) †	0.69 (0.47, 1.00)
Poultry					
Q2	0.94 (0.79, 1.12)	1.64 (1.10, 2.45) †	0.98 (0.69, 1.39)	1.01 (0.74, 1.38)	0.74 (0.51, 1.07)
Q3	0.81 (0.67, 0.97) †	0.82 (0.52, 1.29)	1.05 (0.73, 1.49)	0.85 (0.59, 1.21)	0.75 (0.51, 1.12)
Q4	0.62 (0.52, 0.75) †	0.59 (0.37, 0.94) †	0.61 (0.41, 0.89) †	0.67 (0.47, 0.96) †	0.72 (0.49, 1.06)
Fish					
Q2	1.01 (0.84, 1.21)	1.82 (1.19, 2.78) †	0.68 (0.47, 0.97) †	1.35 (0.99, 1.84)	0.70 (0.47, 1.04)
Q3	0.72 (0.60, 0.87) †	0.91 (0.57, 1.46)	0.74 (0.52, 1.05)	0.79 (0.56, 1.13)	0.72 (0.48, 1.07)
Q4	0.68 (0.56, 0.82) †	0.76 (0.47, 1.24)	0.65 (0.45, 0.94) †	0.60 (0.41, 0.87) †	1.10 (0.76, 1.59)
Eggs					
Q2	1.15 (0.96, 1.38)	1.10 (0.70, 1.70)	1.78 (1.25, 2.56) †	0.93 (0.67, 1.31)	1.00 (0.67, 1.47)
Q3	1.05 (0.88, 1.26)	1.01 (0.65, 1.57)	1.26 (0.86, 1.85)	0.81 (0.57, 1.14)	1.14 (0.78, 1.68)
Q4	1.23 (1.03, 1.48) †	1.48 (0.97, 2.27)	1.57 (1.07, 2.31) †	1.08 (0.78, 1.50)	1.32 (0.90, 1.94)
Dairy					
T1	1.08 (0.89, 1.30)	1.54 (1.01, 2.35) †	1.21 (0.86, 1.72)	1.47 (1.05, 2.05) †	0.69 (0.45, 1.08)
T2	0.82 (0.67, 1.00) †	0.75 (0.45, 1.26)	0.86 (0.59, 1.25)	0.93 (0.60, 1.42)	0.67 (0.42, 1.06)
T3	0.87 (0.72, 1.07)	1.51 (1.00, 2.29) †	0.60 (0.38, 0.93) †	1.09 (0.73, 1.63)	0.49 (0.29, 0.82) †
Nuts					
T1	1.00 (0.84, 1.20)	3.01 (2.03, 4.47) †	0.51 (0.34, 0.77) †	1.63 (1.20, 2.21) †	0.87 (0.60, 1.26)
T2	0.77 (0.64, 0.92)	1.69 (1.09, 2.62) †	0.83 (0.59, 1.17)	0.87 (0.60, 1.24)	0.79 (0.54, 1.16)
T3	0.65 (0.54, 0.78) †	1.40 (0.87, 2.24)	0.77 (0.54, 1.09)	0.80 (0.55, 1.17)	0.48 (0.30, 0.75) †

[a]: expressed as OR (95% CI). Q = quartile, reference = Q1; T = tertile, reference = T0 (non-consumer). Adjusted for age, gender, residential area, education level, current employment, income level, physical activity, smoking, alcohol intake, sleep duration status, energy, disease history, obesity, and central obesity. †: p value < 0.05.

3.4. Association between Food Consumptions and Cognitive Domains

The lowest scores of global cognitive function and cognitive domains were observed in the bottom consumption level of rice, legumes, fresh vegetables, fresh fruit, pork, and fish, and in the top consumption level of wheat, among the four consumption levels of the above foods ($p < 0.001$). Moreover, participants who consumed dairy had higher scores of global cognitive function and indexes of cognitive domains other than memory compared to the non-consumers ($p < 0.001$) (Table 4).

Table 4. Global cognitive function score and cognitive domain subscores of participants according to consumption levels of food subgroups [a].

Foods	Global Cognitive Function	Cognition Domain Scores					
		MIS	EIS	VIS	LIS	AIS	OIS
Rice							
Q1	19.55 ± 6.17	10.00 ± 4.59	7.61 ± 3.34	4.97 ± 1.75	4.36 ± 1.35	12.09 ± 4.31	5.23 ± 1.22
Q2	22.03 ± 5.74	11.19 ± 4.00	9.04 ± 3.13	5.49 ± 1.56	4.59 ± 1.36	13.19 ± 3.95	5.57 ± 0.92
Q3	22.68 ± 6.44	11.80 ± 3.95	9.17 ± 3.45	5.44 ± 1.85	4.65 ± 1.45	13.90 ± 3.85	5.60 ± 0.88
Q4	22.05 ± 6.22	11.40 ± 4.09	9.06 ± 3.24	5.17 ± 1.91	4.40 ± 1.50	13.59 ± 3.69	5.59 ± 0.84

Table 4. Cont.

Foods	Global Cognitive Function	Cognition Domain Scores					
		MIS	EIS	VIS	LIS	AIS	OIS
Wheat							
Q1	22.71 ± 6.63	11.77 ± 4.02	9.28 ± 3.51	5.40 ± 1.90	4.54 ± 1.51	13.67 ± 4.00	5.60 ± 0.87
Q2	21.95 ± 5.76	11.18 ± 3.89	8.92 ± 3.13	5.41 ± 1.70	4.59 ± 1.37	13.38 ± 3.77	5.63 ± 0.81
Q3	21.82 ± 5.92	11.09 ± 4.23	8.88 ± 3.20	5.31 ± 1.74	4.56 ± 1.39	13.39 ± 3.90	5.59 ± 0.92
Q4	19.68 ± 6.31	10.27 ± 4.60	7.71 ± 3.38	4.95 ± 1.74	4.30 ± 1.40	12.22 ± 4.27	5.15 ± 1.24
Tubers							
Q1	21.07 ± 6.74 *	11.07 ± 4.22 *	8.45 ± 3.61 *	5.08 ± 1.93	4.33 ± 1.50	12.74 ± 4.22	5.38 ± 1.08
Q2	21.81 ± 6.28	11.24 ± 4.19	8.85 ± 3.33	5.35 ± 1.76	4.56 ± 1.44	13.35 ± 3.89	5.51 ± 0.97
Q3	21.74 ± 6.10	11.03 ± 4.30	8.79 ± 3.27	5.35 ± 1.72	4.60 ± 1.35	13.28 ± 4.01	5.55 ± 0.95
Q4	21.49 ± 5.88	10.93 ± 4.20	8.68 ± 3.19	5.28 ± 1.69	4.51 ± 1.38	13.25 ± 3.97	5.53 ± 0.97
Legumes							
Q1	19.47 ± 6.68	9.94 ± 4.67	7.74 ± 3.52	4.70 ± 1.95	4.08 ± 1.52	11.95 ± 4.34	5.26 ± 1.19
Q2	21.44 ± 6.36	10.98 ± 4.41	8.64 ± 3.42	5.25 ± 1.73	4.57 ± 1.40	13.16 ± 4.06	5.47 ± 1.02
Q3	22.16 ± 5.88	11.52 ± 3.78	9.01 ± 3.20	5.50 ± 1.64	4.57 ± 1.38	13.44 ± 3.81	5.54 ± 0.91
Q4	23.02 ± 5.50	11.82 ± 3.74	9.39 ± 3.05	5.61 ± 1.64	4.77 ± 1.29	14.08 ± 3.57	5.70 ± 0.76
Fresh vegetables							
Q1	20.37 ± 6.29	10.28 ± 4.62	8.16 ± 3.28	5.05 ± 1.75	4.30 ± 1.48	12.35 ± 4.11	5.39 ± 1.12
Q2	20.61 ± 6.45	10.52 ± 4.39	8.24 ± 3.49	5.14 ± 1.82	4.38 ± 1.43	12.53 ± 4.26	5.41 ± 1.08
Q3	21.91 ± 6.18	11.44 ± 3.94	8.88 ± 3.35	5.31 ± 1.76	4.55 ± 1.40	13.49 ± 3.82	5.48 ± 0.97
Q4	23.23 ± 5.67	12.04 ± 3.67	9.49 ± 3.13	5.55 ± 1.74	4.77 ± 1.32	14.27 ± 3.60	5.69 ± 0.75
Fresh fruit							
Q1	19.62 ± 6.48	10.31 ± 4.56	7.70 ± 3.43	4.78 ± 1.89	4.15 ± 1.54	12.08 ± 4.22	5.25 ± 1.16
Q2	21.02 ± 6.01	10.73 ± 4.18	8.46 ± 3.25	5.11 ± 1.77	4.43 ± 1.39	12.96 ± 3.87	5.51 ± 0.97
Q3	22.66 ± 6.05	11.66 ± 3.86	9.28 ± 3.26	5.54 ± 1.71	4.68 ± 1.37	13.71 ± 3.87	5.59 ± 0.93
Q4	22.81 ± 5.94	11.58 ± 4.14	9.34 ± 3.21	5.63 ± 1.60	4.74 ± 1.29	13.87 ± 3.89	5.63 ± 0.86
Pork							
Q1	19.98 ± 6.11	10.17 ± 4.57	7.97 ± 3.23	5.04 ± 1.76	4.28 ± 1.46	12.24 ± 4.20	5.32 ± 1.15
Q2	21.30 ± 6.29	11.02 ± 4.05	8.60 ± 3.38	5.22 ± 1.79	4.49 ± 1.45	12.96 ± 3.98	5.44 ± 1.07
Q3	22.18 ± 6.35	11.19 ± 4.26	9.02 ± 3.43	5.42 ± 1.76	4.59 ± 1.38	13.52 ± 4.04	5.58 ± 0.91
Q4	22.66 ± 5.96	11.89 ± 3.81	9.18 ± 3.25	5.38 ± 1.78	4.63 ± 1.37	13.92 ± 3.68	5.64 ± 0.78
Beef or mutton							
Q1	20.38 ± 6.61	10.65 ± 4.52	8.03 ± 3.50	5.03 ± 1.83	4.29 ± 1.47	12.32 ± 4.37	5.34 ± 1.13
Q2	20.40 ± 6.14	10.60 ± 4.44	8.14 ± 3.31	5.00 ± 1.78	4.31 ± 1.43	12.57 ± 4.07	5.42 ± 1.01
Q3	22.18 ± 5.80	11.18 ± 4.06	9.14 ± 3.09	5.41 ± 1.74	4.67 ± 1.37	13.83 ± 3.60	5.59 ± 0.91
Q4	23.16 ± 5.75	11.82 ± 3.70	9.52 ± 3.15	5.60 ± 1.67	4.74 ± 1.33	14.05 ± 3.54	5.66 ± 0.79
Poultry							
Q1	20.25 ± 6.22	10.57 ± 4.36	7.97 ± 3.37	5.09 ± 1.78	4.32 ± 1.43	12.38 ± 4.28	5.34 ± 1.11
Q2	20.41 ± 6.28	10.55 ± 4.42	8.26 ± 3.28	4.92 ± 1.84	4.30 ± 1.49	12.78 ± 3.96	5.38 ± 1.09
Q3	22.32 ± 6.02	11.30 ± 3.89	9.16 ± 3.28	5.47 ± 1.68	4.66 ± 1.33	13.63 ± 3.72	5.57 ± 0.91
Q4	23.11 ± 6.04	11.84 ± 4.08	9.38 ± 3.29	5.58 ± 1.73	4.72 ± 1.38	13.84 ± 3.95	5.68 ± 0.81
Fish							
Q1	20.13 ± 6.05	10.50 ± 4.30	7.92 ± 3.24	5.07 ± 1.72	4.25 ± 1.40	12.10 ± 4.25	5.34 ± 1.13
Q2	20.64 ± 6.23	10.31 ± 4.49	8.36 ± 3.28	5.14 ± 1.76	4.41 ± 1.46	12.72 ± 4.05	5.45 ± 1.02
Q3	22.71 ± 6.12	11.56 ± 4.16	9.30 ± 3.27	5.56 ± 1.66	4.73 ± 1.37	13.84 ± 3.85	5.59 ± 0.91
Q4	22.61 ± 6.21	11.88 ± 3.74	9.18 ± 3.43	5.29 ± 1.92	4.61 ± 1.40	13.96 ± 3.64	5.58 ± 0.89
Eggs							
Q1	21.53 ± 6.48	11.01 ± 4.30	8.76 ± 3.39 *	5.14 ± 1.93	4.45 ± 1.47	13.14 ± 4.01	5.54 ± 0.96
Q2	21.92 ± 6.02	11.32 ± 4.03	8.85 ± 3.27	5.35 ± 1.76	4.58 ± 1.38	13.56 ± 3.75	5.52 ± 0.94
Q3	21.63 ± 6.18	11.14 ± 4.25	8.68 ± 3.30	5.37 ± 1.72	4.54 ± 1.42	13.08 ± 4.13	5.48 ± 1.04
Q4	21.04 ± 6.33	10.80 ± 4.32	8.49 ± 3.46	5.20 ± 1.69	4.43 ± 1.40	12.84 ± 4.20	5.43 ± 1.03
Dairy							
T0	20.94 ± 6.46	10.96 ± 4.34	8.32 ± 3.45	5.10 ± 1.83	4.39 ± 1.44	12.82 ± 4.16	5.40 ± 1.06
T1	21.15 ± 6.17	10.55 ± 4.27	8.67 ± 3.29	5.18 ± 1.81	4.44 ± 1.44	12.99 ± 3.87	5.50 ± 0.99
T2	22.79 ± 5.98	11.71 ± 3.82	9.29 ± 3.24	5.58 ± 1.69	4.71 ± 1.38	13.89 ± 3.85	5.65 ± 0.90
T3	23.00 ± 5.36	11.39 ± 4.00	9.58 ± 2.90	5.70 ± 1.50	4.78 ± 1.30	13.95 ± 3.63	5.68 ± 0.76

Table 4. Cont.

Foods	Global Cognitive Function	Cognition Domain Scores					
		MIS	EIS	VIS	LIS	AIS	OIS
Nuts							
T0	20.69 ± 6.16	10.80 ± 4.30	8.15 ± 3.32	5.14 ± 1.72	4.38 ± 1.41	12.46 ± 4.17	5.39 ± 1.08
T1	20.80 ± 6.36	10.36 ± 4.40	8.53 ± 3.39	5.02 ± 1.96	4.37 ± 1.46	13.09 ± 4.00	5.48 ± 0.99
T2	22.27 ± 6.10	11.43 ± 4.06	9.20 ± 3.29	5.35 ± 1.79	4.58 ± 1.42	13.68 ± 3.61	5.55 ± 0.95
T3	23.44 ± 6.03	12.03 ± 3.83	9.59 ± 3.22	5.72 ± 1.62	4.83 ± 1.35	14.32 ± 3.77	5.68 ± 0.80

[a]: MIS = Memory index score, EIS = Executive index score, VIS = Visuospatial index score, LIS = Language index score, AIS = Attention index score, OIS = Orientation index score. Global cognitive function score and cognitive domain scores are expressed as mean ± SD, evaluated by Montreal Cognitive Assessment (MoCA, Beijing Version). Q1–Q4 are consumption levels of foods (except dairy and nuts) grouped by their quartile consumption; T0 = non-consumer group for dairy and nuts, T1–T3 are consumption levels of dairy and nuts grouped by the tertile consumption of consumers, expressed as mean ± SD. *: p value > 0.05, examined by Wilcoxon signed rank test and Kruskal–Wallis H test.

As compared with the bottom consumption level, participants with higher consumption of rice had higher scores of global cognitive function and indexes of cognitive domains, while those with higher consumption of wheat, ranging from the second quartile level to the top level, had lower scores of global cognitive function and EIS ($p < 0.05$) after adjusting for potential factors. The score of global cognitive function, EIS, VIS, and LIS were positively associated with the higher consumption levels of legumes, ranging from the second quartile consumption level to the top level, in comparison to the bottom one ($p < 0.05$). In addition, the scores of global cognitive function and indexes of several types of cognitive domains increased in the top consumption level of fresh vegetables, fresh fruit, pork, poultry, fish, and nuts, compared to the bottom counterpart. No significant association was observed between OIS and an increased consumption level of each selected food in comparison to the corresponding bottom counterpart ($p > 0.05$) (Table 5).

Table 5. Associations of food consumption with global cognitive score and cognitive domain subscores using quantile regression model [a].

Foods	Global Cognitive Function		Cognition Domain Scores										
			MIS		EIS		VIS		LIS		AIS		OIS	
	β	p Value	β	p Value	β	p Value	β	p Value	β	p Value	β	p Value	β	p Value
Rice														
Q2	0.79	0.008	0.51	0.016	0.44	0.002	0.08	0.257	0.00	0.952	−0.10	0.609	0.00	0.963
Q3	2.26	<0.001	1.19	<0.001	1.00	<0.001	0.25	<0.001	0.26	<0.001	1.10	<0.001	0.00	0.564
Q4	0.51	0.056	0.21	0.378	0.49	0.003	−0.19	0.028	−0.12	0.116	0.32	0.109	0.00	1.000
Wheat														
Q2	−0.88	0.003	−0.50	0.004	−0.60	<0.001	0.00	0.952	−0.10	0.194	−0.30	0.087	0.00	1.000
Q3	−1.01	<0.001	−0.37	0.013	−0.47	0.002	−0.19	0.021	−0.03	0.626	−0.45	0.007	0.00	1.000
Q4	−1.16	<0.001	−0.19	0.307	−0.64	<0.001	−0.06	0.531	−0.02	0.787	−0.38	0.106	0.00	1.000
Tubers														
Q2	−0.03	0.917	−0.18	0.299	0.06	0.688	0.00	0.974	0.13	0.092	−0.01	0.973	0.00	0.945
Q3	−0.01	0.964	−0.27	0.267	0.00	0.990	0.04	0.616	0.13	0.062	0.02	0.916	0.00	1.000
Q4	−0.11	0.693	−0.24	0.161	0.07	0.642	−0.01	0.898	0.08	0.269	0.14	0.442	0.00	0.979
Legumes														
Q2	0.68	0.018	0.30	0.153	0.39	0.015	0.32	<0.001	0.28	<0.001	0.36	0.055	0.00	1.000
Q3	1.12	<0.001	0.64	0.002	0.35	0.009	0.47	<0.001	0.19	0.013	0.25	0.186	0.00	1.000
Q4	1.57	<0.001	1.04	<0.001	0.61	<0.001	0.60	<0.001	0.29	<0.001	1.09	<0.001	0.00	1.000
Fresh vegetables														
Q2	0.22	0.462	−0.03	0.868	−0.07	0.672	0.06	0.503	−0.09	0.201	−0.04	0.823	0.00	0.988
Q3	0.65	0.032	0.76	<0.001	0.12	0.458	0.03	0.807	−0.04	0.585	0.75	<0.001	0.00	0.926
Q4	1.58	<0.001	1.14	<0.001	0.64	<0.001	0.27	0.010	0.15	0.041	1.16	<0.001	0.00	1.000
Fresh fruit														
Q2	0.00	1.000	−0.20	0.232	−0.01	0.962	0.07	0.280	0.06	0.325	0.11	0.573	0.00	0.981
Q3	1.54	<0.001	0.76	<0.001	0.79	<0.001	0.44	<0.001	0.26	0.001	0.86	<0.001	0.00	1.000
Q4	1.16	<0.001	0.41	0.054	0.56	<0.001	0.41	<0.001	0.15	0.055	0.83	<0.001	0.00	1.000
Pork														
Q2	1.03	<0.001	0.40	0.032	0.30	0.039	−0.01	0.861	0.22	0.001	0.56	0.003	0.00	1.000
Q3	1.70	<0.001	0.83	<0.001	0.69	<0.001	0.19	0.020	0.22	0.002	0.88	<0.001	0.00	0.874
Q4	1.46	<0.001	1.10	<0.001	0.45	0.014	0.02	0.769	0.11	0.116	0.89	<0.001	0.00	1.000

Table 5. Cont.

Foods	Global Cognitive Function		MIS		EIS		VIS		LIS		AIS		OIS	
	β	p Value	β	p Value	β	p Value	β	p Value	β	p Value	β	p Value	β	p Value
Beef or mutton														
Q2	−0.42	0.169	−0.53	0.069	−0.28	0.150	−0.18	0.066	−0.06	0.437	0.18	0.431	0.00	0.923
Q3	0.42	0.144	−0.14	0.310	0.38	0.004	0.12	0.095	0.20	0.002	0.79	<0.001	0.00	1.000
Q4	0.66	0.016	0.06	0.723	0.20	0.130	0.08	0.260	0.07	0.273	0.42	0.023	0.00	0.969
Poultry														
Q2	0.00	0.993	−0.05	0.780	−0.01	0.939	−0.17	0.021	0.03	0.695	0.42	0.018	0.00	1.000
Q3	0.68	0.010	0.00	1.000	0.26	0.042	0.01	0.875	0.08	0.238	0.38	0.028	0.00	0.994
Q4	1.69	<0.001	0.75	<0.001	0.61	<0.001	0.00	1.000	0.25	<0.001	0.67	<0.001	0.00	1.000
Fish														
Q2	0.09	0.755	−0.08	0.717	0.18	0.286	−0.05	0.507	0.11	0.060	0.69	<0.001	0.00	0.948
Q3	1.51	<0.001	0.74	<0.001	0.64	<0.001	0.26	0.003	0.25	<0.001	1.15	<0.001	0.00	1.000
Q4	1.60	<0.001	0.87	<0.001	0.66	<0.001	0.06	0.545	0.23	0.004	1.33	<0.001	0.00	1.000
Eggs														
Q2	0.01	0.985	0.12	0.493	−0.04	0.775	0.28	<0.001	0.14	0.046	0.34	0.066	0.00	1.000
Q3	0.10	0.682	0.30	0.120	−0.13	0.328	0.21	0.010	0.10	0.110	−0.03	0.846	0.00	1.000
Q4	−0.44	0.127	−0.01	0.957	−0.28	0.088	−0.01	0.877	0.04	0.561	−0.12	0.536	0.00	1.000
Dairy														
T1	−0.86	0.001	−1.00	<0.001	−0.25	0.099	−0.29	<0.001	−0.18	0.020	−0.62	0.001	0.00	1.000
T2	0.26	0.405	−0.08	0.551	0.05	0.757	0.10	0.193	0.10	0.196	−0.10	0.632	0.00	0.998
T3	0.18	0.568	−0.17	0.382	0.22	0.165	0.14	0.068	0.08	0.387	0.10	0.610	0.00	1.000
Nuts														
T1	−0.58	0.048	−0.65	0.003	−0.02	0.899	0.00	1.000	−0.17	0.012	0.41	0.018	0.00	1.000
T2	0.49	0.048	0.25	0.144	0.35	0.008	0.06	0.458	0.02	0.706	0.60	<0.001	0.00	1.000
T3	1.87	<0.001	0.71	<0.001	0.64	<0.001	0.50	<0.001	0.34	<0.001	1.39	<0.001	0.00	1.000

[a]: Q = quartile, reference = Q1; T = tertile, reference = T0 (non-consumer). Adjusted for age, gender, residential area, education level, employment, income level, physical activity, smoking, alcohol intake, sleep duration status, energy, disease history, obesity, and central obesity.

4. Discussion

In our study involving four provincial men and women aged 55 years and above in China without prior AD or related medication for mental disease, we observed that the participants' cognition function, including MCI and its subtypes, as well as global cognitive function and specific domains, varied with different consumption levels of the main selected foods. Moreover, increased consumption levels of rice, legumes, fresh vegetables, and pork were associated with better cognitive function, whereas the inverse association was observed between wheat and egg consumption and cognition.

The prevalence of MCI, ranging from 3.2% to 32.6%, varied in populations of elderly Americans, Finns, French, and Swedish [32–35], and was lower than that of individuals included in this study. This, to some extent, reflects the severe situation of cognition decline among the Chinese population even with differences in the range of participants' ages or the diagnosis criteria of MCI. The MCI progression factors were characterized as older age and worse income level [36]. Similarly, a finding from our study showed that participants with MCI and its subtypes clustered with old age, rural area, and lower monthly income level groups. Previous studies reported that the prevalence of amnestic MCI was significantly higher than that of non-amnestic MCI [37,38], suggesting that MCI with memory impairment was a more common MCI subtype. However, Jungwirth and coworkers reported that the percentage of non-amnestic MCI was 6% higher than that of amnestic MCI (14.86% vs. 9.0%) among 592 Australians at age 75 to 76 years old [39], and Busse et al. [40] showed no obvious difference in the prevalence of these two subtypes, which was similar to our results, just with a prevalence difference of 0.1%. Accordingly, there are inconsistent results in identifying the dominant subtype of MCI.

Epidemiological evidence supported the hypothesis that the diet disparity was significant between normal cognition individuals and MCI ones [21,23], and indicated that a diet characterized by high consumption of fruit, vegetables, nuts, legumes, fish, and low consumption of red meat and poultry, was associated with a decreased risk of cognitive decline [41]. Further, special attention has been devoted to the consumption of fruit, vegetables, fish, and nuts because of their nutrient profiles that are rich in antioxidants or polyunsaturated fatty acids, which are considered to have anti-inflammatory properties, while oxidative stress and inflammation are incentive factors of the cognitive decline process [42]. A cross-sectional study conducted with 1849 Brazilian subjects with an average age of 77.5 years old showed that a daily consumption of vegetables and fruit ≥400 g was associated with a decreased prevalence of cognitive impairment (OR = 0.53, 95% CI: 0.31~0.89). O'Brien et al. followed up 15,467 women aged 70 or older for 6 years and observed that those with a higher long-term nut intake (>5 servings of nuts/week) had a significantly higher score of global cognitive function than that of non-consumers [43]. In the Chinese population, adults with a daily nut consumption of more than 10 g had 40% decreased odds of poor cognitive function (OR = 0.60, 95%CI: 0.43~0.84) among the sample of 4822 participants aged 55 and over [44]; those aged 65 years old and over with at least 1 serving/week of fish tended to have a better global cognitive function, found in a prospective cohort study with a follow-up of 5.3 years of 1566 participants [22]. Generally, the frequent consumption of fruit, vegetables, fish, and nuts was related to relatively healthy cognitive function, which was similar to results from our study that increased consumption of these foods decreased the odds of MCI and some of its subtypes, as well as was positively associated with higher scores of extensive cognitive domains. However, no significant association was found between the consumption of fish, fruit, and vegetables and the risk of cognitive impairment among elderly French people from the Three-City Study [8], as well as others [45,46]. The disparities in populations with distinctive diets might be a potential explanation for these discrepancies. Indeed, it was neglected that there are regional disparities in the subgroups of each food item.

For other food items, meat consumption was generally considered to have an adverse effect on cognitive outcomes due to its high saturated fat content [47,48] which is potentially associated with the overproduction of circulating free fatty acids and systemic inflammation. However, the specific effect of meat consumption on cognitive disorders was often discordant [18]. A longitudinal study of a large cohort with a mean follow-up of 9.8 years and active ascertainment of dementia showed that low meat consumption (≤1 time/week) was associated with an increased risk of cognitive impairment compared with regular consumption (≥4 times/week) [8]. Another study observed a positive association of red meat with entorhinal cortex thickness, which was negatively related to dementia [49]. In our study, we observed that eating adequately varied meat, including pork, beef or mutton, and poultry, was positively associated with a better comprehensive cognitive state. Given that lean meat and poultry are high in protein, which is related to superior cognitive function [50], moderation of meat consumption is probably advised due to the controversial association between meat consumption and cognition, along with the potential risks of overweight and obesity.

A stable blood glucose profile is associated with better cognitive function and a lower risk of cognitive impairments [51]. In general, food with a low glycemic index and low glycemic load (e.g., vegetables, legumes, and whole grains) is less likely to detrimentally impact glucose metabolism and neuronal integrity. Rice and wheat are both acknowledged for their high carbohydrate content and glycemic index, and we found that participants who preferred to consume wheat, mainly as low-fiber wheat products including non-fried noodles, white bread, steamed buns, dumplings, etc., had relatively worse cognitive function and we unexpectedly observed that higher rice consumption was associated with decreased odds of MCI and aMCI-SD in comparison with the bottom level, as well as with better function of most cognitive domains in the current study. Of note, the beneficial effect was seen at a moderate consumption level of the third quartile rather than the top one. Kim et al. [52] also found, among Korean adults aged over 50 years in 2018, that a moderate consumption of cooked white rice was negatively associated with the risk of MCI, adding data supporting a positive link between cognition and rice consumption within a considerable range. Previous studies showed the different associations of rice intake and wheat intake with metabolic syndrome, diabetes, and dyslipidemia among the Chinese population [53,54]. However, few studies have been conducted in the field of the rice–cognition and wheat–cognition relationship. Given the cross-sectional nature of our study, large-scale prospective cohort studies are required to provide stronger evidence. Overall, moderation of rice consumption may be necessary, although the threshold–effect association remains unclear, and further research on it, of course, is required to elicit the potential mechanism in order to identify the optimal recommendations.

This study is the first to separately examine the associations between food consumptions and each subtype of MCI and multiple cognitive domains. We found the selected foods have similar links to various cognitive domains, consistently positive or negative, and a similar relationship of most these foods among subtypes of MCI, but not completely. For instance, the highest consumption level of dairy decreased the prevalence of naMCI-SD or naMCI-MD, whereas it was associated with 50% higher odds of aMCI-SD. This observation suggests that it is favorable to differentiate different subtypes of MCI when identifying the impact of exposures, like dietary factors, on MCI due to differentially regional impairment features of diverse subtypes [55–57]. Only presenting the relationship of exposures, like dietary factors, with MCI might lead to controversy for the potential interactions among distinct subtypes. Apart from this, various MCI subtypes have been proposed to broaden the concept of the pathology of different subtypes of MCI. Given that the transition probabilities from the MCI subtypes with memory impairment to AD were reported to be higher [58], to focus on isolated subtypes of MCI may add value for developing accurate strategies to combat AD.

Our study has several limitations. First, the dietary consumption level was estimated based on an FFQ that covered the past 12 months, which may lead to a recall bias. Second, the relative precision of the estimation of dietary consumption level relied on the self-reported exposure information from people with normal cognition, thus, the reliance on cognitive ability of the FFQ method may not have led to a precise estimate of dietary intake in all similar prospective epidemiological studies. Recall error due to cognitive impairment is thought to bias results towards the null hypothesis [59], nevertheless, we did sensitivity analyses in which we excluded those with the lowest 5% scores of the MoCA and found associations consistent with those modeled by multiple logistic regression. Third, a huge proportion of participants did not consume nuts and dairy, and the consumption of them was relatively low, so we could not clarify the appropriate dose in the association analysis and had difficulty in ranking their consumption. Fourth, although we adjusted carefully for some covariates during the data analysis, residual confounding was still possible. In addition, the cross-sectional nature of our study does not allow us to draw any causal conclusions. The major strengths of this study include the use of the MoCA to evaluate overall cognitive function and domains and recognize the subtypes of MCI, and the use of a relatively unlimited population-based sample from CCSNSD, which imparts the ability to generalize the results to the Chinese population in part.

5. Conclusions

In conclusion, most diet global cognitive benefits were observed to be associated with the preexisting consumption of foods in the present study, and adaptation to a higher consumption of rice, legumes, fresh vegetables, fresh fruit, meat, and nuts may be primarily considered as the benefits. Additionally, this study has revealed the heterogeneity of associations between the consumption of certain foods and MCI subtypes, representing value in developing accurate strategies against the progress of cognitive impairment. Further studies, including more cohort studies or randomized clinical trials, are needed to confirm these observations.

Supplementary Materials: The following are available online at https://www.mdpi.com/article/10.3390/nu13041341/s1, Table S1: Food grouping used in the dietary consumption analysis, Table S2: Characteristics and prevalence of MCI and its subtypes among Chinese adults aged 55 years and above in four provinces in CCSNSD 2018–2019, Table S3: Differences in global cognitive scores and cognitive domain subscores by characteristics among Chinese adults aged 55 years and above in four provinces in CCSNSD 2018–2019.

Author Contributions: Writing—Original draft preparation, Q.H.; Writing—Review and editing, X.J., J.Z., and Z.W.; methodology, Q.H.; data analysis, Q.H.; project administration, Z.W. and B.Z.; supervision, H.W.; investigation, F.H., L.W., and H.J. All authors have read and agreed to the published version of the manuscript.

Funding: This research was supported by the Ministry of Finance of China, the National Key R&D Program of China, Precision Medicine Project–Cohort Study on Nervous System Diseases (2017YFC0907700), Community-based Cohort Study on Nervous System Diseases (2017YFC0907701). All funders had no role in the design, analysis, or writing of this article.

Institutional Review Board Statement: The study was reviewed and approved by the Institutional Review Board of National Institute for Nutrition and Health (No. 2017020, 6 November 2017).

Informed Consent Statement: Written informed consent was obtained for each participant before the survey.

Data Availability Statement: No additional data are available.

Acknowledgments: The present study uses data from the CCSNSD. We thank all of the participants and staff involved in the surveys.

Conflicts of Interest: The funders had no role in the design of the study; in the collection, analyses, or interpretation of data; in the writing of the manuscript, or in the decision to publish the results.

References

1. Nichols, E.; Szoeke, C.E.I.; Vollset, S.E.; Abbasi, N.; Abd-Allah, F.; Abdela, J.; Aichour, M.T.E.; Akinyemi, R.O.; Alahdab, F.; Asgedom, S.W.; et al. Global, regional, and national burden of Alzheimer's disease and other dementias, 1990–2016: A systematic analysis for the Global Burden of Disease Study 2016. *Lancet Neurol.* **2019**, *18*, 88–106. [CrossRef]
2. Jia, L.; Du, Y.; Chu, L.; Zhang, Z.; Li, F.; Lyu, D.; Li, Y.; Li, Y.; Zhu, M.; Jiao, H.; et al. Prevalence, risk factors, and management of dementia and mild cognitive impairment in adults aged 60 years or older in China: A cross-sectional study. *Lancet Public Health* **2020**, *5*, e661–e671. [CrossRef]
3. Davis, M.; O'Connell, T.; Johnson, S.; Cline, S.; Merikle, E.; Martenyi, F.; Simpson, K. Estimating Alzheimer's Disease Progression Rates from Normal Cognition Through Mild Cognitive Impairment and Stages of Dementia. *Curr. Alzheimer Res.* **2018**, *15*, 777–788. [CrossRef]
4. Ding, D.; Zhao, Q.; Guo, Q.; Meng, H.; Wang, B.; Luo, J.; Mortimer, J.A.; Borenstein, A.R.; Hong, Z. Prevalence of mild cognitive impairment in an urban community in China: A cross-sectional analysis of the Shanghai Aging Study. *Alzheimer's Dement.* **2015**, *11*, 300–309 e302. [CrossRef]
5. Liu-Seifert, H.; Schumi, J.; Miao, X.; Tian, Y.; Rabbia, M.; Andersen, S.W.; Wilson, S.; Li, W.; Entsuah, R. Disease Modification in Alzheimer's Disease: Current Thinking. *Ther. Innov. Regul. Sci.* **2020**, *54*, 396–403. [CrossRef] [PubMed]
6. Flanagan, E.; Lamport, D.; Brennan, L.; Burnet, P.; Calabrese, V.; Cunnane, S.C.; Wilde, M.C.; Dye, L.; Farrimond, J.A.; Emerson Lombardo, N.; et al. Nutrition and the ageing brain: Moving towards clinical applications. *Ageing Res. Rev.* **2020**, *62*, 101079. [CrossRef]
7. Solfrizzi, V.; Custodero, C.; Lozupone, M.; Imbimbo, B.P.; Valiani, V.; Agosti, P.; Schilardi, A.; D'Introno, A.; La Montagna, M.; Calvani, M.; et al. Relationships of Dietary Patterns, Foods, and Micro- and Macronutrients with Alzheimer's Disease and Late-Life Cognitive Disorders: A Systematic Review. *J. Alzheimer's Dis* **2017**, *59*, 815–849. [CrossRef]
8. Ngabirano, L.; Samieri, C.; Feart, C.; Gabelle, A.; Artero, S.; Duflos, C.; Berr, C.; Mura, T. Intake of Meat, Fish, Fruits, and Vegetables and Long-Term Risk of Dementia and Alzheimer's Disease. *J. Alzheimers Dis.* **2019**, *68*, 711–722. [CrossRef] [PubMed]
9. Loef, M.; Walach, H. Fruit, vegetables and prevention of cognitive decline or dementia: A systematic review of cohort studies. *J. Nutr. Health Aging* **2012**, *16*, 626–630. [CrossRef]
10. Ritchie, K.; Carriere, I.; Ritchie, C.W.; Berr, C.; Artero, S.; Ancelin, M.L. Designing prevention programmes to reduce incidence of dementia: Prospective cohort study of modifiable risk factors. *Br. Med. J.* **2010**, *341*, c3885. [CrossRef] [PubMed]
11. Hughes, T.F.; Andel, R.; Small, B.J.; Borenstein, A.R.; Mortimer, J.A.; Wolk, A.; Johansson, B.; Fratiglioni, L.; Pedersen, N.L.; Gatz, M. Midlife fruit and vegetable consumption and risk of dementia in later life in Swedish twins. *Am. J. Geriatr. Psychiatry* **2010**, *18*, 413–420. [CrossRef]
12. Barberger-Gateau, P.; Raffaitin, C.; Letenneur, L.; Berr, C.; Tzourio, C.; Dartigues, J.F.; Alperovitch, A. Dietary patterns and risk of dementia: The Three-City cohort study. *Neurology* **2007**, *69*, 1921–1930. [CrossRef] [PubMed]
13. Devore, E.E.; Kang, J.H.; Breteler, M.M.; Grodstein, F. Dietary intakes of berries and flavonoids in relation to cognitive decline. *Ann. Neurol.* **2012**, *72*, 135–143. [CrossRef]
14. Lamport, D.J.; Saunders, C.; Butler, L.T.; Spencer, J.P. Fruits, vegetables, 100% juices, and cognitive function. *Nutr. Rev.* **2014**, *72*, 774–789. [CrossRef] [PubMed]
15. Zhang, Y.; Chen, J.; Qiu, J.; Li, Y.; Wang, J.; Jiao, J. Intakes of fish and polyunsaturated fatty acids and mild-to-severe cognitive impairment risks: A dose-response meta-analysis of 21 cohort studies. *Am. J. Clin. Nutr.* **2016**, *103*, 330–340. [CrossRef] [PubMed]

16. Li, M.; Shi, Z. A Prospective Association of Nut Consumption with Cognitive Function in Chinese Adults aged 55+ China Health and Nutrition Survey. *J. Nutr. Health Aging* **2019**, *23*, 211–216. [CrossRef]
17. Taylor, M.K.; Sullivan, D.K.; Swerdlow, R.H.; Vidoni, E.D.; Morris, J.K.; Mahnken, J.D.; Burns, J.M. A high-glycemic diet is associated with cerebral amyloid burden in cognitively normal older adults. *Am. J. Clin. Nutr.* **2017**, *106*, 1463–1470. [CrossRef]
18. Zhang, H.; Hardie, L.; Bawajeeh, A.O.; Cade, J. Meat Consumption, Cognitive Function and Disorders: A Systematic Review with Narrative Synthesis and Meta-Analysis. *Nutrients* **2020**, *12*, 1528. [CrossRef]
19. Petersen, R.C. Mild cognitive impairment as a diagnostic entity. *J. Intern. Med.* **2004**, *256*, 183–194. [CrossRef]
20. Zhao, X.; Yuan, L.; Feng, L.; Xi, Y.; Yu, H.; Ma, W.; Zhang, D.; Xiao, R. Association of dietary intake and lifestyle pattern with mild cognitive impairment in the elderly. *J. Nutr. Health Aging* **2015**, *19*, 164–168. [CrossRef] [PubMed]
21. Dong, L.; Xiao, R.; Cai, C.; Xu, Z.; Wang, S.; Pan, L.; Yuan, L. Diet, lifestyle and cognitive function in old Chinese adults. *Arch. Gerontol. Geriatr.* **2016**, *63*, 36–42. [CrossRef]
22. Qin, B.; Plassman, B.L.; Edwards, L.J.; Popkin, B.M.; Adair, L.S.; Mendez, M.A. Fish intake is associated with slower cognitive decline in Chinese older adults. *J. Nutr.* **2014**, *144*, 1579–1585. [CrossRef]
23. Yuan, L.; Liu, J.; Ma, W.; Dong, L.; Wang, W.; Che, R.; Xiao, R. Dietary pattern and antioxidants in plasma and erythrocyte in patients with mild cognitive impairment from China. *Nutrition* **2016**, *32*, 193–198. [CrossRef]
24. Julayanont, P.; Brousseau, M.; Chertkow, H.; Phillips, N.; Nasreddine, Z.S. Montreal Cognitive Assessment Memory Index Score (MoCA-MIS) as a predictor of conversion from mild cognitive impairment to Alzheimer's disease. *J. Am. Geriatr. Soc.* **2014**, *62*, 679–684. [CrossRef]
25. Lu, J.; Li, D.; Li, F.; Zhou, A.; Wang, F.; Zuo, X.; Jia, X.F.; Song, H.; Jia, J. Montreal cognitive assessment in detecting cognitive impairment in Chinese elderly individuals: A population-based study. *J. Geriatr. Psychiatry Neurol.* **2011**, *24*, 184–190. [CrossRef]
26. Petersen, R.C. Mild Cognitive Impairment. *Continuum* **2016**, *22*, 404–418. [CrossRef] [PubMed]
27. Winblad, B.; Palmer, K.; Kivipelto, M.; Jelic, V.; Fratiglioni, L.; Wahlund, L.O.; Nordberg, A.; Backman, L.; Albert, M.; Almkvist, O.; et al. Mild cognitive impairment—Beyond controversies, towards a consensus: Report of the International Working Group on Mild Cognitive Impairment. *J. Intern. Med.* **2004**, *256*, 240–246. [CrossRef]
28. Ainsworth, B.E.; Haskell, W.L.; Whitt, M.C.; Irwin, M.L.; Swartz, A.M.; Strath, S.J.; O'Brien, W.L.; Bassett, D.R., Jr.; Schmitz, K.H.; Emplaincourt, P.O.; et al. Compendium of physical activities: An update of activity codes and MET intensities. *Med. Sci. Sports Exerc.* **2000**, *32*, S498–S504. [CrossRef] [PubMed]
29. Hirshkowitz, M.; Whiton, K.; Albert, S.M.; Alessi, C.; Bruni, O.; DonCarlos, L.; Hazen, N.; Herman, J.; Katz, E.S.; Kheirandish-Gozal, L.; et al. National Sleep Foundation's sleep time duration recommendations: Methodology and results summary. *Sleep Health* **2015**, *1*, 40–43. [CrossRef] [PubMed]
30. Chen, C.; Lu, F.C. The guidelines for prevention and control of overweight and obesity in Chinese adults. *Biomed. Environ. Sci. BES* **2004**, *17*, 1–36. [PubMed]
31. *National Health and Family Planning Commission of the People's Republic of China*; Criteria of Weight for Adults, WS/T 428-2013; Standards Press of China: Beijing, China, 2013.
32. Manly, J.J.; Bell-McGinty, S.; Tang, M.X.; Schupf, N.; Stern, Y.; Mayeux, R. Implementing diagnostic criteria and estimating frequency of mild cognitive impairment in an urban community. *Arch. Neurol.* **2005**, *62*, 1739–1746. [CrossRef]
33. Palmer, K.; Backman, L.; Winblad, B.; Fratiglioni, L. Mild cognitive impairment in the general population: Occurrence and progression to Alzheimer disease. *Am. J. Geriatr. Psychiatry* **2008**, *16*, 603–611. [CrossRef] [PubMed]
34. Ritchie, K.; Artero, S.; Touchon, J. Classification criteria for mild cognitive impairment: A population-based validation study. *Neurology* **2001**, *56*, 37–42. [CrossRef] [PubMed]
35. Hanninen, T.; Hallikainen, M.; Tuomainen, S.; Vanhanen, M.; Soininen, H. Prevalence of mild cognitive impairment: A population-based study in elderly subjects. *Acta Neurol. Scand.* **2002**, *106*, 148–154. [CrossRef]
36. Qin, H.Y.; Zhao, X.D.; Zhu, B.G.; Hu, C.P. Demographic Factors and Cognitive Function Assessments Associated with Mild Cognitive Impairment Progression for the Elderly. *Biomed. Res. Int.* **2020**, *2020*, 3054373. [CrossRef]
37. Rao, D.; Luo, X.; Tang, M.; Shen, Y.; Huang, R.; Yu, J.; Ren, J.; Cheng, X.; Lin, K. Prevalence of mild cognitive impairment and its subtypes in community-dwelling residents aged 65 years or older in Guangzhou, China. *Arch. Gerontol Geriatr* **2018**, *75*, 70–75. [CrossRef]
38. Lopez, O.L.; Becker, J.T.; Jagust, W.J.; Fitzpatrick, A.; Carlson, M.C.; DeKosky, S.T.; Breitner, J.; Lyketsos, C.G.; Jones, B.; Kawas, C.; et al. Neuropsychological characteristics of mild cognitive impairment subgroups. *J. Neurol. Neurosurg. Psychiatry* **2006**, *77*, 159–165. [CrossRef]
39. Jungwirth, S.; Weissgram, S.; Zehetmayer, S.; Tragl, K.H.; Fischer, P. VITA: Subtypes of mild cognitive impairment in a community-based cohort at the age of 75 years. *Int. J. Geriatr. Psychiatry* **2005**, *20*, 452–458. [CrossRef] [PubMed]
40. Busse, A.; Hensel, A.; Guhne, U.; Angermeyer, M.C.; Riedel-Heller, S.G. Mild cognitive impairment: Long-term course of four clinical subtypes. *Neurology* **2006**, *67*, 2176–2185. [CrossRef]
41. Feart, C.; Samieri, C.; Barberger-Gateau, P. Mediterranean diet and cognitive health: An update of available knowledge. *Curr. Opin. Clin. Nutr. Metab. Care* **2015**, *18*, 51–62. [CrossRef]
42. Bamberger, M.E.; Harris, M.E.; McDonald, D.R.; Husemann, J.; Landreth, G.E. A cell surface receptor complex for fibrillar beta-amyloid mediates microglial activation. *J. Neurosci.* **2003**, *23*, 2665–2674. [CrossRef]

43. O'Brien, J.; Okereke, O.; Devore, E.; Rosner, B.; Breteler, M.; Grodstein, F. Long-term intake of nuts in relation to cognitive function in older women. *J. Nutr. Health Aging* **2014**, *18*, 496–502. [CrossRef] [PubMed]
44. Pastor-Valero, M.; Furlan-Viebig, R.; Menezes, P.R.; da Silva, S.A.; Vallada, H.; Scazufca, M. Education and WHO recommendations for fruit and vegetable intake are associated with better cognitive function in a disadvantaged Brazilian elderly population: A population-based cross-sectional study. *PLoS ONE* **2014**, *9*, e94042. [CrossRef]
45. Wu, L.; Sun, D.; Tan, Y. Intake of Fruit and Vegetables and the Incident Risk of Cognitive Disorders: A Systematic Review and Meta-Analysis of Cohort Studies. *J. Nutr. Health Aging* **2017**, *21*, 1284–1290. [CrossRef] [PubMed]
46. Devore, E.E.; Grodstein, F.; van Rooij, F.J.; Hofman, A.; Rosner, B.; Stampfer, M.J.; Witteman, J.C.; Breteler, M.M. Dietary intake of fish and omega-3 fatty acids in relation to long-term dementia risk. *Am. J. Clin. Nutr.* **2009**, *90*, 170–176. [CrossRef]
47. Grant, W.B. Diet and risk of dementia: Does fat matter? The Rotterdam Study. *Neurology* **2003**, *60*, 2020–2021. [CrossRef] [PubMed]
48. Tan, B.L.; Norhaizan, M.E. Effect of High-Fat Diets on Oxidative Stress, Cellular Inflammatory Response and Cognitive Function. *Nutrients* **2019**, *11*, 2579. [CrossRef]
49. Staubo, S.C.; Aakre, J.A.; Vemuri, P.; Syrjanen, J.A.; Mielke, M.M.; Geda, Y.E.; Kremers, W.K.; Machulda, M.M.; Knopman, D.S.; Petersen, R.C.; et al. Mediterranean diet, micronutrients and macronutrients, and MRI measures of cortical thickness. *Alzheimer's Dement.* **2017**, *13*, 168–177. [CrossRef]
50. La Rue, A.; Koehler, K.M.; Wayne, S.J.; Chiulli, S.J.; Haaland, K.Y.; Garry, P.J. Nutritional status and cognitive functioning in a normally aging sample: A 6-y reassessment. *Am. J. Clin. Nutr.* **1997**, *65*, 20–29. [CrossRef]
51. Sunram-Lea, S.I.; Owen, L. The impact of diet-based glycaemic response and glucose regulation on cognition: Evidence across the lifespan. *Proc. Nutr. Soc.* **2017**, *76*, 466–477. [CrossRef] [PubMed]
52. Kim, K.Y.; Yun, J.M. Association between diets and mild cognitive impairment in adults aged 50 years or older. *Nutr. Res. Pract.* **2018**, *12*, 415–425. [CrossRef] [PubMed]
53. Huang, L.; Wang, H.; Wang, Z.; Zhang, J.; Zhang, B.; Ding, G. Regional Disparities in the Association between Cereal Consumption and Metabolic Syndrome: Results from the China Health and Nutrition Survey. *Nutrients* **2019**, *11*, 764. [CrossRef] [PubMed]
54. Dong, F.; Howard, A.G.; Herring, A.H.; Popkin, B.M.; Gordon-Larsen, P. White Rice Intake Varies in Its Association with Metabolic Markers of Diabetes and Dyslipidemia Across Region among Chinese Adults. *Ann. Nutr. Metab.* **2015**, *66*, 209–218. [CrossRef]
55. Bangen, K.J.; Clark, A.L.; Werhane, M.; Edmonds, E.C.; Nation, D.A.; Evangelista, N.; Libon, D.J.; Bondi, M.W.; Delano-Wood, L.; Alzheimer's Disease Neuroimaging, I. Cortical Amyloid Burden Differences Across Empirically-Derived Mild Cognitive Impairment Subtypes and Interaction with APOE varepsilon4 Genotype. *J. Alzheimer's Dis.* **2016**, *52*, 849–861. [CrossRef]
56. Guan, H.; Liu, T.; Jiang, J.; Tao, D.; Zhang, J.; Niu, H.; Zhu, W.; Wang, Y.; Cheng, J.; Kochan, N.A.; et al. Classifying MCI Subtypes in Community-Dwelling Elderly Using Cross-Sectional and Longitudinal MRI-Based Biomarkers. *Front. Aging Neurosc.* **2017**, *9*, 309. [CrossRef] [PubMed]
57. Lam, C.L.M.; Yiend, J.; Lee, T.M.C. Imaging and neuropsychological correlates of white matter lesions in different subtypes of Mild Cognitive Impairment: A systematic review. *NeuroRehabilitation* **2017**, *41*, 189–204. [CrossRef]
58. Kida, J.; Nemoto, K.; Ikejima, C.; Bun, S.; Kakuma, T.; Mizukami, K.; Asada, T. Impact of Depressive Symptoms on Conversion from Mild Cognitive Impairment Subtypes to Alzheimer's Disease: A Community-Based Longitudinal Study. *J. Alzheimer's Dis.* **2016**, *51*, 405–415. [CrossRef]
59. Raphael, K. Recall bias: A proposal for assessment and control. *Int. J. Epidemiol.* **1987**, *16*, 167–170. [CrossRef]

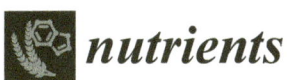

Article

Fruit and Vegetable Intake and Telomere Length in a Random Sample of 5448 U.S. Adults

Larry A. Tucker

College of Life Sciences, Brigham Young University, Provo, UT 84602, USA; tucker@byu.edu;
Tel.: +01-801-422-4927

Abstract: The relationship between fruit and vegetable intake and telomere length was examined using a cross-sectional design and an NHANES random sample of 5448 U.S. adults. Fruit and vegetable (F&V) consumption was assessed using a 24 h recall, and telomere length, an index of cellular aging, was measured using the quantitative polymerase chain reaction method. Telomere length was linearly related to F&V intake when combined (F = 22.7, $p < 0.0001$) and also when separated as fruit (F = 7.2, $p < 0.0121$) or vegetables (F = 15.4, $p < 0.0005$), after adjusting for covariates. Specifically, telomeres were 27.8 base pairs longer for each 100 g (3.5 ounces) of F&V consumed. Because each additional year of chronological age was associated with telomeres that were 14.9 base pairs shorter, when women and men were analyzed together, results indicated that a 100 g (3.5 oz) per day increment in F&V corresponded with 1.9 years less biological aging. When the 75th percentile of F&V intake was compared to the 25th, the difference was 4.4 years of cellular aging. When separated by sex, fruits and vegetables were both related to telomere length in women, but only vegetable intake was predictive of telomere length in men. In conclusion, evidence based on a random sample of U.S. adults indicates that the more the servings of F&V, the longer telomeres tend to be.

Keywords: telomere; diet; carbohydrate; NHANES; antioxidant; inflammation; legume; potato

Citation: Tucker, L.A. Fruit and Vegetable Intake and Telomere Length in a Random Sample of 5448 U.S. Adults. *Nutrients* **2021**, *13*, 1415. https://doi.org/10.3390/nu13051415

Academic Editors: Emiliana Giacomello and Luana Toniolo

Received: 13 March 2021
Accepted: 21 April 2021
Published: 23 April 2021

Publisher's Note: MDPI stays neutral with regard to jurisdictional claims in published maps and institutional affiliations.

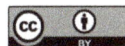

Copyright: © 2021 by the author. Licensee MDPI, Basel, Switzerland. This article is an open access article distributed under the terms and conditions of the Creative Commons Attribution (CC BY) license (https://creativecommons.org/licenses/by/4.0/).

1. Introduction

There are many health benefits associated with vegetable and fruit intake. Unfortunately, approximately 85% of Americans do not consume sufficient amounts of vegetables and over 75% fall short regarding intake of fruits [1]. Consequently, the U.S. report, "Dietary Guidelines for Americans (2015–2020)," recommends that individuals increase their intake of vegetables from all vegetable subgroups. The guidelines also encourage Americans to shift toward consuming more fruits, mostly whole fruits, in nutrient-dense forms [1]. Similarly, the World Health Organization (WHO) recommends that adults consume more than 400 g (>14 oz) of fruits and vegetables per day to improve overall health and reduce the risk of disease [2].

Numerous investigations show that mortality decreases as consumption of vegetables and fruits increases. In a recent meta-analysis that included over 830,000 adults, Wang et al. combined 16 prospective cohort studies with follow-up periods ranging from approximately 5 years to 26 years [3]. Pooled results showed that all-cause mortality was 5–6% lower for each serving of fruits and vegetables, with a threshold of approximately five servings per day. Pooled findings for cardiovascular mortality were comparable [3].

Similarly, in a 2016 Australian cohort study of over 150,000 adults, Nguyen et al. showed that fruit and vegetable intake was associated significantly with reduced risk of all-cause mortality [4]. With an average follow-up period of 6.2 years, the investigation pointed out that the highest risk reduction was seen with seven servings of fruits and vegetables per day [4].

Vegetable and fruit intake could decrease mortality and reduce biologic aging by preserving telomeres. Telomeres are the DNA protein caps that provide stability and shield the ends of chromosomes [5]. When cells divide, a portion of the telomeric DNA does not replicate. Therefore, mitosis causes telomeres to gradually shorten. Because somatic cells experience a finite number of cell divisions, telomere length is highly related to chronological age [6]. It reflects a person's telomere length when born and subsequent telomere breakdown. Hence, the shortening of telomeres is a mechanism and an index of cell aging [7,8].

Adults vary considerably within physiological, motor, cognitive, sensory, health, and other areas of function as chronological age increases. Vast differences exist within these domains even among adults of the same chronological age. Although chronological age is a good index of the health and function of adults, the length of telomeres can quantify biological aging beyond the reach of the calendar.

Because telomeres shorten with the passage of time, are highly variable across individuals, are good predictors of a number of age-sensitive diseases and conditions, and are well-established within critical biological processes, telomere length is considered a meaningful measure of biological aging, as shown in a review by Mather et al. [9]. However, some studies indicate that telomere length is not a significant predictor of biological aging [10,11].

Evidence supporting the use of telomeres as an index of cell aging is plentiful. Cawthon et al. studied older adults for 15 years [12]. Results showed that individuals with shorter telomeres had 1.9-fold greater all-cause mortality compared to those with longer telomeres. Differences in mortality from heart disease was 3.2-fold greater for those with the shorter telomeres [12]. Similarly, in a prospective investigation by Bakaysa and associates [13], Swedish twins who had shorter telomeres compared to their co-twin had approximately 3-fold higher mortality over 7 years compared to the co-twin [13]. Finally, in a sample of almost 700 Italians, Ehrlenbach et al. found that shorter telomeres at baseline were predictive of greater all-cause mortality over 10 years [14]. Specifically, those who survived during the 10 years of follow-up had telomeres that were approximately 50% longer (median) than those who died.

Scientists have investigated the relationship between telomere length and consumption of fruits and vegetables with varying results. In an investigation based on 455 normotensive men living in China, Lian et al. showed that higher vegetable intake was associated with longer telomeres [15]. Fruit intake was not related to telomere length, however. Marcon et al. uncovered similar findings [16]. Specifically, as vegetable intake increased, telomeres increased in length, but again, fruit consumption was not related to telomere length. However, Lee et al. studied 1958 middle-aged and older Korean adults and found the opposite [17]. These researchers showed that fruit intake was predictive of longer telomeres, but vegetable consumption was not. Conversely, Bethancourt et al. found that neither fruits nor vegetables were predictive of telomere length in 1459 young adult Filipino men [18]. These disparate findings do not appear to be a result of differences in statistical control of covariates. However, the mixed findings could be a result of differences in factors such as culture, lifestyle, and medical systems.

The effect of fruits and vegetables on telomere length is not clear, especially in U.S. adults. To date, little research has focused on this research question using large samples of U.S. adults. Hence, the aim of this investigation was to evaluate the degree to which consumption of fruits and vegetables accounts for differences in telomere length in an NHANES sample of over 5000 men and women representing the adult population of the U.S. An ancillary aim was to evaluate the degree to which demographic and lifestyle variables influence the relationship between intake of vegetables and fruits and the length of telomeres. Lastly, vegetable intake was defined using multiple definitions. Specifically, vegetable consumption was studied with and without legumes included, and with and without the inclusion of potatoes.

2. Materials and Methods

The present investigation was conducted employing a cross-sectional design and data collected as part of the ongoing National Health and Nutrition Examination Survey

(NHANES) in the United States. Overseen by the U.S. Centers for Disease Control and Prevention, NHANES has been conducted for many decades to provide ongoing estimates of the health and nutrition status of non-institutionalized individuals living in the United States. A multifaceted sampling design is employed by NHANES to enable the findings to be generalized throughout the United States [19]. Specifically, NHANES uses a four-stage sampling design with random selection employed at each stage. First counties are selected, followed by city blocks, then households are chosen, and lastly individuals are selected for participation [19].

The length of leukocyte telomeres was measured by NHANES during a four-year period in the United States only, 1999–2002. During this four-year period, multiple subcategories were oversampled to afford more exact estimates, including low-income individuals, Mexican Americans, Non-Hispanic Black Americans, individuals ages 60 or older, and teenagers 12–19 years old [19].

For the present study, adults were asked to give a blood sample for DNA analysis. A total of 76% consented and gave a useable sample. To maximize confidentiality, NHANES assigned all adults 85 years old and older the age of 85. Hence, participants that were 85 years or older were excluded from the sample. Subjects with missing data or extreme results (±3 standard deviations from the mean) were also excluded from the sample [20–23]. A total of 5448 adults, 2935 women and 2647 men, were included in the analyses. Written informed consent was acquired from each participant. The Ethics Review Board (ERB) approved the data collection protocol. The ethical approval code for NHANES data collection from 1999–2002 was #98-12 [24].

2.1. Measures

More than a dozen variables were measured in the present study: fruit intake, vegetable consumption (including and excluding potatoes, and including and excluding legumes and pulses), estimated energy intake, leukocyte telomere length, age, sex, race, body mass index (BMI), smoking, physical activity, and alcohol use.

2.1.1. Fruits and Vegetables

Dietary assessments were performed in private settings within an NHANES Mobile Examination Center (MEC). A computer-assisted procedure, managed by a qualified NHANES interviewer, was employed to gather the dietary data [25]. A standardized interview protocol was followed for each participant [26]. Food probes were part of the interview format. All the interviewers spoke at least two languages and each had a degree in nutrition or home economics. Each dietary assessment focused on foods and beverages consumed during the previous 24 h (midnight to midnight). Numerous investigations have employed the 24 h recall system managed by NHANES to collect data on dietary intake in adults [27–29].

Concurrent validity of the NHANES 24 h diet assessment has been established through numerous studies. For example, results derived using the NHANES 24 h recall are predictive of non-alcoholic fatty liver disease [30], total mortality [31], cardiovascular mortality [32], cancer mortality [33], and coronary heart disease [34], to name a few.

Consumption of fruits and vegetables served as the exposure variables of the present study. Fruit intake was measured in grams. Fruit drinks and juices were not counted as part of the fruit intake total. Vegetable consumption, cooked or raw, was also measured in grams, and included starchy vegetables. However, in separate analyses, potatoes and potato soups were excluded from the vegetable group, as recommended by the World Health Organization [2] and a number of independent investigations [35–37]. Similarly, consumption of legumes and pulses were analyzed as part of the vegetable group and also separately. According to the United Kingdom Eatwell Plate program, pulses are not a standard vegetable [38]. The Eatwell Plate program states, " . . . while pulses contain fibre, they don't give the same mixture of vitamins, minerals and other nutrients as fruit and vegetables" [38].

Intake of fruits and vegetables was reported separately and combined. Additionally, because intake of specific foods tends to increase as energy intake increases, two methods were employed to quantify fruit and vegetable consumption. First, intake was expressed simply as grams consumed per day, not accounting for differences in energy intake. Second, intake of fruits and vegetables was standardized based on energy intake. In short, fruit and vegetable intakes were expressed as grams consumed per 1000 kcal.

2.1.2. Energy Intake

Underreporting energy or kilocalorie (kcal) intake is a common problem when food consumption is self-reported [39]. Hence, the Mifflin resting metabolic rate formula (RMR) [40], combined with a measure of physical activity level (PAL) [41], were used to estimate energy expenditure and energy intake [42]. PAL was assessed using four NHANES questions, each describing a higher level of physical activity [41]. Each of the four levels of physical activity was assigned a PAL value: 1.45, 1.55, 1.65, and 1.75, respectively. Multiplied together, resting metabolic rate and physical activity level were used to approximate total energy consumption, as reported in other research [43].

2.1.3. Telomere Length

The outcome variable of the present study was leukocyte telomere length, an indicator of the biological age of humans. Leukocyte telomeres are the most commonly used telomeres in research. From time to time, other tissues are used, such as colon, skin, nerves, muscle, and mucosa, but these tissues are much less common for the study of telomeres. According to Demanelis et al., variations in the lengths of telomeres based on tissue types, and the extent of the associations between tissue type telomere lengths can be ascribed to differences in both internal (e.g., cell division rate and history, telomere maintenance) and external (e.g., response to environmental exposures) factors across tissues [44]. Telomeres derived from blood (leukocytes) are used most often because they are the best all-around substitute for telomeres in other tissues [44].

The length of telomeres was evaluated with care to minimize measurement error, as described by NHANES and others [45–47]. The interassay coefficient of variation was 6.5% [47]. The relative telomere to single copy gene (T/S) ratios were transformed to base pairs using the formula: $3274 + 2413 \times (T/S)$ [47].

2.1.4. Weight and Height

A digital scale was employed to assess body weight. During the measurement, the subject wore only underclothes, a disposable paper gown, and foam slippers [48]. A mounted stadiometer with an adjustable headboard was employed to assess height [48]. Weight and height were utilized to figure body mass index (BMI), defined below.

2.1.5. Sociodemographic Covariates

There were three sociodemographic covariates included in the present study: age, sex, and race. Chronological age ranged from 20 to 84 years. To maximize confidentiality, all participants older than 85 years were recorded as 85 by NHANES, so individuals older than 84 were not included in this study. NHANES defined sex using two categories, female or male. NHANES defined race and ethnicity using five categories: Non-Hispanic White, Non-Hispanic Black, Mexican American, Other Race or Multi-Racial (Other), and Other Hispanic.

2.1.6. Lifestyle Covariates

Four lifestyle factors were used as covariates and were controlled statistically in some models: BMI, alcohol use, total physical activity, and smoking. BMI was employed to index body weight independent of height. BMI was determined employing the formula: weight in kilograms divided by height in meters squared, kg/m^2 [49]. Categories based on standard cut-off points were used: underweight (<18.5), normal weight (≥18.5 and <25.0), overweight (≥25.0 and <30.0), obese (≥30.0), or missing.

Alcohol consumption was indexed using three categories—abstainers, moderate drinkers, and heavy drinkers—as described by NHANES [50]. The NHANES question (ALQ130) was used to assess the number of alcoholic drinks consumed by participants.

To assess participation in physical activity (PA), MET (metabolic equivalent) minutes per week during the past 30 days were calculated. Adults indicated their involvement in 62 separate PAs, if any, and if the activity was moderate or vigorous in intensity, frequency of participation over the past 30 days, and the amount of time spent in the PA. Less than 10 min of PA was counted as 0. A MET score was estimated for each PA reported and total MET-min per week were estimated by NHANES for each adult by employing the physical activity compendium [51].

Smoking was indexed using pack-years, which was calculated as the number of cigarettes smoked per day multiplied by the years smoked, divided by 20 [52].

2.2. Statistical Analysis

NHANES participants are unique because they are selected randomly from the U.S. adult population. Each participant is assigned an individual sample weight, allowing that person to represent other individuals with similar characteristics. Statistical outcomes were founded on the sophisticated sampling design of NHANES, which included strata, clusters, and sample weights. Hence, statistical results reported in this paper represent the civilian, non-institutionalized, adult population of the United States.

Although the sample size of this investigation was large (n = 5448), degrees of freedom (df) were small in comparison. Because a multi-stage sampling design was employed by NHANES, degrees of freedom for each analysis were computed as the number of clusters (n = 57) minus the number of strata (n = 28), or 29 df [53].

SAS SurveyMeans was used to compute weighted means and SurveyFreq was used to estimate weighted frequencies, each generalizable to the U.S. population. Fruit and vegetable intakes were each indexed using two variables, intake in grams, and grams consumed per 1000 kcal. The extent of the linear relationships between fruit, vegetable, potato, and legume intakes and telomere length were calculated using regression analysis and the SAS SurveyReg procedure [53]. Regression estimates were adjusted based on sampling weights. The SAS SurveyReg procedure and partial correlation were utilized to determine the degree that associations between fruit and vegetable consumption and telomere length were influenced by the covariates [53]. Regression coefficients were used to calculate the number of telomere base pairs associated with each year of age, and to determine the number of base pairs associated with each serving of F&V. Statistical significance was based on $p < 0.05$. The statistical analyses were conducted employing SAS Version 9.4 (SAS Institute, Inc., Cary, NC, USA).

3. Results

There were 5448 adults in the sample. Mean age (±SE) of the sample was 46.5 (±0.4) years. Mean telomere length was 5824 (±39) base pairs, average fruit intake was 78.9 (±2.8) grams per day, and mean vegetable consumption (without potatoes or legumes) was 93.8 (±3.2) grams per day. Potato intake averaged 50.6 (±1.4) grams per day, and consumption of legumes and pulses averaged 24.2 (±1.7) grams per day. Mean (±SE) estimated energy intake was 2410 (±12) kilocalories per day. Table 1 shows the mean (±SE) and percentile values of the continuous variables of the investigation when all the participants were included.

Table 1. Descriptive characteristics of the key variables in U.S. women and men (n = 5448).

Variable	Mean	SE	Percentile 25th	Percentile 50th	Percentile 75th
Age (years)	46.5	0.4	33.0	44.4	58.0
Telomere length (base pairs)	5824	38.9	5380	5743	6185
Body mass index (BMI)	28.3	0.2	23.7	27.1	31.6
Fruit intake (g)	78.9	2.8	0	0	130.9
Fruit intake (g per 1000 kcal)	35.0	1.4	0	0	55.3
Vegetable intake (g) [†]	93.7	3.2	0	43.1	146.0
Vegetable intake (g per 1000 kcal) [†]	40.9	1.4	0	18.2	61.7
Fruit and vegetable intake (g)	169.3	5.1	0	117.8	264.0
F&V intake (g per 1000 kcal)	74.9	2.2	0	47.3	113.6
Potato intake (g)	50.6	1.4	0	0	74.9
Potato intake (g per 1000 kcal)	20.7	0.6	0	0	30.1
Legume intake (g) [‡]	24.2	1.7	0	0	0
Legume intake (g per 1000 kcal) [‡]	10.3	0.7	0	0	0
Veg, potato, and legume intake (g)	169.4	3.7	22.3	120.5	252.9
Veg, potato, and legume intake (g per 1000 kcal)	72.2	1.7	9.2	49.9	109.8
Body weight (kg)	80.6	0.5	65.8	78.1	91.9
Physical activity (MET-min)	132.9	11.7	0	0	135.8
Energy intake (kilocalories)	2410	11.9	2035	2383	2742
Smoking (pack-years)	2.9	0.2	0	0	0

[†] The vegetable food group did not include potatoes or legumes or pulses unless otherwise stated. [‡] Legume and pulse intake not combined with any other vegetable. F&V = fruit and vegetable intake combined. Veg = vegetables. MET-min was MET-minutes of PA per week. The dietary intake results reflect consumption per 24 h.

In the present study, sex, race, BMI, and alcohol use were treated as categorical variables. Of the 5448 participants, 52.9% (±0.7) were female, 70.2% (±1.9) were Non-Hispanic White, 12.1% (±1.4%) were Non-Hispanic Black, 7.6% (±0.9) were Mexican American, 3.6% (±0.6%) placed themselves within the category labeled Other Race or Multi-Racial, and 6.5% (±1.6%) identified themselves as Other Hispanic. For the BMI categories, 31.7% (±1.1) were obese, 34.0% (±1.1) were overweight, 31.5% (±0.8) fit within the normal category, 2.0% (±0.3) were considered underweight, and 0.8% (±0.2) had missing data. For the alcohol use variable, 35.5% (±2.7) indicated that they were alcohol abstainers, 32.2% (±1.7%) were labeled moderate drinkers, and 32.3% (±1.4) were found to be heavy drinkers.

3.1. Age and Telomere Length

Age and telomere length were inversely related (F = 421.0, R^2 = 0.156, r = −0.39, $p < 0.0001$). For each year of age, telomeres were 14.9 base pairs shorter, determined using the regression coefficient. Beyond the linear term, age^2 was unrelated to telomere length (F = 0.1, p = 0.8234). Adjusting statistically for age^2 separately or combined with age had no effect on the relationship between fruit and vegetable intake and telomere length.

3.2. Intake of Fruits and Vegetables Combined and Telomeres

As displayed in Table 2, with data from women and men combined, telomere length was linearly related to fruit and vegetable (F&V) intake (F = 22.7, $p < 0.0001$). After adjusting for differences in age, sex, and race, telomeres were 27.8 base pairs longer for each 100 g (3.5 ounces) of F&V consumed. After controlling for the sociodemographic covariates (age, sex, and race) and the lifestyle covariates (BMI, physical activity, alcohol use, and smoking pack-years), telomeres were 24.7 base pairs longer for each 100 g (3.5 ounces) of F&V consumed (F = 20.3, $p < 0.0001$).

Table 2. Relationship between fruit and vegetable intake and telomere length in U.S. women and men combined.

Exposure Variable	Model	Regression Coefficient	SE	R^2 (%)	F	p
Fruit and vegetable intake (100 g) [†]	1	27.8	5.8	16.8	22.7	<0.0001
	2	24.7	5.5	17.5	20.3	<0.0001
Fruit a vegetable intake (100 g per 1000 kcal) [†]	1	66.9	13.1	16.8	25.9	<0.0001
	2	57.6	11.9	17.4	23.3	<0.0001
Fruit intake (100 g)	1	26.9	10.1	16.4	7.2	0.0121
	2	23.1	9.5	17.2	6.0	0.0206
Fruit intake (100 g per 1000 kcal)	1	74.9	22.8	16.6	10.8	0.0027
	2	63.1	21.5	17.3	8.7	0.0063
Vegetable intake (100 g) [†]	1	32.5	8.3	16.6	15.4	0.0005
	2	28.9	8.0	17.4	13.2	0.0011
Vegetable intake (100 g per 1000 kcal) [†]	1	71.4	14.0	16.6	25.9	<0.0001
	2	59.1	12.8	17.3	21.3	<0.0001
Potato intake (100 g)	1	−5.8	8.6	16.2	0.5	0.5038
	2	−5.1	9.0	17.2	0.3	0.5732
Potato intake (100 g per 1000 kcal)	1	−6.8	22.9	16.2	0.1	0.7688
	2	−9.8	24.0	17.1	0.2	0.6861
Legume and pulse intake (100 g)	1	2..4	12.8	16.2	0.0	0.8533
	2	−0.6	13.1	17.0	0.0	0.9629
Legume and pulse intake (100 g per 1000 kcal)	1	5.0	28.5	16.1	0.0	0.8627
	2	−5.6	29.2	17.0	0.0	0.8498
Vegetable and potato intake (100 g)	1	16.9	4.9	16.4	12.1	0.0016
	2	14.9	4.6	17.2	10.6	0.0029
Vegetable and potato intake (100 g per 1000 kcal)	1	50.2	11.5	16.4	19.2	0.0001
	2	41.1	10.5	17.2	15.3	0.0005
Veg., potato, and legume intake (100 g)	1	15.1	4.7	16.4	10.2	0.0033
	2	12.4	4.5	17.2	7.5	0.0107
Veg., potato, and legume intake (100 g per 1000 kcal)	1	34.7	10.7	16.2	10.5	0.0030
	2	25.5	10.7	17.1	5.7	0.0235

[†] Vegetable intake did not include potato or legume consumption unless otherwise noted. Model 1 included statistical adjustment for differences in age, sex, and race. Model 2 included adjustment for differences in age, sex, race, BMI, physical activity, smoking, and alcohol use. R^2 represents the variance accounted for by the full model. Interpretation is as follows: Regarding fruit consumption, for each 100 g (3.5 ounce) higher intake of fruit, after adjusting for differences in age, sex, and race, telomeres were 26.9 base pairs longer, on average (F = 7.2, p = 0.0121).

When F&V intake was expressed as grams consumed per 1000 kcal, the relationship was stronger than when calculated simply as grams eaten (F = 25.9, p < 0.0001). Specifically, after adjusting for differences in the sociodemographic covariates, for each F&V consumption increment of 100 g (3.5 ounces) per 1000 kcal, telomeres were 66.9 base pairs longer. With all the covariates controlled, telomeres were 57.6 base pairs longer, on average (F = 23.3, p < 0.0001).

3.3. Fruit Intake and Telomeres

With data from women and men combined, fruit intake was related significantly and positively to leukocyte telomere length. With age, sex, and race controlled statistically, for each 100 g (3.5 ounces) of fruit consumed, telomeres were 26.9 base pairs longer, on average (F = 7.2, p = 0.0121). After adjusting for differences in the sociodemographic covariates (age, sex, race) and the lifestyle covariates (physical activity, smoking, BMI, and alcohol use), the association between fruit intake and telomere length remained significant and positive.

Specifically, for each 100 g (3.5 ounce) higher intake of fruits, telomeres were 23.1 base pairs longer (F = 6.0, p = 0.0206), on average.

Instead of expressing fruit intake as total grams consumed, reporting grams consumed per 1000 kcal generally strengthened the relationship between fruit intake and telomere length. After adjusting for the three sociodemographic covariates, for each 100 g (3.5 ounces) consumed per 1000 kcal, telomeres were 74.9 base pairs longer, on average (F = 10.8, p = 0.0027). After controlling for the sociodemographic and lifestyle covariates together, the association remained strong and significant (F = 8.7, p = 0.0063). Specifically, for each 100 g (3.5 ounces) of fruit eaten per 1000 kcal, telomeres were 63.1 base pairs longer, on average (Table 2).

3.4. Vegetable Intake and Telomeres

Vegetable intake, especially with potatoes excluded, was a significant predictor of telomere length, with data from women and men analyzed together. Telomeres were 32.5 base pairs longer for each 100 g (3.5 ounces) of vegetables consumed, after controlling for age, sex, and race (F = 15.4, p = 0.0005). Further, they were 28.9 base pairs longer after adjusting for all the covariates simultaneously (F = 13.2, p = 0.0011). With age, sex, and race controlled, telomeres were 71.4 base pairs longer for each 100 g (3.5 ounces) per 1000 kcal consumed (F = 25.9, p < 0.0001). Similarly, with the lifestyle covariates controlled, along with the sociodemographic covariates, telomeres were 59.1 base pairs longer for each 100 g (3.5 ounces) per 1000 kcal consumed (F = 21.3, p < 0.0001).

3.5. Fruit and Vegetable Intake

Fruit intake and vegetable consumption were positively related to each other. Specifically, with no covariates in the model, fruit intake accounted for 2.9% of the variance in vegetable intake (p < 0.0001) and vice versa. After adjusting for differences in age, sex, and race, the fruit and vegetable relationship demonstrated 2.5% overlapping variance (p < 0.0001). Both fruit intake (F = 5.0, p = 0.0341) and vegetable consumption (F = 12.1, p = 0.0016) were predictive of telomere length when placed into the same competitive regression model.

3.6. Intake of Legumes and Potatoes and Telomeres

As shown in Table 2, none of the relationships between legume and pulse consumption and telomere length were significant. Additionally, all the relationships between potato intake and telomere length were inverse and none were significant. However, when vegetable intake included potato consumption, the relationship with telomere intake remained positive and significant, although weaker than when vegetable intake excluded potato consumption. Similarly, when vegetable consumption included legume intake, the relationship was weakened, but it remained statistically significant.

3.7. Fruits, Vegetables, and Telomeres in U.S. Women Only

Table 3 shows the relationships between fruit and vegetable consumption, with and without potato and legume intake, and telomere length in U.S. women. With fruit and vegetable intakes combined, women with the highest intakes had the longest telomeres. Fruit intake was predictive of telomere length with age and race controlled (model 1) and also after adjusting for the other covariates, model 2. With vegetable intake expressed as grams per 1000 kcal, intake was positively associated with telomere length, in both models 1 and 2. However, when expressed as grams of vegetables consumed (not per 1000 kcal), intake was related to telomeres in model 1 but not in model 2. In U.S. women, vegetable intake, when combined with potato consumption, was positively associated with telomere length. Potato and legume intakes, when considered separately, were not predictive of telomere length in U.S. women, as shown in Table 3.

Table 3. Relationship between fruit and vegetable intake and telomere length in U.S. women only.

Exposure Variable	Model	Regression Coefficient	SE	R² (%)	F	p
Fruit and vegetable intake (100 g) [†]	1	33.6	7.8	15.3	18.7	0.0002
	2	28.8	7.4	16.3	15.1	0.0005
Fruit and vegetable intake (100 g per 1000 kcal) [†]	1	75.5	16.7	15.5	20.5	<0.0001
	2	63.5	16.3	16.3	15.2	0.0005
Fruit intake (100 g)	1	45.3	13.9	15.2	10.6	0.0029
	2	39.9	12.3	16.2	10.5	0.0030
Fruit intake (100 g per 1000 kcal)	1	100.8	28.3	15.4	12.7	0.0013
	2	85.8	25.1	16.3	11.6	0.0019
Vegetable intake (100 g) [†]	1	27.7	13.2	14.7	4.4	0.0449
	2	21.5	13.7	15.8	2.5	0.1274
Vegetable intake (100 g per 1000 kcal) [†]	1	50.6	17.6	14.8	8.3	0.0074
	2	33.5	17.0	15.8	3.9	0.0583
Potato intake (100 g)	1	1.1	19.2	14.4	0.0	0.9525
	2	4.2	21.0	15.6	0.0	0.8436
Potato intake (100 g per 1000 kcal)	1	22.0	42.7	14.4	0.3	0.6094
	2	20.8	46.6	15.6	0.2	0.6588
Legume and pulse intake (100 g)	1	16.3	16.9	14.4	0.9	0.3424
	2	13.7	18.2	15.6	0.6	0.4578
Legume and pulse intake (100 g per 1000 kcal)	1	28.2	33.7	14.4	0.7	0.4087
	2	18.3	35.2	15.6	0.3	0.6065
Vegetable and potato intake (100 g)	1	21.2	7.9	14.7	7.1	0.0123
	2	17.9	7.9	15.8	5.1	0.0315
Vegetable and potato intake (100 g per 1000 kcal)	1	54.9	17.6	14.7	9.8	0.0040
	2	42.8	18.3	15.8	5.5	0.0267
Veg., potato, and legume intake (100 g)	1	20.6	7.3	14.7	8.0	0.0083
	2	16.9	7.0	15.8	5.9	0.0212
Veg., potato, and legume intake (100 g per 1000 kcal)	1	40.8	17.1	14.6	5.7	0.0239
	2	30.0	16.3	15.7	3.4	0.0754

[†] Vegetable intake did not include potato and legume consumption unless otherwise noted. Model 1 included statistical adjustment for differences in age and race. Model 2 included adjustment for differences in age, race, BMI, physical activity, smoking, and alcohol use. R^2 represents the variance accounted for by the full model. Interpretation is as follows: Regarding vegetable consumption, including potato intake, for each 100 g (3.5 ounce) higher intake, after adjusting for differences in age and race, telomeres were 21.2 base pairs longer, on average (F = 7.1, p = 0.0123).

3.8. Fruits, Vegetables, and Telomeres in U.S. Men Only

Table 4 displays the associations between fruit and vegetable intake, without and with legume intake and potato consumption, and telomere length in U.S. men only. In all models, fruit and vegetable consumption, when combined, was associated with telomere length. The significant relationships persisted whether or not the sociodemographic or the sociodemographic and lifestyle covariates were controlled. Similarly, vegetable consumption was significantly and positively related to telomere length in models 1 and 2, as displayed in Table 4. When potatoes were combined with vegetables, the relationship was significant in model 1 but not in model 2. Likewise, when potatoes and legumes were combined with vegetable consumption, intake levels were not associated with telomere length. Additionally, unlike U.S. women, fruit intake was not predictive of telomere length within any of the models in U.S. men, except when combined with vegetable consumption (F&V). Lastly, potato intake and legume consumption, when considered separately, were not related to telomere length in any of the models in U.S. men.

Table 4. Relationship between fruit and vegetable intake and telomere length in U.S. men only.

Exposure Variable	Model	Regression Coefficient	SE	R^2 (%)	F	p
Fruit and vegetable intake (100 g) [†]	1	22.4	7.0	19.0	10.1	0.0034
	2	20.4	7.0	19.8	8.4	0.0070
Fruit and vegetable intake (100 g per 1000 kcal) [†]	1	53.2	15.2	18.8	12.3	0.0015
	2	45.8	15.2	19.5	9.0	0.0054
Fruit intake (100 g)	1	9.3	10.4	18.7	0.8	0.3747
	2	6.7	9.7	19.5	0.5	0.4925
Fruit intake (100 g per 1000 kcal)	1	34.4	24.2	18.7	2.0	0.1661
	2	25.5	22.4	19.4	1.3	0.2649
Vegetable intake (100 g) [†]	1	37.3	10.5	19.3	12.8	0.0013
	2	35.0	10.8	10.8	10.4	0.0031
Vegetable intake (100 g per 1000 kcal) [†]	1	102.7	25.4	19.3	16.2	0.0004
	2	93.0	26.4	20.0	12.3	0.0015
Potato intake (100 g)	1	−10.1	14.5	19.0	0.5	0.4909
	2	−9.7	14.2	19.8	0.5	0.5031
Potato intake (100 g per 1000 kcal)	1	−35.3	43.0	18.9	0.7	0.4198
	2	−37.0	42.3	19.8	0.8	0.3893
Legume and pulse intake (100 g)	1	−4.4	14.0	18.9	0.1	0.7570
	2	−7.3	14.6	19.6	0.3	0.6177
Legume and pulse intake (100 g per 1000 kcal)	1	−16.0	34.5	18.8	0.2	0.6456
	2	−27.4	35.9	19.6	0.6	0.4514
Vegetable and potato intake (100 g)	1	13.5	7.9	18.9	2.9	0.0992
	2	12.1	8.2	19.7	2.2	0.1517
Vegetable and potato intake (100 g per 1000 kcal)	1	43.3	20.9	18.8	4.3	0.0463
	2	36.5	22.2	19.6	2.7	0.1107
Veg., potato, and legume intake (100 g)	1	11.2	7.1	19.0	2.5	0.1258
	2	9.1	7.5	19.8	1.5	0.2309
Veg., potato, and legume intake (100 g per 1000 kcal)	1	28.6	18.6	18.7	2.4	0.1362
	2	20.3	20.2	19.5	1.0	0.3239

[†] Vegetable intake did not include potato or legume consumption unless otherwise noted. Model 1 included statistical adjustment for differences in age and race. Model 2 included adjustment for differences in age, race, BMI, physical activity, smoking, and alcohol use. R^2 represents the variance accounted for by the full model. Interpretation is as follows: Regarding fruit and vegetable consumption combined (grams), for each 100 g (3.5 ounce) higher intake, after adjusting for differences in age and race, telomeres were 22.4 base pairs longer, on average (F = 10.1, p = 0.0034).

4. Discussion

The principal goal of this investigation was to ascertain the association between fruit and vegetable (F&V) intake and leukocyte telomere length in a randomly selected sample of 5448 women and men who represented the non-institutionalized, civilian U.S. adult population. An ancillary aim was to evaluate the associations between potato consumption, and legume intake, and telomere length. Another objective was to assess the extent to which a number of sociodemographic and lifestyle covariates affected the relationships between fruit and vegetable intake and telomere length.

There were six key findings in this investigation. First, using the data for women and men combined, the relationship between F&V intake and telomere length was significant, positive, and meaningful, whether fruits and vegetables were evaluated together or separately. Second, consumption of potatoes, when considered separate from other vegetables, was not related to telomere length. Third, legume and pulse intake, when analyzed separate from other vegetables, was not related to the length of telomeres. Fourth, statistical control of the sociodemographic and lifestyle covariates had little effect on the relationships. Fifth, when the sample was delimited to U.S. women only, fruit intake and vegetable consumption were each related to biological aging. Sixth, when focusing on U.S. men only, vegetable intake was positively associated with telomere length, but fruit consumption was not.

In general, the more F&V consumed, the longer the telomere length tended to be. Intake of fruits and vegetables was directly related to telomere length. The associations were linear. After adjusting for differences in all the covariates (age, sex, race, smoking, physical activity, alcohol use, and BMI), regression analysis showed that each 100 g (3.5 ounce) increment of F&V consumption (combined) was predictive of telomeres that were 24.7 base pairs longer, on average (Table 2). Given each year of chronological age was associated with leukocyte telomeres that were 14.9 base pairs shorter, on average, each increment of 100 g (3.5 ounces) was associated with 1.7 fewer years of biological aging (24.7 ÷ 14.9 = 1.7 years).

Focusing on F&V intake combined, the U.S. 75th percentile (264 g) and the 25th percentile (0 g) differed by 264 g. Given each 100 g (3.5 ounce) increment in consumption was linked to telomeres there were 24.7 base pairs longer (Table 2), and given each 14.9 base pair differential was associated with 1.0 year of cellular aging, the difference between the 75th and 25th percentiles represented a difference of approximately 4.4 years of biological aging (100 g F&V = 24.7 base pairs; difference between the 75th and 25th percentiles = 264 g of F&V; 264 g ÷ 100 g = 2.64; 24.7 base pairs × 2.64 = 65.2 base pairs; 65.2 ÷ 14.9 = 4.4 years). Most would consider a biological aging difference of 4.4 years meaningful.

Level of consumption of cooked and raw vegetables (excluding potatoes and legumes) was a good predictor of biological aging. After controlling for all the covariates, for each 100 g of vegetables consumed, telomere base pairs were 28.9 base pairs longer, on average. Interpretation of these findings by comparing the 75th (146 g) and 25th (0 g) percentiles of intake indicated that adults at the 75th percentile had approximately 2.8 fewer years of biological aging, on average, than those at the 25th percentile of vegetable intake (146 ÷ 100 = 1.46; 1.46 × 28.9 = 42.2; 42.2 ÷ 14.9 = 2.8 years).

Intake of fruits was also a predictor of telomere length in the combined sample. The more fruits that were consumed, the longer the telomeres tended to be. After adjusting for all the covariates, for each 100 g (3.5 ounces) of fruits eaten, telomere base pairs were 23.1 base pairs longer, on average. Interpretation of these findings by comparing the 75th (130.9 g) and 25th (0 g) percentiles of intake showed that adults at the 75th percentile had approximately 2.0 fewer years of cellular aging, on average, than those at the 25th percentile of fruit consumption (130.9 ÷ 100 = 1.31; 1.31 × 23.1 = 30.3; 30.3 ÷ 14.9 = 2.0 years).

Each F&V consumption variable was expressed using two forms: (1) grams, (2) grams per 1000 kcal. Intake based on grams was straightforward. However, consumption was also standardized based on energy intake (g per 1000 kcal) to help offset the fact that adults who consume more total kilocalories tend to eat more fruits and vegetables. Indexing intake based on energy consumption allowed intake to be viewed as a proportion of total consumption (relative intake), rather than absolute intake (grams). In the present study, the relationships between F&V intake and telomere length were generally stronger when intake was standardized based on energy intake (g per 1000 kcal) compared to when the energy intake of the participant was ignored (grams).

A number of investigations have studied the link between intake of various foods and their relationships with telomere length. For example, consumption of sugar-sweetened soda was predictive of shorter telomeres. Specifically, for each 8 ounce serving per day, adults had 1.8 years of increased cellular aging, on average [54]. Similarly, for each 200 kcal of nuts and seeds consumed per day, adults had 1.7 years of decreased biological aging [55]. Furthermore, when adults with the highest quartile of fiber intake were compared to those in the lowest quartile, the cellular aging difference was almost 5 years [6]. Given the results of the present study, consumption of fruits and vegetables seems to compare inversely with sugar-sweetened soda, and positively with nuts and seeds, and dietary fiber, for potential protection against biological aging.

F&V consumption, treated separately or combined, was linearly related to telomere length in the present study. However, intake of particular foods does not happen in isolation. For example, in this investigation, adults who ate significant amounts of fruits and vegetables probably also ate higher levels of fiber and whole grains [1,56]. Fiber and whole grain intakes are connected to reduced risk of mortality and disease [57,58]. Consumption of fruits and vegetables is also associated with decreased disease and mortality [1,59]. Diets high in fiber and whole grains, and diets with large amounts of fruits and vegetables, tend to go hand-in-hand [56]. In short, some of the aging benefits associated with eating large amounts of fruits and vegetables, as seen in this study, might be partly a result of consuming higher levels of fiber and whole grains and perhaps other healthy foods.

When separated by sex, the relationships between both fruit and vegetable intakes and biological aging remained significant for women. However, for men, vegetable consumption was related to telomere length, but fruit intake was not. Why there was a difference between men and women is not clear. In both groups, differences in vegetable intake accounted for more variance in telomere length than fruit consumption.

Adjusting statistically for differences in age, sex, and race, reduced the likelihood that these sociodemographic factors influenced the results. Additionally, controlling for differences in physical activity, smoking, alcohol use, and BMI, minimized the influence of these lifestyle covariates. In general, controlling statistically for the lifestyle factors, in addition to the sociodemographic variables, weakened the relationship between fruits and vegetables and telomere length by an additional 15%. With all the covariates controlled, the findings showed the association between F&V intake and biological aging, as if all participants had the same age, sex, race, physical activity level, smoking habit, alcohol drinking behavior, and body mass index. Hence, it appears that only a small portion of the association between F&V and biological aging can be attributed to differences in these lifestyle factors.

In 2017, Rafie et al. reviewed several dietary studies that focused on the association between various foods, groups of foods, and patterns of eating, and telomere length [60]. Results were not consistent. A total of 13 investigations in the review targeted the relationship between fruit and/or vegetable intake and telomere length [60]. Five of the studies reported significant, positive associations. However, the other eight investigations failed to find significant relationships between fruits and/or vegetables and biological aging. The mixed results could be partly due to the varying methods used to classify fruits and vegetables, especially the latter. The current study is a good example. When potato intake was included as part of the vegetable group, the relationship was weakened significantly. In fact, when isolated, the potato food group was inversely associated with telomere length and the relationship was not significant. Similarly, the legume food group, which is sometimes considered part of the vegetable group, was not significantly related to biological aging when isolated from the vegetable group. In the present investigation, when the vegetable group was analyzed with both potatoes and legumes included, the relationship with telomere length was attenuated substantially, but it remained significant. Given the results of the present study, when developing a dietary pattern most predictive of reduced biologic aging, potatoes and legumes should probably not be included with the vegetable group.

Why were higher consumption levels of fruits and vegetables predictive of less biological aging (i.e., longer telomeres)? Although the exact mechanism is not known, it is likely that reduced inflammation and oxidative stress account for many of the differences [61–64]. Research indicates that telomere length serves as an index of the cumulative oxidative stress and inflammation of progenitor cells [5,65]. In other words, oxidative stress shortens telomeres [66]. On the other hand, F&V intake seems to preserve telomeres and reduce cell aging by reducing inflammation and oxidative stress. The benefits are not limited to adults. Research by Garcia-Calzon et al. shows that total dietary antioxidant capacity is related to leukocyte telomere length in children and adolescents [67].

Several systematic reviews indicate that fruit and vegetable intake reduces established markers of inflammation and oxidative stress [68–71]. Zhu cites numerous studies showing that phenolics in fruits and vegetables are the principal bioactive agents known to benefit health [70]. Moreover, in a meta-analysis by Hosseini et al., fruit and vegetable intake significantly reduced several inflammatory biomarkers, particularly tumor necrosis factor-alpha and C-reactive protein (CRP) [68]. Fruit and vegetable consumption was also associated with higher levels of gamma delta T cells (γ δ-T cells). Additionally, numerous investigations discussed by Hosseini et al. indicate that F&V intake positively affects immune cell function [68]. Independent of vegetable consumption, fruit intake also seems to have valuable effects on markers of systemic inflammation, although some studies have reported no effects [68,71].

In summary, fruits and vegetables include high levels of phytochemicals, which have significant antioxidant and anti-inflammatory properties [68–71]. By increasing antioxidants and anti-inflammatory levels in the body, F&V likely slow the biological aging process, which is manifested by longer leukocyte telomeres. Potato and legume intakes may be less related to telomere length compared to other vegetables because they seem to contain fewer phytochemicals and antioxidant properties [2,38]. Additionally, although speculative, potatoes may be unrelated to telomere length because they are often prepared with or garnished with a significant amount of fat, particularly saturated fat, in the United States. In short, it may not be the potatoes but the condiments they are consumed with that result in no relationship with telomere length.

There were multiple limitations associated with the current study. Perhaps of most importance, because NHANES used a cross-sectional design, cause-and-effect inferences cannot be made. Second, adults who indicated that they consumed lots of F&V could represent adults who have behaviors that are healthier than others. As a result of this potential problem, adjustments were made statistically to control for potential mediating factors, including sociodemographic and lifestyle variables. These covariates had little impact on the key associations. However, other variables, not assessed in this investigation, could account for some of the significant relationships unveiled in this investigation. Additionally, energy intake was estimated. Use of doubly labeled water would have been a better method to estimate energy intake, but it was not available. Additionally, the present investigation used telomere length as a single measure of biological aging. Other indices of aging were not evaluated. Lastly, telomerase activity was not assessed.

This study also possessed multiple strengths. For example, the sample was large, including almost 5500 adults of all races. Additionally, the age range was broad, including adults 20 to 84 years old. Second, because subjects were randomly selected, results are representative of the non-institutionalized, adult population of the U.S. Third, many sociodemographic and lifestyle measures were statistically adjusted for, reducing their influence on the associations of interest. Fourth, a high-quality laboratory was used to assess the length of leukocyte telomeres. In short, valid and reliable procedures were employed to generate the telomere information. Consequently, chronological age was a meaningful predictor of telomere length, as one would expect.

Although the present investigation noted a significant relationship between fruit and vegetable consumption and longer telomeres in U.S. women, and vegetable intake and less biological aging in U.S. men, there remains much to learn about the relationships. To date, most research focusing on diet and telomere length has been cross sectional. Although long-term randomized controlled trials studying changes in telomeres are not feasible, prospective cohort studies would be valuable. Prospective telomere investigations lasting decades would help to determine whether abundant fruit and vegetable consumption reduces risk of developing short telomeres.

5. Conclusions

Consumption of fruits and vegetables, considered separately and combined, was linearly related to telomere length in a large, random sample of women and men, when considered together. After adjusting for a number of sociodemographic and lifestyle covariates, for each 100 g (3.5 ounces) of fruit eaten per day, telomeres reflected 1.6 fewer years of biological aging. Similarly, for each 100 g (3.5 ounces) of vegetables consumed per day (excluding potatoes and legumes), the length of telomeres signified 1.9 fewer years of cellular aging. Comparing the U.S. 75th percentile to the 25th percentile of fruit and vegetable intake was predictive of 4.4 years of reduced cellular aging. On the other hand, potato intake and consumption of legumes and pulses were not related to telomere length. When the sample was delimited to U.S. women, both fruits and vegetables were inversely associated with biological aging. However, in U.S. men, vegetable intake was related to telomere length, but fruit consumption was not. Overall, this investigation highlights the higher levels of biological aging associated with adults who do not eat significant amounts of fruits and vegetables, especially the latter. Results of this study support the Dietary Guidelines for Americans (2015–2020), which encourage adults to eat large amounts of fruits and vegetables each day as part of a high-quality diet.

Funding: This research received no external funding.

Institutional Review Board Statement: This study was conducted according to the guidelines of the Declaration of Helsinki, and The Ethics Review Board (ERB) of the National Center for Health Statistics, approved the NHANES data collection protocol. The ethical approval code for NHANES data collection from 1999–2002 was #98-12.

Informed Consent Statement: Written informed consent was obtained from all subjects involved in this study.

Data Availability Statement: All data supporting the finding are posted online as part of the National Health and Nutrition Examination Survey (NHANES). The data are free and can be found at the following website: https://wwwn.cdc.gov/nchs/nhanes/Default.aspx (accessed on 22 April 2021).

Conflicts of Interest: The author declares no conflict of interest.

References

1. U.S. Department of Health and Human Services; The U.S. Department Agriculture. *2015–2020 Dietary Guidelines for Americans*, 8th ed.; U.S. Department of Health and Human Services: Washington, DC, USA; The U.S. Department Agriculture: Washington, DC, USA, 2015.
2. World Health Organization, Healthy Diet. Available online: https://www.who.int/news-room/fact-sheets/detail/healthy-diet (accessed on 10 March 2021).
3. Wang, X.; Ouyang, Y.; Liu, J.; Zhu, M.; Zhao, G.; Bao, W.; Hu, F.B. Fruit and vegetable consumption and mortality from all causes, cardiovascular disease, and cancer: Systematic review and dose-response meta-analysis of prospective cohort studies. *BMJ* **2014**, *349*, g4490. [CrossRef]
4. Nguyen, B.; Bauman, A.; Gale, J.; Banks, E.; Kritharides, L.; Ding, D. Fruit and vegetable consumption and all-cause mortality: Evidence from a large Australian cohort study. *Int. J. Behav. Nutr. Phys. Act.* **2016**, *13*, 9. [CrossRef]
5. Aviv, A. Leukocyte telomere length: The telomere tale continues. *Am. J. Clin. Nutr.* **2009**, *89*, 1721–1722. [CrossRef]
6. Tucker, L.A. Dietary Fiber and Telomere Length in 5674 U.S. Adults: An NHANES Study of Biological Aging. *Nutrients* **2018**, *10*, 400. [CrossRef]
7. Harley, C.B.; Vaziri, H.; Counter, C.M.; Allsopp, R.C. The telomere hypothesis of cellular aging. *Exp. Gerontol.* **1992**, *27*, 375–382. [CrossRef]
8. Kimura, M.; Hjelmborg, J.V.; Gardner, J.P.; Bathum, L.; Brimacombe, M.; Lu, X.; Christiansen, L.; Vaupel, J.W.; Aviv, A.; Christensen, K. Telomere length and mortality: A study of leukocytes in elderly Danish twins. *Am. J. Epidemiol.* **2008**, *167*, 799–806. [CrossRef]
9. Mather, K.A.; Jorm, A.F.; Parslow, R.A.; Christensen, H. Is telomere length a biomarker of aging? A review. *J. Gerontol. A Biol. Sci. Med. Sci.* **2011**, *66*, 202–213. [CrossRef]
10. Mather, K.A.; Jorm, A.F.; Milburn, P.J.; Tan, X.; Easteal, S.; Christensen, H. No associations between telomere length and age-sensitive indicators of physical function in mid and later life. *J. Gerontol. A Biol. Sci. Med. Sci.* **2010**, *65*, 792–799. [CrossRef] [PubMed]
11. Martin-Ruiz, C.M.; Gussekloo, J.; van Heemst, D.; von Zglinicki, T.; Westendorp, R.G. Telomere length in white blood cells is not associated with morbidity or mortality in the oldest old: A population-based study. *Aging Cell* **2005**, *4*, 287–290. [CrossRef]
12. Cawthon, R.M.; Smith, K.R.; O'Brien, E.; Sivatchenko, A.; Kerber, R.A. Association between telomere length in blood and mortality in people aged 60 years or older. *Lancet* **2003**, *361*, 393–395. [CrossRef]

13. Bakaysa, S.L.; Mucci, L.A.; Slagboom, P.E.; Boomsma, D.I.; McClearn, G.E.; Johansson, B.; Pedersen, N.L. Telomere length predicts survival independent of genetic influences. *Aging Cell* **2007**, *6*, 769–774. [CrossRef]
14. Ehrlenbach, S.; Willeit, P.; Kiechl, S.; Willeit, J.; Reindl, M.; Schanda, K.; Kronenberg, F.; Brandstatter, A. Influences on the reduction of relative telomere length over 10 years in the population-based Bruneck Study: Introduction of a well-controlled high-throughput assay. *Int. J. Epidemiol.* **2009**, *38*, 1725–1734. [CrossRef] [PubMed]
15. Lian, F.; Wang, J.; Huang, X.; Wu, Y.; Cao, Y.; Tan, X.; Xu, X.; Hong, Y.; Yang, L.; Gao, X. Effect of vegetable consumption on the association between peripheral leucocyte telomere length and hypertension: A case-control study. *BMJ Open* **2015**, *5*, e009305. [CrossRef]
16. Marcon, F.; Siniscalchi, E.; Crebelli, R.; Saieva, C.; Sera, F.; Fortini, P.; Simonelli, V.; Palli, D. Diet-related telomere shortening and chromosome stability. *Mutagenesis* **2012**, *27*, 49–57. [CrossRef]
17. Lee, J.Y.; Jun, N.R.; Yoon, D.; Shin, C.; Baik, I. Association between dietary patterns in the remote past and telomere length. *Eur. J. Clin. Nutr.* **2015**, *69*, 1048–1052. [CrossRef]
18. Bethancourt, H.J.; Kratz, M.; Beresford, S.A.A.; Hayes, M.G.; Kuzawa, C.W.; Duazo, P.L.; Borja, J.B.; Eisenberg, D.T.A. No association between blood telomere length and longitudinally assessed diet or adiposity in a young adult Filipino population. *Eur. J. Nutr.* **2017**, *56*, 295–308. [CrossRef]
19. NHANES. *The National Health and Nutrition Examination Survey: Sample Design, 1999–2006*; U.S. Department of Health and Human Services: Washington, DC, USA, 1999–2006.
20. Ruan, D. *Intelligent Data Mining: Techniques and Applications*; Springer: Berlin, Germany; New York, NY, USA, 2005; 517p.
21. Bertges, D.J.; Zwolak, R.M.; Deaton, D.H.; Teigen, C.; Tapper, S.; Koslow, A.R.; Makaroun, M.S. Current hospital costs and medicare reimbursement for endovascular abdominal aortic aneurysm repair. *J. Vasc. Surg.* **2003**, *37*, 272–279. [CrossRef]
22. McCann, S.J. Personality and American state differences in obesity prevalence. *J. Psychol.* **2011**, *145*, 419–433. [CrossRef]
23. Takeda, K.; Mishiba, M.; Sugiura, H.; Nakajima, A.; Kohama, M.; Hiramatsu, S. Evaluated reference intervals for serum free thyroxine and thyrotropin using the conventional outliner rejection test without regard to presence of thyroid antibodies and prevalence of thyroid dysfunction in Japanese subjects. *Endocr. J.* **2009**, *56*, 1059–1066. [CrossRef] [PubMed]
24. NHANES. National Center of Health Statistics Research Ethics Review Board (ERB) Approval. Available online: http://www.cdc.gov/nchs/nhanes/irba98.htm (accessed on 8 April 2021).
25. NHANES. *MEC in-Person Dietary Interviewers Procedures Manual*; U.S. Department of Health and Human Services, Center for Disease Control and Prevention: Washington, DC, USA, 2002.
26. NHANES. Dietary Interview, Individual Foods. Available online: https://wwwn.cdc.gov/Nchs/Nhanes/2001-2002/DRXIFF_B.htm (accessed on 8 April 2021).
27. Haddad, E.H.; Tanzman, J.S. What do vegetarians in the United States eat? *Am. J. Clin. Nutr.* **2003**, *78*, 626S–632S. [CrossRef] [PubMed]
28. Kant, A.K.; Graubard, B.I.; Mattes, R.D. Association of food form with self-reported 24-h energy intake and meal patterns in US adults: NHANES 2003–2008. *Am. J. Clin. Nutr.* **2012**, *96*, 1369–1378. [CrossRef]
29. Tucker, L.A. Caffeine consumption and telomere length in men and women of the National Health and Nutrition Examination Survey (NHANES). *Nutr. Metab.* **2017**, *14*, 10. [CrossRef]
30. Christensen, K.; Lawler, T.; Mares, J. Dietary Carotenoids and Non-Alcoholic Fatty Liver Disease among US Adults, NHANES 2003–2014. *Nutrients* **2019**, *11*, 1101. [CrossRef]
31. Kappeler, R.; Eichholzer, M.; Rohrmann, S. Meat consumption and diet quality and mortality in NHANES III. *Eur. J. Clin. Nutr.* **2013**, *67*, 598–606. [CrossRef]
32. Wolffenbuttel, B.H.R.; Heiner-Fokkema, M.R.; Green, R.; Gans, R.O.B. Relationship between serum B12 concentrations and mortality: Experience in NHANES. *BMC Med.* **2020**, *18*, 307. [CrossRef]
33. Deng, F.E.; Shivappa, N.; Tang, Y.; Mann, J.R.; Hebert, J.R. Association between diet-related inflammation, all-cause, all-cancer, and cardiovascular disease mortality, with special focus on prediabetics: Findings from NHANES III. *Eur. J. Nutr.* **2017**, *56*, 1085–1093. [CrossRef] [PubMed]
34. Liao, Y.; Cooper, R.S.; McGee, D.L. Iron status and coronary heart disease: Negative findings from the NHANES I epidemiologic follow-up study. *Am. J. Epidemiol.* **1994**, *139*, 704–712. [CrossRef]
35. Schulze, M.B.; Fung, T.T.; Manson, J.E.; Willett, W.C.; Hu, F.B. Dietary patterns and changes in body weight in women. *Obesity* **2006**, *14*, 1444–1453. [CrossRef]
36. Mozaffarian, D.; Hao, T.; Rimm, E.B.; Willett, W.C.; Hu, F.B. Changes in diet and lifestyle and long-term weight gain in women and men. *N. Engl. J. Med.* **2011**, *364*, 2392–2404. [CrossRef] [PubMed]
37. Halton, T.L.; Willett, W.C.; Liu, S.; Manson, J.E.; Stampfer, M.J.; Hu, F.B. Potato and french fry consumption and risk of type 2 diabetes in women. *Am. J. Clin. Nutr.* **2006**, *83*, 284–290. [CrossRef]
38. National Health Service. The Eatwell Plate. Available online: http://www.nhs.uk/Livewell/Goodfood/Pages/eatwell-plate.aspx (accessed on 8 April 2021).
39. Archer, E.; Hand, G.A.; Blair, S.N. Validity of U.S. nutritional surveillance:National Health and Nutrition Examination Survey caloric energy intake data, 1971–2010. *PLoS ONE* **2013**, *8*, e76632. [CrossRef] [PubMed]
40. Mifflin, M.D.; St Jeor, S.T.; Hill, L.A.; Scott, B.J.; Daugherty, S.A.; Koh, Y.O. A new predictive equation for resting energy expenditure in healthy individuals. *Am. J. Clin. Nutr.* **1990**, *51*, 241–247. [CrossRef]

41. NHANES. Data Documentation, Codebook, and Frequencies: Physical Activity (PAQ). Available online: https://wwwn.cdc.gov/Nchs/Nhanes/1999-2000/PAQ.htm#PAQ180 (accessed on 8 April 2021).
42. Institute of Medicine. *Dietary Reference Intakes for Energy, Carbohydrate, Fiber, Fat, Fatty Acids, Cholesterol, Protein, and Amino Acids*; National Academies Press: Washington, DC, USA, 2005.
43. Tucker, L.A. Fiber Intake and Insulin Resistance in 6374 Adults: The Role of Abdominal Obesity. *Nutrients* **2018**, *10*, 237. [CrossRef]
44. Demanelis, K.; Jasmine, F.; Chen, L.S.; Chernoff, M.; Tong, L.; Delgado, D.; Zhang, C.; Shinkle, J.; Sabarinathan, M.; Lin, H.; et al. Determinants of telomere length across human tissues. *Science* **2020**, *369*, 5609. [CrossRef]
45. Needham, B.L.; Adler, N.; Gregorich, S.; Rehkopf, D.; Lin, J.; Blackburn, E.H.; Epel, E.S. Socioeconomic status, health behavior, and leukocyte telomere length in the National Health and Nutrition Examination Survey, 1999–2002. *Soc. Sci. Med.* **2013**, *85*, 1–8. [CrossRef]
46. Cawthon, R.M. Telomere measurement by quantitative PCR. *Nucleic Acids Res.* **2002**, *30*, e47. [CrossRef] [PubMed]
47. NHANES. 2001-2002 Data documentation, Codebook, and Frequencies. Telomere Mean and Standard Deviation. Available online: https://wwwn.cdc.gov/Nchs/Nhanes/2001-2002/TELO_B.htm (accessed on 8 April 2021).
48. NHANES. NHANES Anthropometry Procedures Manual. Available online: https://www.cdc.gov/nchs/data/nhanes/nhanes_13_14/2013_Anthropometry.pdf (accessed on 8 April 2021).
49. ACSM. *ACSM's Guidelines for Exercise Testing and Prescription*, 9th ed.; American College of Sports Medicine: Baltimore, MD, USA, 2014.
50. NHANES. Data Documentation, Codebook, and Frequencies: Alcohol Use. Available online: https://wwwn.cdc.gov/Nchs/Nhanes/2001-2002/ALQ_B.htm (accessed on 8 April 2021).
51. Ainsworth, B.E.; Haskell, W.L.; Whitt, M.C.; Irwin, M.L.; Swartz, A.M.; Strath, S.J.; O'Brien, W.L.; Bassett, D.R., Jr.; Schmitz, K.H.; Emplaincourt, P.O.; et al. Compendium of physical activities: An update of activity codes and MET intensities. *Med. Sci. Sports Exerc.* **2000**, *32*, S498–S504. [CrossRef]
52. NHANES. Data Documentation, Codebook, and Frequencies: Smoking, Cigarette, Tobacco Use. Available online: https://wwwn.cdc.gov/Nchs/Nhanes/2001-2002/SMQ_B.htm (accessed on 8 April 2021).
53. SAS Institute. SAS/STAT User's Guide, The SurveyReg Procedure. Available online: https://support.sas.com/documentation/onlinedoc/stat/142/surveyreg.pdf (accessed on 8 April 2021).
54. Leung, C.W.; Laraia, B.A.; Needham, B.L.; Rehkopf, D.H.; Adler, N.E.; Lin, J.; Blackburn, E.H.; Epel, E.S. Soda and cell aging: Associations between sugar-sweetened beverage consumption and leukocyte telomere length in healthy adults from the National Health and Nutrition Examination Surveys. *Am. J. Public Health* **2014**, *104*, 2425–2431. [CrossRef] [PubMed]
55. Tucker, L.A. Consumption of Nuts and Seeds and Telomere Length in 5582 Men and Women of the National Health and Nutrition Examination Survey (NHANES). *J. Nutr. Health Aging* **2017**, *21*, 233–240. [CrossRef]
56. Tapsell, L.C.; Neale, E.P.; Satija, A.; Hu, F.B. Foods, Nutrients, and Dietary Patterns: Interconnections and Implications for Dietary Guidelines. *Adv. Nutr.* **2016**, *7*, 445–454. [CrossRef]
57. Kim, Y.; Je, Y. Dietary fiber intake and total mortality: A meta-analysis of prospective cohort studies. *Am. J. Epidemiol.* **2014**, *180*, 565–573. [CrossRef]
58. Zhang, B.; Zhao, Q.; Guo, W.; Bao, W.; Wang, X. Association of whole grain intake with all-cause, cardiovascular, and cancer mortality: A systematic review and dose-response meta-analysis from prospective cohort studies. *Eur. J. Clin. Nutr.* **2018**, *72*, 57–65. [CrossRef]
59. Aune, D.; Giovannucci, E.; Boffetta, P.; Fadnes, L.T.; Keum, N.; Norat, T.; Greenwood, D.C.; Riboli, E.; Vatten, L.J.; Tonstad, S. Fruit and vegetable intake and the risk of cardiovascular disease, total cancer and all-cause mortality-a systematic review and dose-response meta-analysis of prospective studies. *Int. J. Epidemiol.* **2017**, *46*, 1029–1056. [CrossRef]
60. Rafie, N.; Golpour Hamedani, S.; Barak, F.; Safavi, S.M.; Miraghajani, M. Dietary patterns, food groups and telomere length: A systematic review of current studies. *Eur. J. Clin. Nutr.* **2017**, *71*, 151–158. [CrossRef]
61. Kordinas, V.; Ioannidis, A.; Chatzipanagiotou, S. The Telomere/Telomerase System in Chronic Inflammatory Diseases. Cause or Effect? *Genes* **2016**, *7*, 60. [CrossRef] [PubMed]
62. Zhang, J.; Rane, G.; Dai, X.; Shanmugam, M.K.; Arfuso, F.; Samy, R.P.; Lai, M.K.; Kappei, D.; Kumar, A.P.; Sethi, G. Ageing and the telomere connection: An intimate relationship with inflammation. *Ageing Res. Rev.* **2016**, *25*, 55–69. [CrossRef] [PubMed]
63. Jurk, D.; Wilson, C.; Passos, J.F.; Oakley, F.; Correia-Melo, C.; Greaves, L.; Saretzki, G.; Fox, C.; Lawless, C.; Anderson, R.; et al. Chronic inflammation induces telomere dysfunction and accelerates ageing in mice. *Nat. Commun.* **2014**, *2*, 4172. [CrossRef] [PubMed]
64. Babizhayev, M.A.; Savel'yeva, E.L.; Moskvina, S.N.; Yegorov, Y.E. Telomere length is a biomarker of cumulative oxidative stress, biologic age, and an independent predictor of survival and therapeutic treatment requirement associated with smoking behavior. *Am. J. Ther.* **2011**, *18*, e209–e226. [CrossRef] [PubMed]
65. Houben, J.M.; Moonen, H.J.; van Schooten, F.J.; Hageman, G.J. Telomere length assessment: Biomarker of chronic oxidative stress? *Free Radic. Biol. Med.* **2008**, *44*, 235–246. [CrossRef] [PubMed]
66. von Zglinicki, T. Oxidative stress shortens telomeres. *Trends Biochem. Sci.* **2002**, *27*, 339–344. [CrossRef]
67. Garcia-Calzon, S.; Moleres, A.; Martinez-Gonzalez, M.A.; Martinez, J.A.; Zalba, G.; Marti, A. Dietary total antioxidant capacity is associated with leukocyte telomere length in a children and adolescent population. *Clin. Nutr.* **2015**, *34*, 694–699. [CrossRef]

68. Hosseini, B.; Berthon, B.S.; Saedisomeolia, A.; Starkey, M.R.; Collison, A.; Wark, P.A.B.; Wood, L.G. Effects of fruit and vegetable consumption on inflammatory biomarkers and immune cell populations: A systematic literature review and meta-analysis. *Am. J. Clin. Nutr.* **2018**, *108*, 136–155. [CrossRef]
69. Lapuente, M.; Estruch, R.; Shahbaz, M.; Casas, R. Relation of Fruits and Vegetables with Major Cardiometabolic Risk Factors, Markers of Oxidation, and Inflammation. *Nutrients* **2019**, *11*, 2381. [CrossRef]
70. Zhu, F.; Du, B.; Xu, B. Anti-inflammatory effects of phytochemicals from fruits, vegetables, and food legumes: A review. *Crit. Rev. Food Sci. Nutr.* **2018**, *58*, 1260–1270. [CrossRef]
71. Joseph, S.V.; Edirisinghe, I.; Burton-Freeman, B.M. Fruit Polyphenols: A Review of Anti-inflammatory Effects in Humans. *Crit. Rev. Food Sci. Nutr.* **2016**, *56*, 419–444. [CrossRef]

Review

Seafood Intake as a Method of Non-Communicable Diseases (NCD) Prevention in Adults

Dominika Jamioł-Milc [1,*], Jowita Biernawska [2], Magdalena Liput [3], Laura Stachowska [4] and Zdzisław Domiszewski [5]

1. Department of Human Nutrition and Metabolomics, Pomeranian Medical University in Szczecin, 71-460 Szczecin, Poland
2. Department of Anaesthesiology and Intensive Therapy, Pomeranian Medical University, 71-242 Szczecin, Poland; jowita.biernawska@pum.edu.pl
3. Department of Pharmacognosy and Natural Medicines, Pomeranian Medical University in Szczecin, 70-111 Szczecin, Poland; mliput@pum.edu.pl
4. Department of Biochemical Sciences, Pomeranian Medical University in Szczecin, 71-460 Szczecin, Poland; laura.stachowska@pum.edu.pl
5. Department of Food Industry Processes and Facilities, Koszalin University of Technology, 75-620 Koszalin, Poland; zdzislaw.domiszewski@tu.koszalin.pl
* Correspondence: dominika.jamiol@pum.edu.pl; Tel.: +48-91-441-48-06; Fax: +48-91-441-48-07

Abstract: Seafood (fish in particular) is one of the main food groups in nutrition models with proven health benefits. Seafood has long been considered a very valuable dietary component, mainly due to presence of n-3 polyunsaturated fatty acids (n-3 PUFA) but it is also an important source of protein (including collagen), anserine, taurine, iodine, selenium, vitamin A, vitamin K, vitamin D, tocopherols, B vitamins and astaxanthin. Considering the beneficial effects of these ingredients on blood pressure, lipid profile and the inflammatory process, seafood should be an essential component of the diet. Non-communicable diseases (NCD) such as cardiovascular diseases, cancer, diabetes and mental disorder, chronic respiratory diseases are common diseases associated with advanced age. Promotion of a healthy lifestyle (including proper nutritional behavior) and prevention of diseases are the most effective and efficient ways to decrease premature mortality from NCD and to maintain mental health and well-being. This review article shows the potential preventive and therapeutic effects of seafood with an emphasis on fish. Our narrative review presents the results of systematic reviews and meta-analysis.

Keywords: diet; seafood; elderly people; health; non-communicable diseases

1. Introduction

Seafood includes fish or shellfish, divided into crustaceans and molluscs. Crustaceans include shrimp, lobsters, crabs, crayfish, and molluscs include scallops, oysters, clams, and squid [1]. The most important national and international nutritional guidelines recommend the regular consumption of fish [2,3]. Seafood (fish in particular) is one of the main food groups in nutrition models with proven with health benefits, such as the Mediterranean diet [4] and Dietary Approaches to Stop Hypertension dietary pattern [5].

The consumption of fish in the USA has not changed over almost two decades (1999–2016) [6]. There are variations in the amount of fish consumed both within and between populations. Consumption of fish in many Western populations differs. It can be divided in three groups regarding the frequency of consumption and each group is represented by approximately one third of the studied populations.

The first group includes people who do not eat fish at all, the second group includes people who consume fish up to once a week, and the representatives of the third group eat fish more often than once a week. The differences in fish consumption are undoubtedly due to personal and environmental factors (e.g., culture, place of residence, family habits, socioeconomic status) [7]. In the European and US populations surveyed (86,467 participants from the US, Estonia, Finland, Greece, Italy, and the Netherlands), the average fish consumption ranged from 0.19 servings/day (19 g/day) to 0.75 servings/day (75 g/day). Overall, participants in the European cohorts had a higher fish consumption than the US cohorts [8]. It has been estimated approximately 37% of elderly (range 72–83 years) eat one serving of fish less than once a week, 29% 1 serving/weekly, approx. 27% 2–3 servings/weekly, and only 6% more than four servings/weekly (results from one French cohort and four US cohorts) [9].

The mean consumption of eicosapentaenoic acid and docosahexaenoic acid (EPA and DHA) ranged from 89 to 563 mg/day and was generally adequate to fish consumption. The exception was for the Greek population which had a relatively higher fish consumption than EPA + DHA consumption, suggesting a predominant consumption of white non-greasy fish. Overall, participants in the European cohorts consumed more fish than the US cohorts [8].

As World Health Organization (WHO) experts concluded, promotion of a healthy lifestyle (including proper nutritional behavior) and prevention of diseases are the most effective and efficient ways to decrease premature mortality from non-communicable diseases (NCD) and to maintain mental health and well-being [10]. It is recommended to eat at least two servings of fish per week, one of which should be oily fish [2]. Seafood is of interest as a dietary component with potential beneficial effects in preventing the development of chronic NCD due to the presence of long-chain n-3 fatty acids (especially in oily marine fish), essential amino acids, vitamins and minerals and ingredients with antioxidant activity [11–14]. Considering the beneficial effects of these ingredients on blood pressure, lipid profile and the inflammatory process, seafood should be an essential component of the diet. Meanwhile, the consumption of this group of products varies globally. Several epidemiological studies have shown that higher fish consumption is associated with lower rates of cardiovascular diseases (CVD), coronary heart disease (CHD), and cerebrovascular mortality (including mortality from stroke, myocardial infarction and sudden cardiac death) [15–17].

The World Health Organization (WHO) estimates that the global elderly population will increase from 12% to 22% by 2050 [18]. It has been estimated that non-communicable diseases (NCD) such as cardiovascular diseases, cancer, diabetes and mental disorder, chronic respiratory diseases, which are common diseases associated with advanced age [19], are the leading cause of death in the world (over 70% of all deaths worldwide in 2016). Probability of premature mortality from NCD in the age group of 30–70 years old ranges between 8% and 31%, depending on geographical localization [10]. NCD are an economic burden on the economy, especially in developing countries [20].

Therefore, it is very important to introduce early prophylaxis in order to prevent age-related diseases, to minimize the risk or slow down their development, thus affecting well-being of older adults [19].

This narrative review briefly describes the nutrients and bioactive components found in seafood. It shows the potential preventive and therapeutic effects of seafood with an emphasis on fish based on 14 systematic reviews and meta-analysis published in 2007–2020. The systematic reviews and meta-analysis are considered to be the most powerful assessing tools [21].

2. Nutrients and Bioactive Compound

Seafood has long been considered a very valuable dietary component, mainly due to presence of n-3 polyunsaturated fatty acids (n-3 PUFA) but it is also an important source of protein (including collagen), anserine, taurine, iodine, selenium, vitamin A, vitamin K, vitamin D, tocopherols, B vitamins and astaxanthin [11,22–26].

2.1. Eicosapentaenoic Acid and Docosahexaenoic Acid

Eicosapentaenoic acid (EPA) and docosahexaenoic acid (DHA), which are included in the so-called long-chain acids (n-3 LC PUFA) have particularly health beneficial properties [22]. EPA and DHA acid show a beneficial effect on endothelial dysfunctions, anti-inflammatory properties [27–30], and reducing blood viscosity [31]. N-3 fatty acids lower the level of lipids [32], blood pressure [33] and decrease the risk of cognitive decline [34]. Vitamin D and selenium also present in fish, can enhance the neuroprotective effects of long-chain n-3 fatty acids [34]. Selenium (especially in the form of selenoproteins) and vitamin D are involved in several processes within central nervous system [35–37]. Vitamin D receptors are present in numerous tissues, including brain cells. Vitamin D is an important factor in regulation of the development and functioning of nerve cells. It probably plays a role similar to that of neurosteroids, influencing intracellular metabolism. The active form of vitamin D is involved in the synthesis and release of nerve growth factor (NGF—neurotrophic factors influencing neuron differentiation) and increases the levels of glial cell line-derived neurotrophic factor (GDNF). It also modifies the expression of (i) genes encoding the enzyme choline acetyltransferase (CAT) which participates in the synthesis of acetylcholine neurotransmitter, and (ii) genes associated with GABA-ergic neurotransmission. The hormonal form of vitamin D (1.25-(OH)2 D3) as well as selenium influence calcium ion pathways in the neuronal environment by altering the calcium ion homeostasis. Vitamin D activates the glutamyl transpeptidase enzyme activity and thereby stimulates the synthesis of glutathione. Selenium, selenoproteins and vitamin D protect the cells of the central nervous system against oxidative damage [36,37]. The long-chain docosapentaenoic acid (22:5n-3) is also present in seafood. It is believed that both the circulating and tissue level of this fatty acid may have a beneficial cardiovascular effect [38].

The richest sources of EPA and DHA are mainly fatty fish (including mackerel, salmon, herring, sardines, sprats, farmed trout). Depending on the fishing season, these fish contain from 1.4 to 2.5 g of EPA and DHA in 100 g of muscle tissue [22,39]. As a rule, the lowest EPA and DHA content in oily fish occurs during spawning (March–April) and winter migration, i.e., when the fish are not feeding [40]. However, the highest content occurs after the period of abundant foraging, which most often occurs in the autumn months, between September and October [39].

Farmed seafood is wrongly viewed as being nutritionally inferior to wild seafood. Taking into account EPA and DHA, farmed fish, both marine and freshwater, are often a richer source of fatty acids. This is due to the higher fat content of the feed, which is often based on fishmeal or fish oil rich in EPA and DHA. Farmed seafood also have a less intensive lifestyle compared to their wild counterparts, therefore their fat content is higher [41,42].

Interestingly, a decrease in the content of n-3 LC PUFA (DHA, EPA) in farmed fish has been observed for several years, as a result of replacing fishmeal and fish oil with vegetable oils in feeds [43,44].

Seasonal fluctuations in the content of lipids and n-3 PUFAs occur in both marine fish [45] and freshwater fish [46,47] and are related to fish development cycle (lipid metabolism) and food (availability and composition of the food) [48].

When comparing content of EPA and DHA in seafood, only absolute content of acids per 100 g of the product should be taken into account. The weight of 100 g of muscle tissue of farmed salmon contains 1.36 g of EPA and DHA, while in wild salmon—0.76 g. Observed differences result from higher lipid content in muscle tissue of farmed fish [43]. The lowest content of EPA and DHA, 80–160 mg/100 g, is found in lean fish (cod, pollock, hake) and mollusks such as octopus and cuttlefish.

Assuming that the daily requirement of DHA + EPA is 500 mg [49], it is enough to eat only 20–75 g of oily fish to provide this amount of acids. It does not seem to be a large amount, so it can be easily included in diet even for people who do not prefer fish dishes.

2.2. Astaxanthin and Tocopherols

Astaxanthin (AX) is a red pigment from the carotenoid group, which does not have the properties of provitamin A. The marine products such as alga, shrimp, crabs, trout, krill, lobster, crayfish, salmon and salmon roe are the source of AX [50,51]. It is used as a feed ingredient for farmed fish and as a food coloring [23]. Among salmonids, the content of astaxanthin ranges from 3 to 37 mg/kg and the highest content was estimated in free-living species where the content was at the level of 26–38 mg/kg flesh [23,52]. Thus, a 200 g serving of salmon provides about 1–7 mg of astaxanthin. In a randomized, double-blind, placebo-controlled trial conducted in healthy subjects aged 35–69 years, no side effects were found with a daily intake of 6 mg of astaxanthin (*H. pluvialis* algae extract) [53].

Among carotenoids, astaxanthin most effectively protects cells, lipids and lipoproteins of cell membranes against oxidative damage (fluorometric assay: BODIPY 665/676 or BODIPY 581/591 C11 as an indicators; AMVN as a peroxyl radical generator; Trolox as a calibrator). Astaxanthin was more effective than fish oil in modulating the immune system response and reducing the risk of vascular and inflammatory diseases. The antioxidant activity of astaxanthin is 10 times more than zeaxanthin, lutein, canthaxanthin, β-carotene and 100 times higher than α-tocopherol [23]. Oxidative stress and inflammation are pathophysiological features of atherosclerotic cardiovascular disease and cancer [54].

α-, β-, γ-, and δ-tocopherol, fat-soluble vitamin, which are present in seafood also have antioxidant properties [24]. The vitamin E content in fish is higher than that of meat or poultry and varies between species and tissues (higher amounts in dark muscle). The content ranges from 0.1 mg/100 g in some wild fish species to 3–4 mg/100 g in aquaculture fish and depends on diet, season, age, and size. For example, in cod, which is a lean fish, the level is 0.3 mg/100 g. In seafood the level of tocopherols decreases as a result of freezing storage for 6 months and of cooking [24].

The presence of other vitamins and selenium in seafood enhances the pro-health effect of tocopherols [55]. Vitamin E has been proposed for the prevention against colon, prostate and breast cancers, some cardiovascular diseases, ischemia, cataract, arthritis and certain neurological disorders [56].

2.3. Protein

In case of the lean fish, the main ingredients are proteins, which are a great source of amino acids (AA), including nutritionally essential (EAA), nonessential (NEAA), conditionally essential (CEAA), as well as functional amino acids (FAAs) [57,58]. The latter includes arginine, cystine, leucine, methionine, tryptophan, tyrosine, aspartate, glutamic acid, glycine, proline and taurine [58].

FAAs perform a variety of functions in the human body, including regulation of gene expression, cell signaling via kinase pathways, stimulation of brown adipose tissue development and thermogenesis, appetite and body composition, modulation of immune responses and prevention of infectious disease, reproduction, hormone secretion and endocrine status, antioxidative defense and removal of toxic substances, anti-inflammatory mechanisms, regulation of apoptosis and aging, neurological function and behavior (including neuroprotective effects), regulation of blood flow and cardiovascular function (e.g., NO synthesis) and recovery from injury. Accordingly, FAAs show great potential in the prevention and treatment of metabolic diseases, e.g., obesity, diabetes, cardiovascular disorders, intrauterine growth restriction, infertility, intestinal and neurological dysfunction, and infectious disease [58].

The content of these amino acids in different species of fish varies, resulting in the following range of content for arginine 0.1–6.5 g/100 g protein; leucine 0.1–10.4 g/100 g protein; methionine 0.02–4.0 g/100 g protein; tyrosine 0.03–8.4 g/100 g protein; tryptophan 0.1–6.5 g/100 g protein; cystine 0.03–0.6 g/100 g protein; aspartate 0.1–12.3 g/100 g protein; glutamic acid 0.2–16.5 g/100 g protein; glycine 0.1–13.7 g/100 g protein; proline 0.07–9.6 g/100 g protein [59].

Interestingly, a diet based on lean fish (such as cod) provides more certain amino acids (alanine, arginine, aspartic acid, glycine, methionine, and lysine) compared to a diet in which the lean fish is replaced with lean poultry, beef, veal or pork. In studies involving insulin-resistant men and women, it was found that cod protein diet improves insulin sensitivity compared with other lean animal protein sources. This effect is probably dependent on the amino acid composition, e.g., lower branched-chain amino acids (BCAAs) and higher arginine content [60]. An increase in sex hormone-binding globulin [61] and high-density lipoprotein 2 (HDL2) cholesterol concentrations [61,62] was also observed.

Collagen (mainly type I collagen) is the most abundant protein of intramuscular connective tissue in fish [63] and mostly is composed of amino acids such as glycine, valine, proline, and alanine [64]. Collagen obtained from fish skins, fish bones and scales is used in the pharmaceutical, cosmetic and food industries. Glycine has been shown to, in addition to reducing the symptoms associated with arthritis, have a beneficial effect on the growth of nails and hair [64].

2.4. Taurine and Anserine

Taurine is classified as an amino acid with antioxidant properties, but it is not built into the structure of proteins. Among foods, taurine is the most abundant in seafood (up to 800 mg/100 g in scallops), compared to 300 mg/100 g in turkey [65]. Cooking seafood in water causes its greatest losses [66].

Interestingly, in patients with metabolic syndrome, obesity, type II diabetes and cardiovascular diseases, lower plasma taurine concentrations were observed compared to healthy subjects. The decline in plasma and tissue taurine levels is also associated with the aging process [13].

The physiological function of taurine and its derivatives is very complex and has beneficial properties on many systems: cardiovascular, digestive, endocrine, immune, muscular, neurological, reproductive, and visual systems. Taurine provides antioxidant protection for cells and tissues, including the brain. As a component of bile salts, it is involved in the absorption of fat and fat-soluble vitamins and in the elimination of cholesterol via the fecal route. In addition, it stimulates the development of the nervous system and shows anti-inflammatory and antiapoptotic properties. The taurine derivative, *n*-chlorotaurine participates in defense mechanisms against pathogens: viruses, bacteria, fungi and parasites [11].

Anserine is a carnosine-like dipeptide [67] abundant in fish skeletal muscles e.g., salmon, tuna, trout [68]. For humans, it is an exogenous compound [69] and is metabolized into carnosine [70]. Physiological role includes H^+ buffering, antioxidation and modulation of muscle contractility [68,70].

Human clinical trials have shown anserine to be beneficial for metabolic (reduced blood glucose), ageing-associated neurological (cognitive and memory), inflammation, immunological, cardiovascular and renal functions and also enhance muscular strength [11].

3. Potential Health Benefits

3.1. Cardiovascular Diseases and Mortality

Cardiovascular diseases are the leading cause of death in the United States. Mortality after the onset of heart failure (HF) is estimated at almost 50% within 5 years of the diagnosis [71]. As the incidence of obesity, diabetes and hypertension is increasing, the incidence of HF is projected to increase in the coming years. Coronary artery disease (CHD) and hypertension are the main causes of HF, therefore reduction of the risk of CHD and hypertension may reduce the incidence of HF [72].

Some studies have shown geographical differences in the effect of fish consumption on mortality risk. An inverse relationship has been observed in studies on the Asian population [73,74], while some Western studies have not shown a relationship and even reported a higher risk associated with high fish consumption [75–77].

Zhong et al., after 30 years of follow-up (mean follow-up 19 years) and a group of 29,682 American adults (mean ± standard deviation (SD) age was 53.7 ± 15.7 years at baseline), found that higher consumption of processed meat, unprocessed red meat or poultry but not fish, is significantly associated with a higher risk CVD occurrences [78]. The median (interquartile range (IQR)) intake in servings per week was 1.6 (0.9–3.4) for fish. The association between fish consumption and the incidence of CVD was stronger for participants who consumed significant amounts of protein in their diet than those who consumed less protein (HR, 0.96 (95% confidence interval (CI): 0.93–0.99) compared to 1.02 (95% CI: 0.99–1.05); p for interaction = 0.002) [68]. Additional intake of two servings of fish per week was not significantly associated with CVD incidence (HR, 1.00 (95% CI: 0.98–1.02); 30-years adjusted absolute risk difference (ARD), 0.12% (95% CI: −0.40% to 0.65%) and with all-cause mortality (HR, 0.99 (95% CI: 0.97–1.01); 30-years adjusted ARD, −0.34% (95% CI, −0.88% to 0.20%) [78]. There was no significant difference between the consumption of oily and non-oily fish with regard to CVD incidents and all-cause mortality [78]. However, in a 10-year follow-up with sensitivity analysis, the authors observed a statistically significant inverse relationship between fish consumption and total mortality (all causes of death) [78].

Two meta-analyses showed a weak inverse correlation between fish consumption and the risk of developing CVD or mortality [79,80]. Jayedi et al. analyzed 14 studies with 911 348 participants (age range 30–84; follow-up duration of 5–30 years) and found that increase of 20 g/day in fish intake was significantly and inversely associated with the risk of total CVD mortality and inversely associated with the risk of all-cause mortality. Interestingly, the shape of the association varied depending on geographical region (linear—Asian studies or U-shaped—Western studies) [79]. The association between 20 g/day increase in fish consumption and all-cause mortality was significant only among Asian studies (RR = 0.97; 95% CI: 0.96–0.98; I^2 = 0%, $P_{heterogeneity}$ = 0.49, n = 5) compared to Western studies (RR = 0.99; 95% CI: 0.97–1.01; I^2 = 80.3%, $P_{heterogeneity}$ < 0.0001, n = 8). It was also significant only in the subgroup of studies with follow-up duration <13 years (RR = 0.97; 95% CI: 0.96–0.99; I^2 = 57 5%, $P_{heterogeneity}$ = 0.02, n = 8) compared to >13 years of follow-up (RR = 1.00; 95% CI: 0.98, 1.01; I^2 = 76.7%, $P_{heterogeneity}$ = 0.001, n = 6) [79]. A relatively rapid decrease in risk was observed with an increase in fish consumption of over ~60 g/day ($P_{non-linear}$ < 0.0001) [79].

Djousse et al. [80] found that higher fish consumption and higher dietary or plasma EPA/DHA levels were associated with an approximately 15% lower risk of HF compared to the corresponding lower exposure category [80]. There is also evidence of a linear and inverse relationship between fish consumption and the risk of HF. There was a 5% lower risk of HF [RR: 0.95 (95% CI: 0.93–0.98)] with a higher fish consumption of 15 g/day (equivalent to one additional fish per week). In the pooled analysis between the highest versus lowest category of fish intake, a higher intake of fish was associated with a 15% (95% CI: 1% to 27%; I^2 = 8%) lower risk of HF. Sensitivity analysis based on geographical location, showed that in USA pooled RR is 0.69 (95% CI: 0.54–0.89). Heterogeneity has not been demonstrated [80].

In turn, Zhao et al. [81] showed a significant inverse relationship between the consumption of fish and the risk of all-cause mortality at the consumption of 60–80 g/day. Further increase of the amount did not affect the RR value [81].

3.2. Metabolic Syndrome and T2DM

Metabolic syndrome is a serious public health problem in Western countries. Its incidence has risen rapidly over the past two decades. According to data from the National Health and Nutrition Examination Survey (NHANES), approximately one-third of American adults suffer from this syndrome [82,83].

Meta-analysis of relative risk from three prospective cohort studies (7860 participants; 18–69 years old) indicated a significant inverse association between fish consumption and development of metabolic syndrome comparing the highest and the lowest category of intake (RR: 0.71, 95% CI: 0.58, 0.87; I^2 = 60.7%, p = 0.08). The increment of one serving of fish/week reduces metabolic syndrome risk by 6% (RR: 0.94; 95% CI: 0.90, 0.98; I^2 = 66.3%, p = 0.052) [84].

The meta-analysis of 16 studies (overall number of participants 679,763) with a minimum and maximum follow-up period of 4 and 23 years, respectively (11.5 years an average), indicated that seven times increase in fatty fish consumption reduces the risk of T2DM (RR 0.89; CI = 0.801, 0.987; I^2 = 0) [85]. The same study found no significant effect of lean fish and shell fish consumption on T2DM. Interestingly, among the Asians and Australians three times higher consumption of marine n-3 fatty acids reduces the risk of diabetes (RR 0.857, CI 0.79–0.93) [85].

3.3. Cancer

In particular, oily fish are a good source of n-3 fatty acids which may have anticancer properties against various types of cancer [86]. Meta-analysis by Tavani et al. [87] showed an inverse relationship between the consumption of n-3 polyunsaturated fatty acids and ovarian cancer [87]. However, the pooled analysis of fish consumption and cancer risk did not show such a trend.

The meta-analyses based on two case–control studies indicated an increased risk of endometrial cancer associated with total fish consumption (OR: 1.88; 95% CI: 1.20–2.98). However, as the authors note, the evidence is limited and inconsistent [88].

Kolahdooz et al. [86] in their meta-analysis defined "the total fish" as "canned tuna and dark-meat fish such as sardines (also classified as fatty fish), other types of fish (also classified as nonfatty fish), fish sticks, and seafood such as prawns and crabs" [86]. Analysis based on overall six studies (16 886 patients, at the age of 18–79 years old) such as population based case–control studies and hospital-based case-control studies showed an inverse relation between total fish consumption and the risk of ovarian cancer (RR: 0.84; 95% CI: 0.68, 1.03; $P_{heterogeneity}$ = 0.003) [86].

Dose-response analysis of 13 cohort studies indicated that overall RR for the fish intake of 120 g/day was 1.07 (95% CI: 0.94–1.21) with moderate heterogeneity (I^2 = 33.3%), therefore null association between fish intake and risk of breast cancer was observed. Additionally, subgroup analysis showed a similar tendency taking into account factors such as age, menopausal status, region, duration of follow-up and study type [89].

Similar results were obtained by Zheng et al. [90] in meta-analysis of 11 studies (687,770 participants) estimating the pooled relative risk between the highest versus lowest category of fish intake (RR 1.03, 95% confidence interval 0.93 to 1.14; I^2 = 54%). Dose–response analysis also showed no association with risk of breast cancer for 15 g/day increase of intake (RR 1.00, 95% CI 0.97 to 1.03) [90].

In pooled analysis with 52,683 patients (range 18–97 years old; 9–22 years of follow-up) Wu et al. did not observe a statistically significant relationship between seafood intake and the risk of prostate cancer regardless of stage or grade for the following consumption categories: below 5 g/day, 5–40 g/day and above 40 g/day (RR 1.04 (0.98–1.09); I^2 = 25%). No separate analysis was performed for lean and fatty fish [91].

Another meta-analysis (49,661 participants) showed no strong evidence of a protective influence of fish consumption on prostate cancer incidence (even in subgroup analyzes for factors such as race, fish type and method of preparation, grade and stage cancer). A statistically significant 63% lower risk was found for prostate cancer-specific mortality comparing the highest versus lowest categories of fish intake (RR: 0.37; 95% CI: 0.18, 0.74). However, the results were based on only four cohort studies and there was significant heterogeneity in the results between studies (test for heterogeneity P = 0.001) [92].

Colorectal cancer is the third most common cancer in men (10.0% of all cancer cases) and the second most common cancer in women (9.2% of all cancer cases) worldwide [93]. An 11% decrease of risk of colorectal cancer was observed for fish intake (RR for 100 g/day = 0.89 (95% CI = 0.80–0.99, I^2 = 0%, $P_{heterogeneity}$ = 0.52)) based on 11 studies [93]. The association of fish intake and colon or rectal cancer risk were not significant, with RR = 0.91

(CI 0.80–1.03, I^2 = 0%, $P_{heterogeneity}$ = 0.76, 11 studies) and RR 0.84 (0.69–1.02; I^2 = 15%, $P_{heterogeneity}$ = 0.31, 10 studies), respectively [93].

3.4. Cognitive Impairment

Zhang et al. in meta-analysis defined standard serving as 105 g. The sample of 21941 participants (55–94 years old; 2–9.6 years of follow-up) from four independent cohorts were included; four trials and five trials reported the association between fish consumption and various risk of adverse cognitive outcomes, respectively, dementia and Alzheimer's disease (AD).

Overall RRs and 95% confidence intervals (CIs) were one-by-one investigated for an increment of fish (one serving/week). A dose–response meta-analysis showed that risk of dementia and AD was significantly reduced for an increment of one serving/week, respectively, RR 0.95 (95% CI: 0.90, 0.99; p = 0.042, I^2 = 63.4%) and RR 0.93; (95% CI: 0.90, 0.95; p = 0.003, I^2 = 74.8%). Both results had no publication bias.

Whereas, for participants who had no fish consumption, relative risks (RRs) of AD were 0.79 (95% CI: 0.66, 0.95), 0.74 (95% CI: 0.62, 0.89), and 0.71 (95% CI: 0.62, 0.81) for 2, 3 and 4 servings fish/week, respectively. However, no significant curvilinear association with risk of dementia was observed (p = 0.176) [94].

Recently published umbrella meta-analysis of 34 meta-analyses on prospective observational studies indicated additional 100 g/day increment in fish consumption was associated with a lower risk of all-cause mortality (summary relative risk SRR: 0.92; 95% CI: 0.87, 0.97), cardiovascular mortality (SRR: 0.75; 95% CI: 0.65, 0.87), coronary heart disease (SRR: 0.88; 95% CI: 0.79, 0.99), myocardial infarction (SRR: 0.75; 95% CI: 0.65, 0.93), stroke (SRR: 0.86; 95% CI: 0.75, 0.99), heart failure (SRR: 0.80; 95% CI: 0.67, 0.95), depression (SRR: 0.88; 95% CI: 0.79, 0.98), and liver cancer (SRR: 0.65; 95% CI: 0.48, 0.87) [95]. These outcomes were evaluated as moderate-quality evidence [95]. The results of described studies are summarized in Table 1.

Table 1. Summary of significant potential health benefits of fish consumption in previous meta-analysis.

References	Studies (N)	Participants (n)	Outcome	RR (95% CI)/SRR *
Jayedi et al. (2018) [79]	14	911,348	All-cause mortality	0.97 (0.96–0.98)
Djousse et al. (2012) [80]	5	170,131	Heart failure	0.95 (0.93–0.98)
Zhao et al. (2016) [81]	12	672,389	All-cause mortality	0.94 (0.90–0.98)
Kim et al. (2015) [84]	9	7860	Metabolic syndrome	0.71 (0.58–0.87)
Muley et al. (2014) [85]	16	679,763	T2DM	0.89 (0.801–0.987)
Kolahdooz et al. (2010) [86]	6	16,886	Ovarian cancer	0.84 (0.68–1.03)
Bandera et al. (2007) [88]	5	10,543	Endometrial cancer	1.88 (1.20–2.98)
Wu et al. (2016) [89]	13	758,359	Breast cancer	1.07 (0.94–1.21)
Zheng et al. (2013) [90]	11	687,770	Breast cancer	1.03 (0.93–1.14)
Wu et al. (2016) [91]		52,683	Prostate cancer	1.04 (0.98–1.09)
Szymański et al. (2010) [92]		49,661	Prostate cancer	0.37 (0.18–0.74)
Vieira et al. (2017) [93]	11	3944	Colorectal cancer	0.89 (0.80–0.99)
Zhang et al. (2016) [94]	4	21,099	Dementia	0.95 (0.90–0.99)
	5	21,941	Alzheimer's disease	0.93 (0.90–0.95)
Jayedi et al. (2020) [95]	38	153,998	All-cause mortality	0.92 * (0.87–0.97)
	8	11,720	Cardiovascular mortality	0.75 * (0.65–0.87)
	22	16,732	Coronary heart disease	0.88 * (0.79–0.99)
	11	8468	Myocardial infarction	0.75 * (0.65–0.93)
	20	14,360	Stroke	0.86 * (0.75–0.99)
	8	7945	Heart failure	0.80 * (0.67–0.95)
	8	5732	Depression	0.88 * (0.79–0.98)
	5	1572	Liver cancer	0.65 * (0.48–0.87)

* SRR—summary relative risk. Type 2 Diabetes Mellitus (T2DM).

4. Culinary Determinants of Seafood Health Properties

Thanks to the lipids, seafood has a widespread opinion that it is "good for everything". Despite this opinion, there are studies showing a positive correlation between fish consumption and the risk of developing cancer of the prostate [96], stomach [97] or even colon [98]. Certain factors, including the method of preparing the fish, the types of fish consumed and the level of local contamination, may determine the impact of fish consumption on health outcomes in different regions [79]. Higher consumption of nonfried fish was inversely associated with the risk of mortality from coronary heart disease, while a nonsignificant trend towards higher risk was observed with increasing consumption of fried fish [99]. Another Australian prospective cohort study indicated that the consumption of uncooked fish was marginal and inversely associated with the risk of CVD mortality in women, while total fish consumption was not related to that risk [100]. There are also different types of fish to consider. Lean fish have lower amounts of *n*-3 fatty acids and are more often deep-fried [99]. Meanwhile, oily fish is generally high in *n*-3 and the results from a population cohort study in China suggest that higher consumption of oily fish may be more strongly associated with a lower risk of death from any cause and CVD compared to nonfatty fish [101]. It should be borne in mind that this correlation is the result of the formation of free radicals during intense heat treatments or the presence of salt that often accompanies seafood products. Both salt and some lipid oxidation products show a strong carcinogenic effect [102,103]. *n*-3 LC PUFA, EPA and DHA, in particular, are characterized by a high level of unsaturation, which promotes oxidation reactions. These reactions can take place both in the enzymatic and nonenzymatic way. The latter are induced mainly by free radicals.

Eating at least one serving a week of fried fish or shellfish (shrimp and oysters) results in a risk ratio for all-cause mortality of 1.07 (1.03 to 1.12) and 1,13 (1.04 to 1.22) for cardiovascular mortality in the US female population (aged 50–79 at study entry, n = 106,966) [104]. On the other hand, in another study involving the Spanish population, no adverse effects were observed [105]. This discrepancy is likely due to the fact that the effect is also dependent on the source of the fried seafood and the frying fat [104]. In the USA, fried food is most often bought, for example, in fast food restaurants, and is prepared in deep oil. Corn oil is commonly used for this purpose. In contrast, in the Mediterranean countries, both olive oil (home-cooked meals) and corn oil (meals prepared in the restaurants) are used for frying [104]. Therefore, it is extremely important to properly select ingredients and cooking methods for the preparation of seafood-based dishes.

The dishes should be prepared using thermal treatment, in which the heat is transferred by convection and/or radiation, i.e., boiling and baking. However, frying, in which heat is transferred by conductivity, should be avoided as it results in a sudden increase in the temperature of the outer parts of seafood [106]. In general, all cooking methods contribute to lipid oxidation [106], however, those in which heat is transferred by convection are characterized by a lower level of oxidation [107].

Elderly people are not advised to eat raw seafood [108], therefore, these dishes should be prepared in the mildest possible conditions. They should also avoid salted, dried and cold-smoked seafood because of its high salt content [14,102].

5. Seafood Safety

5.1. Pollution in Seafood

Environmental pollution has led to contamination of the fish mainly with dioxins and mercury in methylated form (MeHg). Most of the pollutants undergo biogenochemical migration accompanied by the process of bioaccumulation along the subsequent links of the food chain, e.g., in the muscles of fish. It poses a serious health risk to their potential consumers [109].

The adverse health effects associated with chronic exposure to dioxins include carcinogenic, immunotoxic, embryonic and fetotoxic, teratogenic and hepatotoxic effects [110]. In adults, the possible health effects associated with the consumption of MeHg is mainly the increase in oxidative stress. As a consequence, it may lead to, inter alia, atherosclerosis, myocardial infarction, heart rate variability and hypertension [110].

The literature clearly shows that the health benefits of consuming oily fish (2–3 servings per week) far outweigh the potential contamination risks [111,112]. In addition, EPA and DHA are known for their strong antioxidant, anti-inflammatory and pro-extinguishing properties, which mitigate the effects of exposure to such pollutants as polycyclic aromatic hydrocarbons (PAHs) [113], polychlorinated biphenyls (PCB) [114] and 2,3,7,8-Tetrachlorodibenzo-p-Dioxin (TCDD) [115]. There are even countries such as Finland, Sweden and Latvia which allow trade of fish in which permissible level of dioxins has been exceeded (Regulation of European Union (EU) 2016/1139). Tocopherols which are very often found in seafood can also reduce the effects of oxidative stress caused by pollution [116].

The risk related to the presence of contamination can be significantly reduced by choosing seafood from the appropriate fishing areas.

Although the levels of such pollutants as PAHs, dioxins, heavy metals and radionuclides in cod did not exceed the limits set by the EU, fish from the Baltic Sea had the higher content of contaminants compared to fish from the Barents Sea or Greenland [109].

Catch area is also of key importance in the case of mercury contamination in seafood. Depending on the geographical area, the mercury content of tuna varied from 0.03 to 0.82 mg/g [117].

Fish, such as shark and swordfish, which are at the top of the aquatic food chain, often have higher levels of contamination than other fish. That is why choosing the right species is so important to reduce consumption of pollutants. Research by Cammiller et al. [118] showed that the mercury content in bluefin tuna was nearly three times higher than in yellowfin tuna [118].

In addition to the catch area and species, factors such as the age and the season of fishing also play a significant role in the concentration of pollution in the seafood. Although the content of dioxins and dioxin-like compounds in Norwegian herring is generally low, the fish caught in the period between January and February had a higher content of contaminants compared to those caught in the period between April and June. Older specimens were also characterized by a higher accumulation of pollutants than younger specimens [119]. As in the case of lipids and n-3 PUFA, also in the case of contaminants, the physiological state of seafood related to its seasonality plays an important role.

In the spring the contaminants are transferred within herring body along with lipids from the muscle tissue to the gonads during their maturation which leads to decrease of their level. In addition, these fish can transfer also a certain amount of pollutants to their offspring via their gonads. In this way, they eliminate lipid-soluble impurities, thus reducing their toxic effects [119].

Contrary to the popular belief, the level of contamination in farmed seafood is at a similar level or often lower than the one of its wild counterparts [120,121]. Some publications show that wild fish have a lower content of contaminants than farmed fish [122,123]. However, the fat content is ignored in these studies. As it is commonly known, most contaminants are lipophilic, so the studies should include this variable [120]. For this reason, farmed fatty fish have a higher level of contamination compared to farmed lean fish [124,125]. In addition, the fat content within the fillet is not the same, which makes it difficult to compare the content of impurities if different parts of the fillet were analyzed, e.g., the dorsal or the abdominal [126]. Due to the fact that the content of contaminants in feed is strictly limited and controlled [127], this translates into a lower level of contamination in farmed fish. It is estimated that in the future, the level of contamination in salmon fillets will be close to the limit of quantification due to the development of methods of purifying fish oil and replacing it in part with plant ingredients [128,129].

5.2. Seafood Allergy

Certain food hypersensitivity may develop during adulthood. Examples are shellfish and fin fish allergy [130,131] and it may concern, respectively, 2.9% and 0.9% of the US adult population [132]. A meta-analysis showed that 0–2% of adults are hypersensitive to fish and 0–10% to crustaceans [131]. Average age of the adult seafood-allergic patient is 50 years old [1]. In adults over 60 years old, the prevalence of various seafood products allergy is similar to that in younger age groups [132]. Most often, elderly people report hypersensitivity after consuming shellfish (2.6%; 95% CI:2.2–3.0), shrimp (1.6%; 95% CI:1.3–1.9) and mollusks (1.2%; 95% CI:1.0–1.5) [132]. The most commonly reported symptoms are skin, respiratory and gastrointestinal symptoms [1]. In Australia, seafood is the most common cause of fatal food anaphylaxis [133]. Ethnically, the most common seafood allergy is among Caucasians and African-Americans [1].

In the available literature there are controversial opinions about the relationship of radiocontrast, iodine, protamine and seafood allergies [134–138]. The major fish allergen is the low molecular-weight calcium-binding protein (parvalbumin). Allergy to seafood is not related to iodine. Iodinated contrast agents and povidone are the main iodinated drugs used in the radiology procedures and perioperative setting. IgE-mediated, both immediate and delayed hypersensitivities have been documented. However, the allergenic determinants remain unknown. The risk of reactions to radiocontrast ranges from 0.2% to 17%, severe reactions occur in 0.02–0.5% and deaths in 0.0006–0.006% [134]. A systematic review from seven prospective studies showed that the risk of reaction after radiocontrast media injections in patients with a seafood allergy is similar to that in patients with other food allergies or asthma [136,137]. Up to date, there is no evidence to avoid the use of iodinated drugs in seafood allergy.

Protamine is a polypeptide, isolated from salmon fish sperm. It is also used in insulin preparation to prolong the pharmacological effect. The evidence for an IgE-mediated allergy to protamine is very limited. Evidence supporting the increased risk for protamine allergy in fish allergy is lacking [136]. Up to date, there is no evidence to avoid the use of protamine or NPH insulin in fish allergies [134,136,137].

6. Conclusions

This review presented a broad overview of the association of seafood (especially fish) intake with the risk of non-communicable disease based on systematic review and meta-analysis. Although some of the results clearly do not state an impact on health, our review has important implications and indicates the direction of future research.

It is essential to evaluate the impact of intake of different types of fish such as fatty, lean, processed (e.g., smoked, canned, salted fish), methods of cooking fish (e.g., frying, steaming) on health and what potential factors cause these differences in effect in presented studies.

On the other hand, this strong or moderate evidence of the beneficial effects of seafood suggests that promoting a diet based on the regular consumption of different types of seafood should be further strengthened in populations of all ages. However, to get the full benefits of eating seafood, it should be cooked properly so as not to lose its health benefits. Our present review provides evidence that seafood, especially fish intake, indicate the potentially beneficial effects of the antiaging process and well-being in the elderly population. Taking action to reduce the incidence of non-communicable diseases in the elderly group (primarily changing the lifestyle, including nutritional behavior) is a moral and an economic imperative.

Author Contributions: Conceptualization, D.J.-M. and Z.D.; methodology, D.J.-M. and Z.D.; investigation, D.J.-M., Z.D., J.B. and M.L.; writing—original draft preparation, D.J.-M., Z.D., J.B. and M.L.; writing—review and editing, D.J.-M., Z.D., J.B., M.L. and L.S.; visualization, D.J.-M. and L.S.; supervision, Z.D. All authors have read and agreed to the published version of the manuscript.

Funding: This research received no external funding.

Institutional Review Board Statement: Not applicable.

Informed Consent Statement: Not applicable.

Acknowledgments: This research did not receive any specific grant from funding agencies in the public, commercial, or not-for-profit sectors.

Conflicts of Interest: The authors declare no conflict of interest.

References

1. Khan, F.; Orson, F.; Ogawa, Y.; Parker, C.; Davis, C.M. Adult Seafood Allergy in the Texas Medical Center: A 13-Year Experience. *Allergy Rhinol.* **2011**, *2*, e71–e77. [CrossRef] [PubMed]
2. Nesheim, M.C.; Oria, M.; Yih, P.T.; National Research Council; Institute of Medicine; Food and Nutrition Board; Board on Agriculture and Natural Resources; Committee on a Framework for Assessing the Health, Environmental, and Social Effects of the Food System. *Dietary Recommendations for Fish Consumption*; The National Academies Press (USA): Washington, DC, USA, 2015. [CrossRef]
3. Center for Food Safety and Applied Nutrition. Advice about Eating Fish. 2020. Available online: https://www.fda.gov/food/consumers/advice-about-eating-fish (accessed on 18 March 2021).
4. Willett, W.C.; Sacks, F.; Trichopoulou, A.; Drescher, G.; Ferro-Luzzi, A.; Helsing, E.; Trichopoulos, D. Mediterranean Diet Pyramid: A Cultural Model for Healthy Eating. *Am. J. Clin. Nutr.* **1995**, *61*, 1402S–1406S. [CrossRef] [PubMed]
5. Lin, P.-H.; Aickin, M.; Champagne, C.; Craddick, S.; Sacks, F.M.; McCarron, P.; Most-Windhauser, M.M.; Rukenbrod, F.; Haworth, L.; Dash-Sodium Collaborative Research Group. Food Group Sources of Nutrients in the Dietary Patterns of the DASH-Sodium Trial. *J. Am. Diet. Assoc.* **2003**, *103*, 488–496. [CrossRef]
6. Zeng, L.; Ruan, M.; Liu, J.; Wilde, P.; Naumova, E.N.; Mozaffarian, D.; Zhang, F.F. Trends in Processed Meat, Unprocessed Red Meat, Poultry, and Fish Consumption in the United States, 1999–2016. *J. Acad. Nutr. Diet.* **2019**, *119*, 1085–1098. [CrossRef]
7. Papanikolaou, Y.; Brooks, J.; Reider, C.; Fulgoni, V.L. U.S. Adults Are Not Meeting Recommended Levels for Fish and Omega-3 Fatty Acid Intake: Results of an Analysis Using Observational Data from NHANES 2003–2008. *Nutr. J.* **2014**, *13*, 31. [CrossRef]
8. Mozaffarian, D.; Dashti, H.S.; Wojczynski, M.K.; Chu, A.Y.; Nettleton, J.A.; Männistö, S.; Kristiansson, K.; Reedik, M.; Lahti, J.; Houston, D.K.; et al. Genome-Wide Association Meta-Analysis of Fish and EPA+DHA Consumption in 17 US and European Cohorts. *PLoS ONE* **2017**, *12*, e0186456. [CrossRef] [PubMed]
9. Samieri, C.; Morris, M.-C.; Bennett, D.A.; Berr, C.; Amouyel, P.; Dartigues, J.-F.; Tzourio, C.; Chasman, D.I.; Grodstein, F. Fish Intake, Genetic Predisposition to Alzheimer Disease, and Decline in Global Cognition and Memory in 5 Cohorts of Older Persons. *Am. J. Epidemiol.* **2018**, *187*, 933–940. [CrossRef] [PubMed]
10. Noncommunicable Diseases Progress Monitor 2020. Available online: https://www.who.int/publications/i/item/ncd-progress-monitor-2020 (accessed on 17 March 2021).
11. Wu, G. Important Roles of Dietary Taurine, Creatine, Carnosine, Anserine and 4-Hydroxyproline in Human Nutrition and Health. *Amino Acids* **2020**, *52*, 329–360. [CrossRef] [PubMed]
12. Wu, D.; Sun, N.; Ding, J.; Zhu, B.; Lin, S. Evaluation and Structure-Activity Relationship Analysis of Antioxidant Shrimp Peptides. *Food Funct.* **2019**, *10*, 5605–5615. [CrossRef] [PubMed]
13. Seidel, U.; Huebbe, P.; Rimbach, G. Taurine: A Regulator of Cellular Redox Homeostasis and Skeletal Muscle Function. *Mol. Nutr. Food Res.* **2019**, *63*, e1800569. [CrossRef]
14. Kiczorowska, B.; Samolińska, W.; Grela, E.R.; Bik-Małodzińska, M. Nutrient and Mineral Profile of Chosen Fresh and Smoked Fish. *Nutrients* **2019**, *11*, 1448. [CrossRef] [PubMed]
15. Daviglus, M.L.; Stamler, J.; Orencia, A.J.; Dyer, A.R.; Liu, K.; Greenland, P.; Walsh, M.K.; Morris, D.; Shekelle, R.B. Fish Consumption and the 30-Year Risk of Fatal Myocardial Infarction. *N. Engl. J. Med.* **1997**, *336*, 1046–1053. [CrossRef] [PubMed]
16. Albert, C.M.; Hennekens, C.H.; O'Donnell, C.J.; Ajani, U.A.; Carey, V.J.; Willett, W.C.; Ruskin, J.N.; Manson, J.E. Fish Consumption and Risk of Sudden Cardiac Death. *JAMA* **1998**, *279*, 23–28. [CrossRef]
17. Yuan, J.M.; Ross, R.K.; Gao, Y.T.; Yu, M.C. Fish and Shellfish Consumption in Relation to Death from Myocardial Infarction among Men in Shanghai, China. *Am. J. Epidemiol.* **2001**, *154*, 809–816. [CrossRef]
18. Hu, D.; Yan, W.; Zhu, J.; Zhu, Y.; Chen, J. Age-Related Disease Burden in China, 1997–2017: Findings from the Global Burden of Disease Study. *Front. Public Health* **2021**, *9*. [CrossRef]
19. Partridge, L.; Deelen, J.; Slagboom, P.E. Facing up to the Global Challenges of Ageing. *Nature* **2018**, *561*, 45–56. [CrossRef] [PubMed]
20. Lee, J.T.; Hamid, F.; Pati, S.; Atun, R.; Millett, C. Impact of Noncommunicable Disease Multimorbidity on Healthcare Utilisation and Out-Of-Pocket Expenditures in Middle-Income Countries: Cross Sectional Analysis. *PLoS ONE* **2015**, *10*, e0127199. [CrossRef] [PubMed]
21. Murad, M.H.; Asi, N.; Alsawas, M.; Alahdab, F. New Evidence Pyramid. *BMJ Evid. Based Med.* **2016**, *21*, 125–127. [CrossRef]
22. Tørris, C.; Småstuen, M.C.; Molin, M. Nutrients in Fish and Possible Associations with Cardiovascular Disease Risk Factors in Metabolic Syndrome. *Nutrients* **2018**, *10*, 952. [CrossRef]
23. Ambati, R.R.; Phang, S.M.; Ravi, S.; Aswathanarayana, R.G. Astaxanthin: Sources, Extraction, Stability, Biological Activities and Its Commercial Applications—A Review. *Mar. Drugs* **2014**, *12*, 128–152. [CrossRef]

24. Afonso, C.; Bandarra, N.M.; Nunes, L.; Cardoso, C. Tocopherols in Seafood and Aquaculture Products. *Crit. Rev. Food Sci. Nutr.* **2016**, *56*, 128–140. [CrossRef]
25. Watanabe, F.; Bito, T. Vitamin B12 Sources and Microbial Interaction. *Exp. Biol. Med. (Maywood)* **2018**, *243*, 148–158. [CrossRef]
26. Powers, H.J. Riboflavin (Vitamin B-2) and Health. *Am. J. Clin. Nutr.* **2003**, *77*, 1352–1360. [CrossRef]
27. de Mello, V.D.F.; Schwab, U.; Kolehmainen, M.; Koenig, W.; Siloaho, M.; Poutanen, K.; Mykkänen, H.; Uusitupa, M. A Diet High in Fatty Fish, Bilberries and Wholegrain Products Improves Markers of Endothelial Function and Inflammation in Individuals with Impaired Glucose Metabolism in a Randomised Controlled Trial: The Sysdimet Study. *Diabetologia* **2011**, *54*, 2755–2767. [CrossRef]
28. Rangel-Huerta, O.D.; Aguilera, C.M.; Mesa, M.D.; Gil, A. Omega-3 Long-Chain Polyunsaturated Fatty Acids Supplementation on Inflammatory Biomakers: A Systematic Review of Randomised Clinical Trials. *Br. J. Nutr.* **2012**, *107* (Suppl. 2), S159–S170. [CrossRef]
29. Robinson, L.E.; Mazurak, V.C. N-3 Polyunsaturated Fatty Acids: Relationship to Inflammation in Healthy Adults and Adults Exhibiting Features of Metabolic Syndrome. *Lipids* **2013**, *48*, 319–332. [CrossRef] [PubMed]
30. von Schacky, C. N-3 Fatty Acids and the Prevention of Coronary Atherosclerosis. *Am. J. Clin. Nutr.* **2000**, *71*, 224S–227S. [CrossRef]
31. Simopoulos, A.P. Omega-3 Fatty Acids and Cardiovascular Disease: The Epidemiological Evidence. *Environ. Health Prev. Med.* **2002**, *6*, 203–209. [CrossRef]
32. Bays, H.E.; Tighe, A.P.; Sadovsky, R.; Davidson, M.H. Prescription Omega-3 Fatty Acids and Their Lipid Effects: Physiologic Mechanisms of Action and Clinical Implications. *Expert Rev. Cardiovasc.* **2008**, *6*, 391–409. [CrossRef]
33. Abeywardena, M.Y.; Patten, G.S. Role of Ω3 Long-Chain Polyunsaturated Fatty Acids in Reducing Cardio-Metabolic Risk Factors. *Endocr. Metab. Immune. Disord. Drug Targets* **2011**, *11*, 232–246. [CrossRef]
34. Brookmeyer, R.; Johnson, E.; Ziegler-Graham, K.; Arrighi, H.M. Forecasting the Global Burden of Alzheimer's Disease. *Alzheimers Dement.* **2007**, *3*, 186–191. [CrossRef]
35. Solovyev, N.D. Importance of Selenium and Selenoprotein for Brain Function: From Antioxidant Protection to Neuronal Signalling. *J. Inorg. Biochem.* **2015**, *153*, 1–12. [CrossRef]
36. Wrzosek, M.; Łukaszkiewicz, J.; Wrzosek, M.; Jakubczyk, A.; Matsumoto, H.; Piątkiewicz, P.; Radziwoń-Zaleska, M.; Wojnar, M.; Nowicka, G. Vitamin D and the Central Nervous System. *Pharmacol. Rep.* **2013**, *65*, 271–278. [CrossRef]
37. Rimmelzwaan, L.M.; van Schoor, N.M.; Lips, P.; Berendse, H.W.; Eekhoff, E.M.W. Systematic Review of the Relationship between Vitamin D and Parkinson's Disease. *J. Parkinsons Dis.* **2016**, *6*, 29–37. [CrossRef]
38. Del Gobbo, L.C.; Imamura, F.; Aslibekyan, S.; Marklund, M.; Virtanen, J.K.; Wennberg, M.; Yakoob, M.Y.; Chiuve, S.E.; Dela Cruz, L.; Frazier-Wood, A.C.; et al. ω-3 Polyunsaturated Fatty Acid Biomarkers and Coronary Heart Disease: Pooling Project of 19 Cohort Studies. *JAMA Intern. Med.* **2016**, *176*, 1155–1166. [CrossRef]
39. Bandarra, N.M.; Batista, I.; Nunes, M.L.; Empis, J.M.; Christie, W.W. Seasonal Changes in Lipid Composition of Sardine (Sardina Pilchardus). *J. Food Sci.* **1997**, *62*, 40–42. [CrossRef]
40. Jensen, K.N.; Jacobsen, C.; Nielsen, H.H. Fatty Acid Composition of Herring (Clupea Harengus L.): Influence of Time and Place of Catch on n-3 PUFA Content. *J. Sci. Food AGR* **2007**, *87*, 710–718. [CrossRef]
41. Zheng, X.; Leaver, M.J.; Tocher, D.R. Long-Chain Polyunsaturated Fatty Acid Synthesis in Fish: Comparative Analysis of Atlantic Salmon (*Salmo Salar* L.) and Atlantic Cod (*Gadus Morhua* L.) Delta6 Fatty Acyl Desaturase Gene Promoters. *Comp. Biochem. Physiol. B Biochem. Mol. Biol.* **2009**, *154*, 255–263. [CrossRef]
42. Jensen, I.J.; Mæhre, H.K.; Tømmerås, S.; Eilertsen, K.E.; Olsen, R.L.; Elvevoll, E.O. Farmed Atlantic Salmon (Salmo Salar L.) Is a Good Source of Long Chain Omega-3 Fatty Acids. *Nutr. Bull.* **2012**, *37*, 25–29. [CrossRef]
43. Sprague, M.; Dick, J.R.; Tocher, D.R. Impact of Sustainable Feeds on Omega-3 Long-Chain Fatty Acid Levels in Farmed Atlantic Salmon, 2006–2015. *Sci. Rep.* **2016**, *6*, 21892. [CrossRef]
44. Balzano, M.; Pacetti, D.; Lucci, P.; Fiorini, D.; Frega, N.G. Bioactive Fatty Acids in Mantis Shrimp, Crab and Caramote Prawn: Their Content and Distribution among the Main Lipid Classes. *J. Food Compos. Anal.* **2017**, *59*, 88–94. [CrossRef]
45. Méndez, E.; González, R.M. Seasonal Changes in the Chemical and Lipid Composition of Fillets of the Southwest Atlantic Hake (Merluccius Hubbsi). *Food Chem.* **1997**, *59*, 213–217. [CrossRef]
46. Ågren, J.; Muje, P.; Hänninen, O.; Herranen, J.; Penttilä, I. Seasonal Variations of Lipid Fatty Acids of Boreal Freshwater Fish Species. *Comp. Biochem. Physiol. Part. B Comp. Biochem.* **1987**, *88*, 905–909. [CrossRef]
47. Guler, G.O.; Kiztanir, B.; Aktumsek, A.; Citil, O.B.; Ozparlak, H. Determination of the Seasonal Changes on Total Fatty Acid Composition and ω3/ω6 Ratios of Carp (*Cyprinus Carpio* L.) Muscle Lipids in Beysehir Lake (Turkey). *Food Chem.* **2008**, *108*, 689–694. [CrossRef]
48. Kołakowska, A.; Domiszewski, Z.; Bienkiewicz, G. Effects of biological and technological factors on the utility of fish as a source of n-3 PUFA. In *Omega 3 Fatty Acid Research*; Nova Science Publishers: Hauppauge, NY, USA, 2006; pp. 83–107.
49. EFSA Panel on Dietetic Products, Nutrition and Allergies (NDA). Scientific Opinion on the Tolerable Upper Intake Level of Eicosapentaenoic Acid (EPA), Docosahexaenoic Acid (DHA) and Docosapentaenoic Acid (DPA). *EFSA J.* **2012**, *10*, 2815. [CrossRef]
50. Miyawaki, H.; Takahashi, J.; Tsukahara, H.; Takehara, I. Effects of Astaxanthin on Human Blood Rheology. *J. Clin. Biochem. Nutr.* **2008**, *43*, 69–74. [CrossRef]
51. Park, J.S.; Chyun, J.H.; Kim, Y.K.; Line, L.L.; Chew, B.P. Astaxanthin Decreased Oxidative Stress and Inflammation and Enhanced Immune Response in Humans. *Nutr. Metab.* **2010**, *7*, 18. [CrossRef]

52. Turujman, S.A.; Warner, W.G.; Wei, R.R.; Albert, R.H. Rapid Liquid Chromatographic Method to Distinguish Wild Salmon from Aquacultured Salmon Fed Synthetic Astaxanthin. *J. AOAC Int.* **1997**, *80*, 622–632. [CrossRef]
53. Spiller, G.A.; Dewell, A. Safety of an Astaxanthin-Rich Haematococcus Pluvialis Algal Extract: A Randomized Clinical Trial. *J. Med. Food* **2003**, *6*, 51–56. [CrossRef]
54. Palozza, P.; Torelli, C.; Boninsegna, A.; Simone, R.; Catalano, A.; Mele, M.C.; Picci, N. Growth-Inhibitory Effects of the Astaxanthin-Rich Alga Haematococcus Pluvialis in Human Colon Cancer Cells. *Cancer Lett.* **2009**, *283*, 108–117. [CrossRef] [PubMed]
55. Institute of Medicine (US). Panel on Dietary Antioxidants and Related Compounds. In *Dietary Reference Intakes for Vitamin C, Vitamin E, Selenium, and Carotenoids*; National Academies Press (US): Washington, DC, USA, 2000; ISBN 978-0-309-06949-6.
56. Pham-Huy, L.A.; He, H.; Pham-Huy, C. Free Radicals, Antioxidants in Disease and Health. *Int. J. Biomed. Sci* **2008**, *4*, 89–96.
57. Wu, G. Functional Amino Acids in Growth, Reproduction, and Health. *Adv. Nutr.* **2010**, *1*, 31–37. [CrossRef]
58. Wu, G. Functional Amino Acids in Nutrition and Health. *Amino Acids* **2013**, *45*, 407–411. [CrossRef] [PubMed]
59. Mohanty, B.; Mahanty, A.; Ganguly, S.; Sankar, T.V.; Chakraborty, K.; Rangasamy, A.; Paul, B.; Sarma, D.; Mathew, S.; Asha, K.K.; et al. Amino Acid Compositions of 27 Food Fishes and Their Importance in Clinical Nutrition. *J. Amino Acids* **2014**, *2014*, e269797. [CrossRef] [PubMed]
60. Ouellet, V.; Marois, J.; Weisnagel, S.J.; Jacques, H. Dietary Cod Protein Improves Insulin Sensitivity in Insulin-Resistant Men and Women: A Randomized Controlled Trial. *Diabetes Care* **2007**, *30*, 2816–2821. [CrossRef] [PubMed]
61. Lacaille, B.; Julien, P.; Deshaies, Y.; Lavigne, C.; Brun, L.D.; Jacques, H. Responses of Plasma Lipoproteins and Sex Hormones to the Consumption of Lean Fish Incorporated in a Prudent-Type Diet in Normolipidemic Men. *J. Am. Coll. Nutr.* **2000**, *19*, 745–753. [CrossRef] [PubMed]
62. Beauchesne-Rondeau, E.; Gascon, A.; Bergeron, J.; Jacques, H. Plasma Lipids and Lipoproteins in Hypercholesterolemic Men Fed a Lipid-Lowering Diet Containing Lean Beef, Lean Fish, or Poultry. *Am. J. Clin. Nutr.* **2003**, *77*, 587–593. [CrossRef] [PubMed]
63. Moreno, H.M.; Montero, M.P.; Gómez-Guillén, M.C.; Fernández-Martín, F.; Mørkøre, T.; Borderías, J. Collagen Characteristics of Farmed Atlantic Salmon with Firm and Soft Fillet Texture. *Food Chem.* **2012**, *134*, 678–685. [CrossRef] [PubMed]
64. Shavandi, A.; Hou, Y.; Carne, A.; McConnell, M.; Bekhit, A.E.-D.A. Marine Waste Utilization as a Source of Functional and Health Compounds. *Adv. Food Nutr. Res.* **2019**, *87*, 187–254. [CrossRef]
65. Laidlaw, S.A.; Grosvenor, M.; Kopple, J.D. The Taurine Content of Common Foodstuffs. *JPEN J. Parenter. Enter. Nutr.* **1990**, *14*, 183–188. [CrossRef]
66. Spitze, A.R.; Wong, D.L.; Rogers, Q.R.; Fascetti, A.J. Taurine Concentrations in Animal Feed Ingredients; Cooking Influences Taurine Content. *J. Anim. Physiol. Anim. Nutr.* **2003**, *87*, 251–262. [CrossRef]
67. Bertinaria, M.; Rolando, B.; Giorgis, M.; Montanaro, G.; Guglielmo, S.; Buonsanti, M.F.; Carabelli, V.; Gavello, D.; Daniele, P.G.; Fruttero, R.; et al. Synthesis, Physicochemical Characterization, and Biological Activities of New Carnosine Derivatives Stable in Human Serum as Potential Neuroprotective Agents. *J. Med. Chem.* **2011**, *54*, 611–621. [CrossRef]
68. Boldyrev, A.A.; Aldini, G.; Derave, W. Physiology and Pathophysiology of Carnosine. *Physiol. Rev.* **2013**, *93*, 1803–1845. [CrossRef]
69. Mannion, A.F.; Jakeman, P.M.; Dunnett, M.; Harris, R.C.; Willan, P.L. Carnosine and Anserine Concentrations in the Quadriceps Femoris Muscle of Healthy Humans. *Eur. J. Appl. Physiol. Occup Physiol.* **1992**, *64*, 47–50. [CrossRef]
70. Everaert, I.; Baron, G.; Barbaresi, S.; Gilardoni, E.; Coppa, C.; Carini, M.; Vistoli, G.; Bex, T.; Stautemas, J.; Blancquaert, L.; et al. Development and Validation of a Sensitive LC-MS/MS Assay for the Quantification of Anserine in Human Plasma and Urine and Its Application to Pharmacokinetic Study. *Amino Acids* **2019**, *51*, 103–114. [CrossRef]
71. Saour, B.; Smith, B.; Yancy, C.W. Heart Failure and Sudden Cardiac Death. *Card. Electrophysiol. Clin.* **2017**, *9*, 709–723. [CrossRef]
72. Meijers, W.C.; de Boer, R.A. Common Risk Factors for Heart Failure and Cancer. *Cardiovasc. Res.* **2019**, *115*, 844–853. [CrossRef]
73. Lee, J.E.; McLerran, D.F.; Rolland, B.; Chen, Y.; Grant, E.J.; Vedanthan, R.; Inoue, M.; Tsugane, S.; Gao, Y.-T.; Tsuji, I.; et al. Meat Intake and Cause-Specific Mortality: A Pooled Analysis of Asian Prospective Cohort Studies. *Am. J. Clin. Nutr.* **2013**, *98*, 1032–1041. [CrossRef]
74. Wang, M.P.; Thomas, G.N.; Ho, S.Y.; Lai, H.K.; Mak, K.H.; Lam, T.H. Fish Consumption and Mortality in Hong Kong Chinese–the LIMOR Study. *Ann. Epidemiol.* **2011**, *21*, 164–169. [CrossRef]
75. Osler, M.; Andreasen, A.H.; Hoidrup, S. No Inverse Association between Fish Consumption and Risk of Death from All-Causes, and Incidence of Coronary Heart Disease in Middle-Aged, Danish Adults. *J. Clin. Epidemiol.* **2003**, *56*, 274–279. [CrossRef]
76. Gillum, R.F.; Mussolino, M.; Madans, J.H. The Relation between Fish Consumption, Death from All Causes, and Incidence of Coronary Heart Disease. the NHANES I Epidemiologic Follow-up Study. *J. Clin. Epidemiol.* **2000**, *53*, 237–244. [CrossRef]
77. Olsen, A.; Egeberg, R.; Halkjær, J.; Christensen, J.; Overvad, K.; Tjønneland, A. Healthy Aspects of the Nordic Diet Are Related to Lower Total Mortality. *J. Nutr.* **2011**, *141*, 639–644. [CrossRef] [PubMed]
78. Zhong, V.W.; Van Horn, L.; Greenland, P.; Carnethon, M.R.; Ning, H.; Wilkins, J.T.; Lloyd-Jones, D.M.; Allen, N.B. Associations of Processed Meat, Unprocessed Red Meat, Poultry, or Fish Intake with Incident Cardiovascular Disease and All-Cause Mortality. *JAMA Intern. Med.* **2020**, *180*, 503–512. [CrossRef]
79. Jayedi, A.; Shab-Bidar, S.; Eimeri, S.; Djafarian, K. Fish Consumption and Risk of All-Cause and Cardiovascular Mortality: A Dose–Response Meta-Analysis of Prospective Observational Studies. *Public Health Nutr.* **2018**, *21*, 1297–1306. [CrossRef]
80. Djoussé, L.; Akinkuolie, A.O.; Wu, J.H.Y.; Ding, E.L.; Gaziano, J.M. Fish Consumption, Omega-3 Fatty Acids and Risk of Heart Failure: A Meta-Analysis. *Clin. Nutr.* **2012**, *31*, 846–853. [CrossRef] [PubMed]

81. Zhao, L.-G.; Sun, J.-W.; Yang, Y.; Ma, X.; Wang, Y.-Y.; Xiang, Y.-B. Fish Consumption and All-Cause Mortality: A Meta-Analysis of Cohort Studies. *Eur. J. Clin. Nutr.* **2016**, *70*, 155–161. [CrossRef]
82. Ford, E.S.; Giles, W.H.; Dietz, W.H. Prevalence of the Metabolic Syndrome among US Adults: Findings from the Third National Health and Nutrition Examination Survey. *JAMA* **2002**, *287*, 356–359. [CrossRef]
83. Mozumdar, A.; Liguori, G. Persistent Increase of Prevalence of Metabolic Syndrome among U.S. Adults: NHANES III to NHANES 1999–2006. *Diabetes Care* **2011**, *34*, 216–219. [CrossRef]
84. Kim, Y.-S.; Xun, P.; He, K. Fish Consumption, Long-Chain Omega-3 Polyunsaturated Fatty Acid Intake and Risk of Metabolic Syndrome: A Meta-Analysis. *Nutrients* **2015**, *7*, 2085–2100. [CrossRef]
85. Muley, A.; Muley, P.; Shah, M. ALA, Fatty Fish or Marine n-3 Fatty Acids for Preventing DM?: A Systematic Review and Meta-Analysis. *Curr. Diabetes Rev.* **2014**, *10*, 158–165. [CrossRef]
86. Kolahdooz, F.; van der Pols, J.C.; Bain, C.J.; Marks, G.C.; Hughes, M.C.; Whiteman, D.C.; Webb, P.M.; Australian Cancer Study (Ovarian Cancer) and the Australian Ovarian Cancer Study Group. Meat, Fish, and Ovarian Cancer Risk: Results from 2 Australian Case-Control Studies, a Systematic Review, and Meta-Analysis. *Am. J. Clin. Nutr.* **2010**, *91*, 1752–1763. [CrossRef]
87. Tavani, A.; Pelucchi, C.; Parpinel, M.; Negri, E.; Franceschi, S.; Levi, F.; La Vecchia, C. N-3 Polyunsaturated Fatty Acid Intake and Cancer Risk in Italy and Switzerland. *Int. J. Cancer* **2003**, *105*, 113–116. [CrossRef]
88. Bandera, E.V.; Kushi, L.H.; Moore, D.F.; Gifkins, D.M.; McCullough, M.L. Consumption of Animal Foods and Endometrial Cancer Risk: A Systematic Literature Review and Meta-Analysis. *Cancer Causes Control* **2007**, *18*, 967–988. [CrossRef] [PubMed]
89. Wu, J.; Zeng, R.; Huang, J.; Li, X.; Zhang, J.; Ho, J.C.-M.; Zheng, Y. Dietary Protein Sources and Incidence of Breast Cancer: A Dose-Response Meta-Analysis of Prospective Studies. *Nutrients* **2016**, *8*, 730. [CrossRef]
90. Zheng, J.-S.; Hu, X.-J.; Zhao, Y.-M.; Yang, J.; Li, D. Intake of Fish and Marine N-3 Polyunsaturated Fatty Acids and Risk of Breast Cancer: Meta-Analysis of Data from 21 Independent Prospective Cohort Studies. *BMJ (Clin. Res. Ed.)* **2013**, *346*, f3706. [CrossRef]
91. Wu, K.; Spiegelman, D.; Hou, T.; Albanes, D.; Allen, N.E.; Berndt, S.I.; van den Brandt, P.A.; Giles, G.G.; Giovannucci, E.; Alexandra Goldbohm, R.; et al. Associations between Unprocessed Red and Processed Meat, Poultry, Seafood and Egg Intake and the Risk of Prostate Cancer: A Pooled Analysis of 15 Prospective Cohort Studies. *Int. J. Cancer* **2016**, *138*, 2368–2382. [CrossRef]
92. Szymanski, K.M.; Wheeler, D.C.; Mucci, L.A. Fish Consumption and Prostate Cancer Risk: A Review and Meta-Analysis. *Am. J. Clin. Nutr.* **2010**, *92*, 1223–1233. [CrossRef]
93. Vieira, A.R.; Abar, L.; Chan, D.S.M.; Vingeliene, S.; Polemiti, E.; Stevens, C.; Greenwood, D.; Norat, T. Foods and Beverages and Colorectal Cancer Risk: A Systematic Review and Meta-Analysis of Cohort Studies, an Update of the Evidence of the WCRF-AICR Continuous Update Project. *Ann. Oncol.* **2017**, *28*, 1788–1802. [CrossRef]
94. Zhang, Y.; Chen, J.; Qiu, J.; Li, Y.; Wang, J.; Jiao, J. Intakes of Fish and Polyunsaturated Fatty Acids and Mild-to-Severe Cognitive Impairment Risks: A Dose-Response Meta-Analysis of 21 Cohort Studies. *Am. J. Clin. Nutr.* **2016**, *103*, 330–340. [CrossRef]
95. Jayedi, A.; Shab-Bidar, S. Fish Consumption and the Risk of Chronic Disease: An Umbrella Review of Meta-Analyses of Prospective Cohort Studies. *Adv. Nutr.* **2020**, *11*, 1123–1133. [CrossRef]
96. Joshi, A.D.; John, E.M.; Koo, J.; Ingles, S.A.; Stern, M.C. Fish Intake, Cooking Practices, and Risk of Prostate Cancer: Results from a Multi-Ethnic Case-Control Study. *Cancer Causes Control* **2012**, *23*, 405–420. [CrossRef]
97. Cai, L.; Zheng, Z.-L.; Zhang, Z.-F. Risk Factors for the Gastric Cardia Cancer: A Case-Control Study in Fujian Province. *World J. Gastroenterol.* **2003**, *9*, 214–218. [CrossRef]
98. Chen, Z.; Wang, P.P.; Woodrow, J.; Zhu, Y.; Roebothan, B.; Mclaughlin, J.R.; Parfrey, P.S. Dietary Patterns and Colorectal Cancer: Results from a Canadian Population-Based Study. *Nutr. J.* **2015**, *14*, 8. [CrossRef] [PubMed]
99. Mozaffarian, D.; Lemaitre, R.N.; Kuller, L.H.; Burke, G.L.; Tracy, R.P.; Siscovick, D.S. Cardiovascular Health Study Cardiac Benefits of Fish Consumption May Depend on the Type of Fish Meal Consumed: The Cardiovascular Health Study. *Circulation* **2003**, *107*, 1372–1377. [CrossRef]
100. Owen, A.J.; Magliano, D.J.; O'Dea, K.; Barr, E.L.M.; Shaw, J.E. Polyunsaturated Fatty Acid Intake and Risk of Cardiovascular Mortality in a Low Fish-Consuming Population: A Prospective Cohort Analysis. *Eur. J. Nutr.* **2016**, *55*, 1605–1613. [CrossRef]
101. Takata, Y.; Zhang, X.; Li, H.; Gao, Y.-T.; Yang, G.; Gao, J.; Cai, H.; Xiang, Y.-B.; Zheng, W.; Shu, X.-O. Fish Intake and Risks of Total and Cause-Specific Mortality in 2 Population-Based Cohort Studies of 134,296 Men and Women. *Am. J. Epidemiol.* **2013**, *178*, 46–57. [CrossRef] [PubMed]
102. Wang, X.-Q.; Terry, P.D.; Yan, H. Review of Salt Consumption and Stomach Cancer Risk: Epidemiological and Biological Evidence. *World J. Gastroenterol.* **2009**, *15*, 2204–2213. [CrossRef]
103. Vieira, S.A.; Zhang, G.; Decker, E.A. Biological Implications of Lipid Oxidation Products. *J. Am. Oil Chem. Soc.* **2017**, *94*, 339–351. [CrossRef]
104. Sun, Y.; Liu, B.; Snetselaar, L.G.; Robinson, J.G.; Wallace, R.B.; Peterson, L.L.; Bao, W. Association of Fried Food Consumption with All Cause, Cardiovascular, and Cancer Mortality: Prospective Cohort Study. *BMJ* **2019**, *364*, k5420. [CrossRef]
105. Guallar-Castillón, P.; Rodríguez-Artalejo, F.; Lopez-Garcia, E.; León-Muñoz, L.M.; Amiano, P.; Ardanaz, E.; Arriola, L.; Barricarte, A.; Buckland, G.; Chirlaque, M.-D.; et al. Consumption of Fried Foods and Risk of Coronary Heart Disease: Spanish Cohort of the European Prospective Investigation into Cancer and Nutrition Study. *BMJ* **2012**, *344*, e363. [CrossRef]
106. Leung, K.S.; Galano, J.-M.; Durand, T.; Lee, J.C.-Y. Profiling of Omega-Polyunsaturated Fatty Acids and Their Oxidized Products in Salmon after Different Cooking Methods. *Antioxidants* **2018**, *7*, 96. [CrossRef]

107. Domiszewski, Z.; Duszyńska, K.; Stachowska, E. Influence of Different Heat Treatments on the Lipid Quality of African Catfish (Clarias Gariepinus). *J. Aquat. Food Prod. Technol.* **2020**, *29*, 886–900. [CrossRef]
108. Kendall, P.; Hillers, V.; Medeiros, L. Food Safety Guidance for Older Adults. *Clin. Infect. Dis. Off. Publ. Infect. Dis. Soc. Am.* **2006**, *42*, 1298–1304. [CrossRef] [PubMed]
109. Karl, H.; Kammann, U.; Aust, M.-O.; Manthey-Karl, M.; Lüth, A.; Kanisch, G. Large Scale Distribution of Dioxins, PCBs, Heavy Metals, PAH-Metabolites and Radionuclides in Cod (Gadus Morhua) from the North Atlantic and Its Adjacent Seas. *Chemosphere* **2016**, *149*, 294–303. [CrossRef] [PubMed]
110. Struciński, P.; Piskorska-Pliszczynska, J.; Góralczyk, K.; Warenik-Bany, M.; Maszewski, S.; Czaja, K.; Ludwicki, J. Dioxins and Food Safety. *Rocz. Państwowego Zakładu Hig.* **2011**, *62*, 3–17.
111. Leventakou, V.; Roumeliotaki, T.; Martinez, D.; Barros, H.; Brantsaeter, A.-L.; Casas, M.; Charles, M.-A.; Cordier, S.; Eggesbø, M.; van Eijsden, M.; et al. Fish Intake during Pregnancy, Fetal Growth, and Gestational Length in 19 European Birth Cohort Studies. *Am. J. Clin. Nutr.* **2014**, *99*, 506–516. [CrossRef] [PubMed]
112. Assessment and Management of Seafood Safety and Quality. Available online: http://www.fao.org/3/y4743e/y4743e0e.htm (accessed on 18 March 2021).
113. Gdula-Argasińska, J.; Czepiel, J.; Woźniakiewicz, A.; Wojtoń, K.; Grzywacz, A.; Woźniakiewicz, M.; Jurczyszyn, A.; Perucki, W.; Librowski, T. N-3 Fatty Acids as Resolvents of Inflammation in the A549 Cells. *Pharm. Rep.* **2015**, *67*, 610–615. [CrossRef]
114. Donat-Vargas, C.; Berglund, M.; Glynn, A.; Wolk, A.; Åkesson, A. Dietary Polychlorinated Biphenyls, Long-Chain n-3 Polyunsaturated Fatty Acids and Incidence of Malignant Melanoma. *Eur. J. Cancer* **2017**, *72*, 137–143. [CrossRef]
115. Turkez, H.; Geyikoglu, F.; Yousef, M.I. Ameliorative Effects of Docosahexaenoic Acid on the Toxicity Induced by 2,3,7,8-Tetrachlorodibenzo-p-Dioxin in Cultured Rat Hepatocytes. *Toxicol. Ind. Health* **2016**, *32*, 1074–1085. [CrossRef]
116. Ireneusz, C.; Joanna, R.-T.; Monika, S.; Dobrzyński, M.; Andrzej, G. Zastosowanie Wysokich Dawek Tokoferolu w Prewencji i Potencjalizacji Działania Dioksyn w Doświadczalnym Zapaleniu. *Postępy Hig. I Med. Doświadczalnej* **2011**, *65*. [CrossRef]
117. Nicklisch, S.C.T.; Bonito, L.T.; Sandin, S.; Hamdoun, A. Mercury Levels of Yellowfin Tuna (Thunnus Albacares) Are Associated with Capture Location. *Environ. Pollut.* **2017**, *229*, 87–93. [CrossRef]
118. Cammilleri, G.; Vazzana, M.; Arizza, V.; Giunta, F.; Vella, A.; Lo Dico, G.; Giaccone, V.; Giofrè, S.V.; Giangrosso, G.; Cicero, N.; et al. Mercury in Fish Products: What's the Best for Consumers between Bluefin Tuna and Yellowfin Tuna? *Nat. Prod. Res.* **2018**, *32*, 457–462. [CrossRef] [PubMed]
119. Frantzen, S.; Måge, A.; Iversen, S.A.; Julshamn, K. Seasonal Variation in the Levels of Organohalogen Compounds in Herring (Clupea Harengus) from the Norwegian Sea. *Chemosphere* **2011**, *85*, 179–187. [CrossRef] [PubMed]
120. Lundebye, A.-K.; Lock, E.-J.; Rasinger, J.D.; Nøstbakken, O.J.; Hannisdal, R.; Karlsbakk, E.; Wennevik, V.; Madhun, A.S.; Madsen, L.; Graff, I.E.; et al. Lower Levels of Persistent Organic Pollutants, Metals and the Marine Omega 3-Fatty Acid DHA in Farmed Compared to Wild Atlantic Salmon (Salmo Salar). *Environ. Res.* **2017**, *155*, 49–59. [CrossRef]
121. Varol, M.; Sünbül, M.R. Comparison of Heavy Metal Levels of Farmed and Escaped Farmed Rainbow Trout and Health Risk Assessment Associated with Their Consumption. *Environ. Sci. Pollut. Res. Int.* **2017**, *24*, 23114–23124. [CrossRef] [PubMed]
122. Hites, R.A.; Foran, J.A.; Carpenter, D.O.; Hamilton, M.C.; Knuth, B.A.; Schwager, S.J. Global Assessment of Organic Contaminants in Farmed Salmon. *Science* **2004**, *303*, 226–229. [CrossRef] [PubMed]
123. Shaw, S.D.; Brenner, D.; Berger, M.L.; Carpenter, D.O.; Hong, C.-S.; Kannan, K. PCBs, PCDD/Fs, and Organochlorine Pesticides in Farmed Atlantic Salmon from Maine, Eastern Canada, and Norway, and Wild Salmon from Alaska. *Environ. Sci. Technol.* **2006**, *40*, 5347–5354. [CrossRef] [PubMed]
124. Nácher-Mestre, J.; Serrano, R.; Benedito-Palos, L.; Navarro, J.; López, F.; Kaushik, S.; Pérez-Sánchez, J. Bioaccumulation of Polycyclic Aromatic Hydrocarbons in Gilthead Sea Bream (*Sparus Aurata* L.) Exposed to Long Term Feeding Trials with Different Experimental Diets. *Arch. Environ. Contam. Toxicol.* **2010**, *59*, 137–146. [CrossRef]
125. van Leeuwen, S.P.J.; Swart, C.P.; van der Veen, I.; de Boer, J. Significant Improvements in the Analysis of Perfluorinated Compounds in Water and Fish: Results from an Interlaboratory Method Evaluation Study. *J. Chromatogr. A* **2009**, *1216*, 401–409. [CrossRef]
126. Bienkiewicz, G.; Domiszewski, Z.; Tokarczyk, G.; Plust, D. Distribution of Lipids and Oxidative Changes Therein in Particularized Parts of Rainbow Trout Fillets. *Zywnosc. Nauka. Technol. Jakosc Food. Sci. Technol. Qual.* **2013**, 20. [CrossRef]
127. Knutsen, H.K.; Alexander, J.; Barregård, L.; Bignami, M.; Brüschweiler, B.; Ceccatelli, S.; Cottrill, B.; Dinovi, M.; Edler, L.; Grasl-Kraupp, B.; et al. Risk for Animal and Human Health Related to the Presence of Dioxins and Dioxin-like PCBs in Feed and Food. *EFSA J.* **2018**, *16*, e05333. [CrossRef]
128. Knutsen, H.K.; Alexander, J.; Barregård, L.; Bignami, M.; Brüschweiler, B.; Ceccatelli, S.; Cottrill, B.; Dinovi, M.; Edler, L.; Grasl-Kraupp, B.; et al. Assessment of a Decontamination Process for Dioxins and PCBs from Fish Meal by Replacement of Fish Oil. *EFSA J.* **2018**, *16*, e05174. [CrossRef]
129. Berntssen, M.H.G.; Sanden, M.; Hove, H.; Lie, Ø. Modelling Scenarios on Feed-to-Fillet Transfer of Dioxins and Dioxin-like PCBs in Future Feeds to Farmed Atlantic Salmon (Salmo Salar). *Chemosphere* **2016**, *163*, 413–421. [CrossRef] [PubMed]
130. Kamdar, T.A.; Peterson, S.; Lau, C.H.; Saltoun, C.A.; Gupta, R.S.; Bryce, P.J. Prevalence and Characteristics of Adult-Onset Food Allergy. *J. Allergy Clin. Immunol. Pract.* **2015**, *3*, 114–115.e1. [CrossRef] [PubMed]

131. Rona, R.J.; Keil, T.; Summers, C.; Gislason, D.; Zuidmeer, L.; Sodergren, E.; Sigurdardottir, S.T.; Lindner, T.; Goldhahn, K.; Dahlstrom, J.; et al. The Prevalence of Food Allergy: A Meta-Analysis. *J. Allergy Clin. Immunol.* **2007**, *120*, 638–646. [CrossRef] [PubMed]
132. Gupta, R.S.; Warren, C.M.; Smith, B.M.; Jiang, J.; Blumenstock, J.A.; Davis, M.M.; Schleimer, R.P.; Nadeau, K.C. Prevalence and Severity of Food Allergies Among US Adults. *JAMA Netw. Open* **2019**, *2*, e185630. [CrossRef]
133. Mullins, R.J.; Wainstein, B.K.; Barnes, E.H.; Liew, W.K.; Campbell, D.E. Increases in Anaphylaxis Fatalities in Australia from 1997 to 2013. *Clin. Exp. Allergy* **2016**, *46*, 1099–1110. [CrossRef]
134. Schabelman, E.; Witting, M. The Relationship of Radiocontrast, Iodine, and Seafood Allergies: A Medical Myth Exposed. *J. Emerg. Med.* **2010**, *39*, 701–707. [CrossRef]
135. Beaty, A.D.; Lieberman, P.L.; Slavin, R.G. Seafood Allergy and Radiocontrast Media: Are Physicians Propagating a Myth? *Am. J. Med.* **2008**, *121*, 158-e1. [CrossRef]
136. Dewachter, P.; Kopac, P.; Laguna, J.J.; Mertes, P.M.; Sabato, V.; Volcheck, G.W.; Cooke, P.J. Anaesthetic Management of Patients with Pre-Existing Allergic Conditions: A Narrative Review. *Br. J. Anaesth.* **2019**, *123*, e65–e81. [CrossRef]
137. Pradubpongsa, P.; Dhana, N.; Jongjarearnprasert, K.; Janpanich, S.; Thongngarm, T. Adverse Reactions to Iodinated Contrast Media: Prevalence, Risk Factors and Outcome-the Results of a 3-Year Period. *Asian Pac. J. Allergy Immunol.* **2013**, *31*, 299–306. [CrossRef] [PubMed]
138. Schlifke, A.; Geiderman, J.M. Seafood Allergy Is a Specific and Unique Contraindication to the Administration of Ionic Contrast Media. *CJEM* **2003**, *5*, 166–168. [CrossRef] [PubMed]

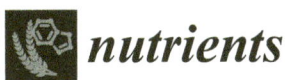

Article

Malnutrition Risk among Older Mexican Adults in the Mexican Health and Aging Study

Jaqueline C. Avila [1,*], Rafael Samper-Ternent [2,3] and Rebeca Wong [2,4]

1. Center for Alcohol and Addiction Studies, School of Public Health, Brown University, Providence, RI 02903, USA
2. Sealy Center on Aging, University of Texas Medical Branch, Galveston, TX 77555, USA; rasamper@utmb.edu (R.S.-T.); rewong@utmb.edu (R.W.)
3. Department of Internal Medicine, Division of Geriatrics, University of Texas Medical Branch, Galveston, TX 77555, USA
4. Department of Preventive Medicine and Population Health, University of Texas Medical Branch, Galveston, TX 77555, USA
* Correspondence: jaqueline_avila@brown.edu

Abstract: Few studies assess the malnutrition risk of older Mexican adults because most studies do not assess nutritional status. This study proposes a modified version of the Mini Nutritional Assessment (MNA) to assess the risk of malnutrition among older Mexicans adults in the Mexican Health and Aging Study (MHAS). Data comes from the 2012, 2015, and 2018 waves of the MHAS, a nationally representative study of Mexicans aged 50 and older. The sample included 13,338 participants and a subsample of 1911 with biomarker values. ROC analysis was used to calculate the cut point for malnutrition risk. This cut point was compared to the definition of malnutrition from the ESPEN criteria, BMI, low hemoglobin, or low cholesterol. Logistic regression was used to assess predictors of malnutrition risk. A score of 10 was the optimal cut point for malnutrition risk in the modified MNA. This cut point had high concordance to identify malnutrition risk compared to the ESPEN criteria (97.7%) and had moderate concordance compared to BMI only (78.6%), and the biomarkers of low hemoglobin (56.1%) and low cholesterol (54.1%). Women, those older than 70, those with Seguro Popular health insurance, and those with fair/poor health were more likely to be malnourished. The modified MNA is an important tool to assess malnutrition risk in future studies using MHAS data.

Keywords: malnutrition; older adults; Mexico; MNA; MHAS

1. Introduction

Malnutrition has been identified as a risk factor for adverse events among older adults. Further, malnutrition among older adults may present before a specific health condition [1], and having malnutrition is associated with poorer health outcomes, longer hospital stays, disability, and mortality [2–4]. Globally, there is a wide range of malnutrition prevalence among community older adults 60 years and older, ranging between 1.3% and 47.8% [5], with the greatest prevalence of malnutrition seen in low and middle-income countries [5]. A study among communities of older adults in 12 countries showed that the prevalence of malnutrition was 5.8% [6].

Low socioeconomic status [7,8] and poor health [9] have been reported as risk factors for malnutrition among older adults. Older adults in Mexico have aged in a health and socioeconomic context where these risk factors are highly prevalent, increasing the risk for malnutrition. First, a significant percentage of older adults in Mexico have low socioeconomic status. In 2012, nearly 10% of the population 50 and older reported 0 years of education and 17% of men and 14% of women did not have health insurance [10]. In addition, older adults in Mexico also have high prevalence of chronic diseases and disability that may add to their risk of malnutrition [10]. In 2012, more than half of the population 50 and older reported fair or poor health status and the prevalence of diabetes was near 20%. Further, 6.4% of men and 9.9% of women reported at least one limitation on Activities of Daily Living (ADL) [10]. Older adults in Mexico experienced the earlier stages of the epidemiologic transition with high prevalence of infectious diseases and childhood malnutrition, and they aged as the transition occurred. These adults, therefore, experience a double disease burden (infectious and chronic) that results in poor outcomes [11,12]. They experience high prevalence of chronic diseases, in addition to high disease-related disability and mortality, due to poor disease management and low access to care.

Despite the greater malnutrition risk of older Mexican adults [13], few studies have focused on the malnutrition risk of this population, and most studies assessing nutritional status focus on the high prevalence of overweight and obesity in this population [14,15]. Although the older Mexican population has high obesity rates, malnutrition and obesity can coexist [16,17].

One of the barriers for the study of malnutrition among older adults in Mexico is that the longest running nationally representative survey of the population 50 and older in Mexico, the Mexican Health and Aging Study (MHAS), does not assess nutritional status directly. The MHAS is a comprehensive population-based study of aging and health in Mexico, thus limiting the opportunity for a full nutritional assessment. Although the MHAS does not apply a full nutritional assessment, it includes several measures that, when used together, result in a modified version of the Mini Nutritional Assessment (MNA). The MNA is a widely used tool to screen the nutritional status of community-dwelling older adults, and it provides a validated and detailed assessment that goes beyond considering BMI and weight loss only [18,19]. Thus, the first objective of this paper is to use MHAS data to propose a modified MNA to identify older Mexican adults at risk for malnutrition. The modified MNA includes determination of a cut point to classify older Mexican adults in the MHAS as at risk for malnutrition. In addition, the modified MNA will be compared with other measures of nutritional status such as objective biomarkers, body mass index (BMI), and the European Society of Parenteral and Enteral Nutrition and Metabolism (ESPEN) criteria. The second objective is to use the modified MNA to assess the main predictors of malnutrition risk among older Mexican adults.

2. Methods

2.1. Data

We used the 2012 wave of the MHAS to conduct this study to provide a nationally representative cross-section of the population aged 50 and older in Mexico. We also used the 2015 and 2018 waves of the MHAS to provide data on mortality for those in the 2012 wave. In addition, we used a subsample of the 2012 cohort that provided a blood sample to measure biomarkers and measured height and weight. The final sample included 13,338 individuals aged 50 and older on whom we had all the information needed to assess nutritional status. The sample size of the subsample for the biomarker analysis was 1911 individuals.

2.1.1. Development of the Modified Mini Nutritional Assessment

Table 1 shows the modifications made to the original short-form MNA to allow it to be used with the MHAS. The original MNA includes measures related to changes in food intake, weight loss, mobility, stress and acute disease, neuropsychological disorders, and BMI over the past three months. In the original MNA, each measure receives a score and these are summed to a total score ranging from 0 to 14 [19,20]. Similar measures capturing the same domains were assessed in the MHAS survey. These measures were scored in the same way as the original MNA and were summed into a total score ranging from 0 to 14.

Table 1. Measures for the Mini Nutritional Assessment Adaptation using MHAS 2012.

Original Mini Nutritional Assessment	Modified MNA Using MHAS
Has food intake declined over the past 3 months due to loss of appetite, digestive problems, chewing or swallowing difficulties?	In the last two years, respondent has eaten less due to loss of appetite, digestive problems, and difficulties chewing or swallowing
0 = Severe decrease in food intake	0 = Most of the time
1 = Moderate decrease in food intake	1 = Sometimes
2 = No decrease in food intake	2 = Hardly ever
Weight loss during the last 3 months	Respondent has experienced weight loss in the past 2 years
0 = Weight loss greater than 3 kg	0 = Decreased 5kg or more
1 = Does not know	1 = Does not know
2 = Weight loss between 1 and 3 kg	2 = N/A
3 = No weight loss	3 = Remained the same or increased 5kg or more
Mobility	Respondent's mobility
0 = Bed or chair bound	0 = Has difficulty getting in and out of bed AND has difficulty walking one block or several blocks
1 = Able to get out of bed/chair but does not go out	1 = Does not have difficulty getting in and out of bed AND has difficulty walking one block or several blocks OR has problems getting in and out of bed AND does not have difficulty walking one block or several blocks
2 = Goes out	2 = Does not have difficulty walking one block or several blocks AND does not have difficulty getting in and out of bed
Has suffered psychological stress or acute disease in the past 3 months?	Respondent has suffered a major event with psychological trauma from accident, crime or natural disaster or has been hospitalized in the past 2 years
0 = Yes	0 = Has suffered a natural disaster that damaged home OR suffered accident, crime, or any similar event OR has been hospitalized in the last 2 years
2 = No	2 = Has not suffered a natural disaster that damaged home AND has not suffered accident, crime, or any similar event AND has not been hospitalized in the last 2 years
Neuropsychological problems	Respondent's current memory status and depressive symptoms
0 = Severe dementia or depression	0 = Has poor memory AND depressive symptoms
1 = Mild dementia	1 = Has a fair memory AND does not have depressive symptoms
2 = No psychological problems	2 = Has a good memory AND does not have depressive symptoms
Body Mass Index (BMI)	BMI (self-report of weight and height)
0 = BMI less than 19	0 = BMI less than 19
1 = BMI 19 to less than 21	1 = BMI 19 to less than 21
2 = BMI 21 to less than 23	2 = BMI 21 to less than 23
3 = BMI 23 or greater	3 = BMI 23 or greater
Screening Score	
12–14 Points: Normal nutritional status	11–14: Normal nutritional status
8–11 point: At risk of malnutrition	
0–7 points: Malnourished	0–10: At risk for malnutrition

One main difference between the MNA and the modified MNA is the time reference: in the MHAS, respondents are asked similar questions but using the previous two years as the point of reference. In addition, there were differences on specific items. For example, the weight loss item in the modified MNA was assessed as change in 5 kg or more instead of 3 kg or more. The MHAS only assessed changes of 5 kg or more and did not assess if there was any change between 1 and 5 kg. Thus, no one received a score of "2" in the modified MNA. The stress and acute disease item was assessed with the closest measure of psychological distress in the MHAS (report of a major event such as accident, crime, or natural disaster), and the closest measure of acute disease (hospitalization). Due to differences in the time span, as well as other differences on specific items asked between the original MNA and the MHAS modification, we did not consider the cut points of malnutrition, at risk for malnutrition, and normal nutrition from the original MNA.

We used receiver operating characteristic (ROC) analysis to calculate the optimal cut point for malnutrition risk. In order to create the ROC curve, we examined the effectiveness of the modified MNA in 2012 to predict mortality by 2018. We calculated the ROC curve based on mortality because this is an outcome highly associated with malnutrition [4] and serves as a close proxy when malnutrition is not assessed. Evidence from a systematic review showed that the original short-form MNA significantly predicted mortality over time among community older adults [21]. The Liu index was used to determine the best cut point based on the maximized sensitivity and specificity. We generated 1000 bootstrap samples to internally validate the cut point of the modified MNA and calculated the area under the curve (AUC), sensitivity, specificity, positive predictive value and negative predictive value at the optimal cut point.

We also conducted logistic regression models to assess the odds of dying with a 1-unit increase in the modified MNA score, as well as the odds of dying for those identified as at risk for malnutrition compared to those with normal nutritional status, based on the cut point determined as described above.

Sensitivity Analysis: Comparison to other nutritional screenings.

After the optimal cut point was defined, we conducted sensitivity analysis to compare the concordance of the modified MNA cut point to other validated measures used to assess nutritional status: the ESPEN criteria, BMI, and biomarkers. This sensitivity analysis was restricted to the subsample with biomarker information. We compared how many of those classified at risk for malnutrition, based on the modified MNA, were also classified as with malnutrition based on these measures.

- ESPEN criteria: The ESPEN criteria categorizes older adults at risk for malnutrition if either of these alternatives is met [22]:

    (1) BMI < 18.5 kg/m^2
    (2) Unintentional weight loss greater than 10% over an indefinite time, or 5% in the past 3 months *in addition* to either of these conditions:
        (2a) BMI < 20 if younger than 70, or BMI < 22 if 70 or older
        (2b) Fat Free Mass Index (FFMI) <15 for women and <17 for men

We used both alternatives to classify older adults using the MHAS data. The BMI values used for the first alternative were obtained using measured height and weight and imputed for missing values by the MHAS research team. In the second alternative, unintentional weight loss was defined as answering yes to the question "weight loss greater than 5 kg in the previous two years" to meet the MNA criteria for weight loss greater than 10% over an indefinite time. We considered that 5 kg or more is more than 10% of weight, given that the mean weight in the MHAS population is 70 kg (SD: 13.7). The second alternative was classified based on the 2a alternative of BMI differences, considering age. This is because FFMI (alternative 2b) is not measured in the MHAS. Individuals who met alternatives 1 or 2 were defined as at risk for malnutrition.

- Biomarkers: We used low cholesterol or low hemoglobin as proxies for malnutrition as previous studies have indicated [23]. Participants with cholesterol ≤160 mg/dL, or hemoglobin ≤12 for women and ≤13 for men were defined as at risk for malnutrition.
- BMI only: We used underweight, defined as BMI <18.5 kg/m^2, as a proxy for malnutrition.

2.1.2. Analysis of Predictors of Malnutrition among Older Mexican Adults

We used a logistic regression model to assess the predictors of malnutrition risk using the modified MNA. We included the following demographic and health covariates associated with malnutrition: sex, age (50–59; 60–69; 70+ years), education (0; 1–6; 7+ years), health insurance status (None; IMSS/ISSTE/Other; Seguro Popular), locality size (less urban if population < 100,000; more urban if population ≥ 100,000), and self-reported health (Excellent/Very good/Good; Fair; Poor).

3. Results

3.1. Accuracy of the Modified MNA

The sample characteristics are described in Supplementary Table S1. Overall, the majority of older Mexican adults were female, ages 50–59, and had 1–6 years of education. Near 15% of the sample did not have health insurance, and 12% reported poor health status.

The results from the ROC analysis showed that the best cut point for the modified MNA score was 10.5, which was rounded down to 10. Those with an MNA score of 0–10 were defined as at risk for malnutrition, and those with scores 11–14 were defined as having normal nutritional status. A total of 40.4% of the sample was classified as at risk for malnutrition. This cut point (0–10) was able to predict mortality by 2018 with moderate to high accuracy. The AUC for having a score of 10 or lower was 0.61, the sensitivity was 60.5%, the specificity was 62.5%, the positive predictive value was 18.8%, and the negative predictive value was 91.7%.

A 1-point increase in the modified MNA scale was associated with a 15% decrease in the 6-year odds of mortality (Odds Ratio (OR): 0.85, 95% Confidence Interval (CI): 0.83; 0.87) (Table 2) and those classified as at risk for malnutrition based on the proposed cut point were 79% more likely to die by 2018 than those with normal nutritional status (OR: 1.79, 95% CI: 1.59; 2.01) (Table 2).

Table 2. Logistic regression models to test the association between the modified MNA as a continuous score, with the proposed cut-point, and 6-year mortality in 2015. 2012 MHAS Sample (n = 13,338) [a].

	Continuous MNA Score		At Risk for Malnutrition (Proposed Cut-Point)	
	OR	95% CI	OR	95% CI
Modified MNA Score	0.85 ***	0.83; 0.87	NA	
Modified MNA Cut-off				
0–10 (At risk for malnutrition)	NA		1.79 ***	1.59; 2.01
11–14				Ref.

[a] Results adjusted by sex, age, locality size, education, health insurance, and self-reported health status. *** p-value < 0.001. NA: Not applicable.

Further, when compared to other measures of nutritional status, the modified MNA cut point had moderate to high concordance. In the subsample with biomarker information, the sensitivity of the modified MNA cut point was 93.2% compared to the ESPEN criteria, 78.6% compared to BMI of underweight, 54.1% compared to the objective marker of low cholesterol, and 56.1% compared to low hemoglobin. The specificity of the cut point was also moderate, close to 60% for all of the measures (Table 3).

Table 3. Concordance of malnutrition risk in the modified MNA compared to other markers of malnutrition in the MHAS 2012 biomarker subsample (n = 1911) [a].

Modified MNA	ESPEN Criteria		BMI Only		Low Cholesterol		Low Hemoglobin	
	Yes (%)	No (%)	Yes (%)	No (%)	Yes (%)	No (%)	Yes (%)	No (%)
At risk for malnutrition	93.2	38.3	78.6	39.3	54.1	38.0	56.1	38.7
Normal nutritional status	6.8	61.7	21.4	60.7	45.9	62.0	43.9	61.3

[a] Results shown in column percentages.

3.2. Predictors of Malnutrition Risk

Results based on the modified MNA (Table 4) showed that women were more likely to have malnutrition than men. Higher odds of malnutrition were associated with older age and with fewer years of educational achievement. Further, older adults with Seguro Popular as health insurance were 17% more likely to be at risk of malnutrition compared to those with other types of health insurance (IMSS/ISSSTE/Other). Self-reported health was strongly associated with malnutrition in the modified MNA, where individuals who reported fair health were 2.4 times more likely to be at risk for malnutrition (OR: 2.39, 95% CI: 2.19; 2.60), and those who reported poor health were 6.8 times more likely to be at risk for malnutrition compared to those with either excellent, very good, or good health (OR: 6.84, 95% CI: 6.02; 7.78).

Table 4. Predictors of Malnutrition Risk in the MHAS 2012.

	At Risk for Malnutrition (Yes vs. No)	
	OR	95% CI
Female (Ref: Male)	1.41 ***	1.30; 1.52
Age (Ref: 50–59)		
60–69	1.23 ***	1.12; 1.35
70+	1.92 ***	1.74; 2.12
Education years (Ref: 0 years)		
1–6	0.86 ***	0.77; 0.95
7+	0.65 ***	0.58; 0.74
Insurance Status (Ref: IMSS, ISSSTE, Other)		
Uninsured	0.92	0.81; 1.04
Seguro Popular	1.17 ***	1.06; 1.28
More Urban (Ref: Less Urban)	1.11 **	1.02; 1.21
Self-reported health (Ref: Excellent, very good or good)		
Fair	2.39 ***	2.19; 2.60
Poor	6.84 ***	6.02; 7.78

** p-value < 0.01; *** p-value < 0.001.

4. Discussion

The results from this study show that the modified MNA, using MHAS data, can be used as an important source of information regarding the nutritional status of older Mexican adults. Our evidence shows that the modified MNA was significantly associated with greater odds of 6-year mortality as a total continuous score, as well as based on the proposed cut point for "at risk for malnutrition".

The proposed cut point had high sensitivity and moderate specificity to predict 6-year mortality. The modified MNA performed with high sensitivity compared to other measures of nutritional status, such as the ESPEN criteria and BMI of underweight only. More than 90% of those classified as at risk for malnutrition with the modified MNA were also classified as malnourished based on the ESPEN criteria. The sensitivity of the modified MNA cut point was lower for the BMI of underweight only, biomarkers of malnutrition (low cholesterol and low hemoglobin), but had moderate concordance with these (78.6%, 54.1% and 56.1%, respectively). The specificity of the modified MNA was also moderate/low compared to these measures.

Based on the modified MNA, we estimate that 40% the MHAS sample is at risk for malnutrition. Evidence from a study of Mexican adults 60 years and older from the U.S./Mexico border that applied the original MNA also showed half of the sample was at risk for malnutrition (50.2%) and that the prevalence of malnutrition was 8.6% for women and 6.3% for men [24]. Another study in Mexico City found that the prevalence of malnutrition risk was 31.8% among Mexican adults 60 years and older using the in-depth assessment of the MNA (not only the screening part used here) [25]. Evidence from a study combining data from community older adults in 12 countries showed that that 31.9% of older adults were at risk for malnutrition [6].

The results of this study show that the predictors of malnutrition risk, in older Mexican adults, include both socioeconomic and health factors. The main predictors of malnutrition risk were having Seguro Popular insurance, having lower education, and reporting fair or poor health. Previous work in Mexico also highlighted that, in addition to similar health risk factors, socioeconomic factors, such as not having a pension, reporting lack of money to live on [25], and illiteracy [24] were also risk factors for malnutrition in this population. Studies in Spain and Italy also showed that low educational level and other measures of low SES were also associated with greater malnutrition risk among older adults, but this effect was largely explained after adjusting for sex and age [7,8]. Studies in the U.S. showed that socioeconomic factors do not appear to be main risk factors for malnutrition among older adults. The main risk factors in the U.S. were declining health status, poor cognition, and eating problems, such as difficulty swallowing [9].

Measuring nutritional status can be demanding in population-based surveys. One of the strengths of this study is that we used data from a nationally representative study of older Mexican adults that does not directly evaluate nutritional status, and we modified the MNA for potential incorporation into research of nutritional status among older adults in Mexico. The results from this study also help identify target populations in Mexico for interventions to potentially decrease the risk of malnutrition.

5. Limitations

Our approach has limitations, such as the inability to assess further nutritional information, such as short-term changes, and whether weight loss was intentional or unintentional. Further, the MNA cut point proposed in this study has low specificity and may overestimate false positives. This low specificity is seen because mortality is only a proxy for malnutrition. This measure would likely be higher if nutritional status was measured with the original MNA and compared to this modified version. Because of this limitation, the proposed cut point should not be used to assess the prevalence of malnutrition in the population but only as a marker for malnutrition risk. In addition, we recommend that, if the MHAS user wants to study malnutrition risk with the cut point of 10, they should acknowledge the limitation of the sensitivity and specificity of the proposed cut point. We recommend that one way to avoid this limitation is to treat the modified MNA as a continuous score.

6. Conclusions

In summary, our study showed that approximately 40% of Mexican adults aged 50 and older are at risk for malnutrition, according to the modified MNA. Further, the main risk factors for malnutrition in this population include dimensions of both socioeconomic and health status. The modified MNA proposed in this study can be used to capture a comprehensive picture of malnutrition risk among older adults in Mexico and can inform future work with the MHAS aiming to incorporate nutritional status, thus contributing with a framework that is replicable by other investigators.

Supplementary Materials: The following are available online at https://www.mdpi.com/article/10.3390/nu13051615/s1, Table S1: Weighted Sample Characteristics of older Mexican adults in the 2012 MHAS.

Author Contributions: Conceptualization, J.C.A., R.S.-T. and R.W.; methodology, J.C.A., R.S.-T. and R.W.; software, J.C.A.; formal analysis, J.C.A.; resources, R.W.; data curation, J.C.A., R.S.-T. and R.W.; writing—original draft preparation, J.C.A.; writing—review and editing, R.S.-T. and R.W.; visualization, J.C.A., R.S.-T. and R.W.; supervision, R.S.-T. and R.W.; project administration, R.W.; funding acquisition, R.W. All authors have read and agreed to the published version of the manuscript.

Funding: The Mexican Health and Aging Study is supported by the National Institute of Health/ National Institute on Aging in the United States (grant number R01AG018016) and the Mexican Statistical Bureau (Instituto Nacional de Estadistica Y Geografia, INEGI) in Mexico.

Institutional Review Board Statement: Not applicable, publicly available data.

Informed Consent Statement: Informed consent was obtained from all subjects involved in the study.

Data Availability Statement: Data from the MHAS is publicly available at mhasweb.org, accessed data 11 May 2021.

Acknowledgments: We thank the University of Texas Medical Branch and the Sealy Center on Aging for providing the logistic support to conduct the study. We also thank David Lopez at the University of Texas Medical Branch for his review of the ROC analysis and study methodology.

Conflicts of Interest: The authors declare no conflict of interest.

References

1. Chavarro-Carvajal, D.; Reyes-Ortiz, C.; Samper-Ternent, R.; Arciniegas, A.J.; Gutierrez, C.C. Nutritional assessment and factors associated to malnutrition in older adults: A cross-sectional study in Bogotá, Colombia. *J. Aging Health* **2015**, *27*, 304–319. [CrossRef]
2. Mowé, M.; Bøhmer, T.; Kindt, E. Reduced nutritional status in an elderly population (>70 y) is probable before disease and possibly contributes to the development of disease. *Am. J. Clin. Nutr.* **1994**, *59*, 317–324. [CrossRef] [PubMed]
3. Norman, K.; Pichard, C.; Lochs, H.; Pirlich, M. Prognostic impact of disease-related malnutrition. *Clin. Nutr. Edinb. Scotl.* **2008**, *27*, 5–15. [CrossRef]
4. Söderström, L.; Rosenblad, A.; Thors Adolfsson, E.; Bergkvist, L. Malnutrition is associated with increased mortality in older adults regardless of the cause of death. *Br. J. Nutr.* **2017**, *117*, 532–540. [CrossRef] [PubMed]
5. World Health Organization. *Evidence Profile: Malnutrition*; Integrated care for older people (ICOPE) guidelines; World Health Organization: Geneva, Switzerland, 2017.
6. Kaiser, M.J.; Bauer, J.M.; Rämsch, C.; Uter, W.; Guigoz, Y.; Cederholm, T.; Thomas, D.R.; Anthony, P.S.; Charlton, K.E.; Maggio, M.; et al. Frequency of malnutrition in older adults: A multinational perspective using the mini nutritional assessment. *J. Am. Geriatr. Soc.* **2010**, *58*, 1734–1738. [CrossRef] [PubMed]
7. Hoogendijk, E.O.; Flores Ruano, T.; Martínez-Reig, M.; López-Utiel, M.; Lozoya-Moreno, S.; Dent, E.; Abizanda, P. Socioeconomic Position and Malnutrition among Older Adults: Results from the FRADEA Study. *J. Nutr. Health Aging* **2018**, *22*, 1086–1091. [CrossRef] [PubMed]
8. Timpini, A.; Facchi, E.; Cossi, S.; Ghisla, M.K.; Romanelli, G.; Marengoni, A. Self-reported socio-economic status, social, physical and leisure activities and risk for malnutrition in late life: A cross-sectional population-based study. *J. Nutr. Health Aging* **2011**, *15*, 233–238. [CrossRef] [PubMed]
9. Fávaro-Moreira, N.C.; Krausch-Hofmann, S.; Matthys, C.; Vereecken, C.; Vanhauwaert, E.; Declercq, A.; Bekkering, G.E.; Duyck, J. Risk Factors for Malnutrition in Older Adults: A Systematic Review of the Literature Based on Longitudinal Data. *Adv. Nutr. Bethesdamd.* **2016**, *7*, 507–522. [CrossRef]
10. Wong, R.; Michaels-Obregon, A.; Palloni, A. Cohort Profile: The Mexican Health and Aging Study (MHAS). *Int. J. Epidemiol.* **2017**, *46*, e2. [CrossRef]
11. Wong, R.; Palloni, A. Aging in Mexico and Latin America. In *International Handbook of Population Aging*; Uhlenberg, P., Ed.; Springer: Dordrecht, The Netherlands, 2009; pp. 231–252.
12. Samper-Ternent, R.; Michaels-Obregon, A.; Wong, R.; Palloni, A. Older adults under a mixed regime of infectious and chronic diseases. *Salud Publica Mex.* **2012**, *54*, 487–495. [CrossRef]

13. Shamah-Levy, T.; Cuevas-Nasu, L.; Mundo-Rosas, V.; Morales-Ruán, C.; Cervantes-Turrubiates, L.; Villalpando-Hernández, S. Health and nutrition status of older adults in Mexico: Results of a national probabilistic survey. *Salud Publica De Mex.* **2008**, *50*, 383–389. [CrossRef] [PubMed]
14. Ruiz-Arregui, L.; Castillo-Martínez, L.; Orea-Tejeda, A.; Mejía-Arango, S.; Miguel-Jaimes, A. Prevalence of self-reported overweight-obesity and its association with socioeconomic and health factors among older Mexican adults. *Salud Publica Mex.* **2007**, *49* (Suppl. 4), S482–S487. [CrossRef]
15. Rodriguez, M.A.; Wong, R. *Aging in Mexico: Obesity. MHAS Fact Sheet 19-1*; Mexican Health and Aging Study: Galveston, TX, USA, 2019.
16. Samper-Ternent, R.; Michaels-Obregon, A.; Wong, R. Coexistence of Obesity and Anemia in Older Mexican Adults. *Ageing Int.* **2011**, *37*, 104–117. [CrossRef]
17. Alemán-Mateo, H.; Esparza-Romero, J.; Romero, R.U.; García, H.A.; Pérez Flores, F.A.; Ochoa Chacón, B.V.; Valencia, M.E. Prevalence of malnutrition and associated metabolic risk factors for cardiovascular disease in older adults from Northwest Mexico. *Arch. Gerontol. Geriatr.* **2008**, *46*, 375–385. [CrossRef] [PubMed]
18. Kaiser, M.J.; Bauer, J.M.; Ramsch, C.; Uter, W.; Guigoz, Y.; Cederholm, T.; Thomas, D.R.; Anthony, P.; Charlton, K.E.; Maggio, M.; et al. Validation of the Mini Nutritional Assessment short-form (MNA-SF): A practical tool for identification of nutritional status. *J. Nutr. Health Aging* **2009**, *13*, 782–788. [CrossRef] [PubMed]
19. Bauer, J.M.; Kaiser, M.J.; Anthony, P.; Guigoz, Y.; Sieber, C.C. The Mini Nutritional Assessment®—Its History, Today's Practice, and Future Perspectives. *Nutr. Clin. Pract.* **2008**, *23*, 388–396. [CrossRef] [PubMed]
20. Rubenstein, L.Z.; Harker, J.O.; Salvà, A.; Guigoz, Y.; Vellas, B. Screening for undernutrition in geriatric practice: Developing the short-form mini-nutritional assessment (MNA-SF). *J. Gerontology. Ser. Abiological. Sci. Med Sci.* **2001**, *56*, M366–M372. [CrossRef] [PubMed]
21. Dent, E.; Visvanathan, R.; Piantadosi, C.; Chapman, I. Nutritional screening tools as predictors of mortality, functional decline, and move to higher level care in older people: A systematic review. *J. Nutr. Gerontol. Geriatr.* **2012**, *31*, 97–145. [CrossRef]
22. Cederholm, T.; Bosaeus, I.; Barazzoni, R.; Bauer, J.; Van Gossum, A.; Klek, S.; Muscaritoli, M.; Nyulasi, I.; Ockenga, J.; Schneider, S.M.; et al. Diagnostic Criteria for Malnutrition—An ESPEN Consensus Statement. *Clin Nutr.* **2015**, *34*, 335–340. [CrossRef]
23. Zhang, Z.; Pereira, S.L.; Luo, M.; Matheson, E.M. Evaluation of Blood Biomarkers Associated with Risk of Malnutrition in Older Adults: A Systematic Review and Meta-Analysis. *Nutrients* **2017**, *9*, 829. [CrossRef]
24. Rodríguez-Tadeo, A.; Wall-Medrano, A.; Gaytan-Vidaña, M.E.; Campos, A.; Ornelas-Contreras, M.; Novelo-Huerta, H.I. Malnutrition risk factors among the elderly from the US-Mexico border: The "one thousand" study. *J. Nutr. Health Aging* **2012**, *16*, 426–431. [CrossRef]
25. Franco-Alvarez, N.; Avila-Funes, J.A.; Ruiz-Arreguí, L.; Gutiérrez-Robledo, L.M. Determinants of malnutrition risk among the older adult community: A secondary analysis of the Health, Wellbeing, and Aging Study (SABE) in Mexico. *Rev. Panam. Salud Publica Pan Am. J. Public Health* **2007**, *22*, 369–375. [CrossRef]

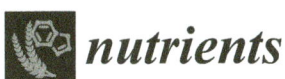

Article

Dietary Diversity and Healthy Aging: A Prospective Study

Jian Zhang [1,2] and Ai Zhao [1,*]

1. Vanke School of Public Health, Tsinghua University, Beijing 100091, China; zhangjian92@pku.edu.cn
2. Department of Nutrition and Food Hygiene, School of Public Health, Peking University, Beijing 100191, China
* Correspondence: aizhao18@tsinghua.edu.cn; Tel.: +86-138-1113-1994

Abstract: Population aging is a global phenomenon. The present study determined the effects of dietary diversity score (DDS) and food consumption on healthy aging. A subset of the data of the China Health and Nutrition Survey was utilized in this study. DDSs were calculated using the dietary data collected in the years 2009 and 2011. A healthy aging score (HAS) was calculated by summing the standardized scores on physical functional limitation, comorbidity, cognitive function, and psychological stress based on the data collected in the year 2015, with a lower HAS indicating a healthier aging process. Life quality was self-reported in the year 2015. This study found that DDS was inversely associated with HAS (T3 vs. T1: β −0.16, 95%CI −0.20 to −0.11, p-trend <0.001). The consumption of meat and poultry, aquatic products, and fruits was inversely associated with HAS, and participants in the highest tertile of staple foods consumption had a higher HAS than those in the lowest tertile. HAS was inversely associated with good self-reported life quality and positively associated with bad life quality. In conclusion, food consumption may influence the aging process, and adherence to a diverse diet is associated with a healthier aging process in elderly people.

Keywords: healthy aging; dietary diversity; physical functional limitation; comorbidity; cognition; psychological stress

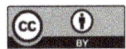

1. Introduction

Population aging is a global phenomenon [1]. In China, people aged 65 years and above made up 13.5% of the total population in 2020 [2] and the proportion is still increasing [3]. Due to the development of the economy and technology, life expectancy continues to increase [4,5]. However, healthy life expectancy increases more slowly than life expectancy [6,7]. It turns out that more older people live in a less healthy state and increasing medical and social resources are needed by the older population [1,6]. Thus, actions to promote a healthier aging process are necessary.

The concept of healthy aging or successful aging was first discussed by Robert J. Havighurst in 1961 [8]. Many of the early definitions of healthy aging were in line with the biomedical model, which was largely based on the absence of disease and disability and classified individuals into healthy and diseased [9,10]. However, as people are living longer, chronic conditions are becoming more common in older people [11], and many individuals have one or more health conditions that are well controlled [12]. In 2009, Young et al. proposed a multidimensional model of healthy aging, emphasizing the coexistence of healthy aging and chronic diseases [13,14]. Young's model covered three domains: physiological (e.g., diseases and functional impairment), psychological (e.g., emotional vitality and cognitive function), and social (e.g., spirituality and adaptation through social support mechanisms) [13]. This model is flexible, and individuals can succeed in some aspects while having limitations in other aspects [13]. To date, there is still no consensus on what healthy aging should comprise [9,12], but the World Health Organization (WHO) proposed physiological and mental capacities as the intrinsic capacity of individuals and the central part of healthy aging [12].

Nutrition is a key determinant of health and well-being throughout the whole lifecycle [15,16]. Some studies have investigated the association between age-related degenerations and some dietary patterns, such as Mediterranean diet score and diet quality index [17]. However, most of these dietary patterns were developed based on data from Western populations, and some food groups included in these patterns are consumed differently among Chinese populations in terms of quantity and the cooking methods used. Thus, the applicability of these patterns in Chinese populations remains unclear. The dietary diversity score (DDS) is an index used to reflect nutrient adequacy [18]. It is widely used in different populations and across all age groups [18]. A diverse diet is a cornerstone of a sufficient and balanced supply of nutrients. Adherence to a diverse diet is recommended by the WHO [19] and the dietary guidelines for Chinese populations [20]. Our previous work showed that higher diet diversity was associated with better memory status in adults [21]. Moreover, prospective studies have suggested that dietary diversity is inversely associated with all-cause mortality in Chinese and Japanese populations [22,23]. However, evidence of dietary diversity in relation to the overall healthy aging process is scarce in the literature. In the present study, we investigated the association of DDS and food consumption with healthy aging using prospective data from elderly Chinese people.

2. Materials and Methods

2.1. Study Design and Study Population

The present study utilized data collected in the China Health and Nutrition Survey (CHNS). The CHNS was a dynamic cohort study. The participants came from twelve geographically diverse areas of China. The first wave of the survey was initiated in 1989, and the last survey—which is open access—was conducted in 2015. Details about the CHNS have previously been published [24]. Prospective data collected in the years 2009, 2011, and 2015 were used in the present study. Baseline information was collected in the years 2009 and 2011, and outcomes (healthy aging) were assessed in the year 2015. The inclusion criteria of the present study included being involved in the year 2009 and/or 2011, involved in the year 2015, and aged 60 to 80 years in the year 2015. The exclusion criteria were having missing information on covariates, being absent from the dietary survey, having missing information on healthy aging indices, answering "don't know" to any questions concerning physical functional limitation and comorbidity, and answering "don't know" to all questions concerning psychological stress. Finally, 3085 participants were included in the analysis (Figure 1).

2.2. Dietary Survey and Dietary Diversity Score

Dietary data collected in the years 2009 and 2011 were used in this study. A total of 35.2% of participants were involved in one wave of the survey and the others were involved in both surveys. Details about the dietary survey process have been published elsewhere [25]. In brief, dietary intakes during three continuous days were recorded with the methods of dietary recall and household food weight inventory. Energy intake was estimated based on the China food composition table [26,27]. Daily food consumption at each wave of survey was expressed as amount per 1000 kcal. For individuals who participated in both waves of the survey, the average intakes across surveys were calculated.

The DDS was developed according to the dietary guidelines for Chinese populations [20]. The dietary guidelines for Chinese populations give suggestions regarding the consumption of ten food groups, including staple foods (cereals, tubers, and beans), vegetables, fruits, eggs, aquatic products, meat and poultry, soybeans and nuts, milk and dairy products, salt, and oil. As salt and oil are essential parts of the Chinese diet, they were excluded when assessing DDS. In the end, the DDS included eight food groups. The consumption of any food from a certain food group in the past 24 h would add one point for that food group. The DDS ranged from 1 to 8. Our previous study reported that a positive trend between the DDS and intakes of most macronutrients and micronutrients in Chinese adults [21]. The average daily DDS was calculated for each participant at each wave. For participants involved in both dietary surveys in the years 2009 and 2011, the average DDS was calculated. The DDS was then grouped into tertiles from low to high (T1: 1.7–3.3, T2: 3.5–4.3, and T3: 4.4–8.0) for further analysis.

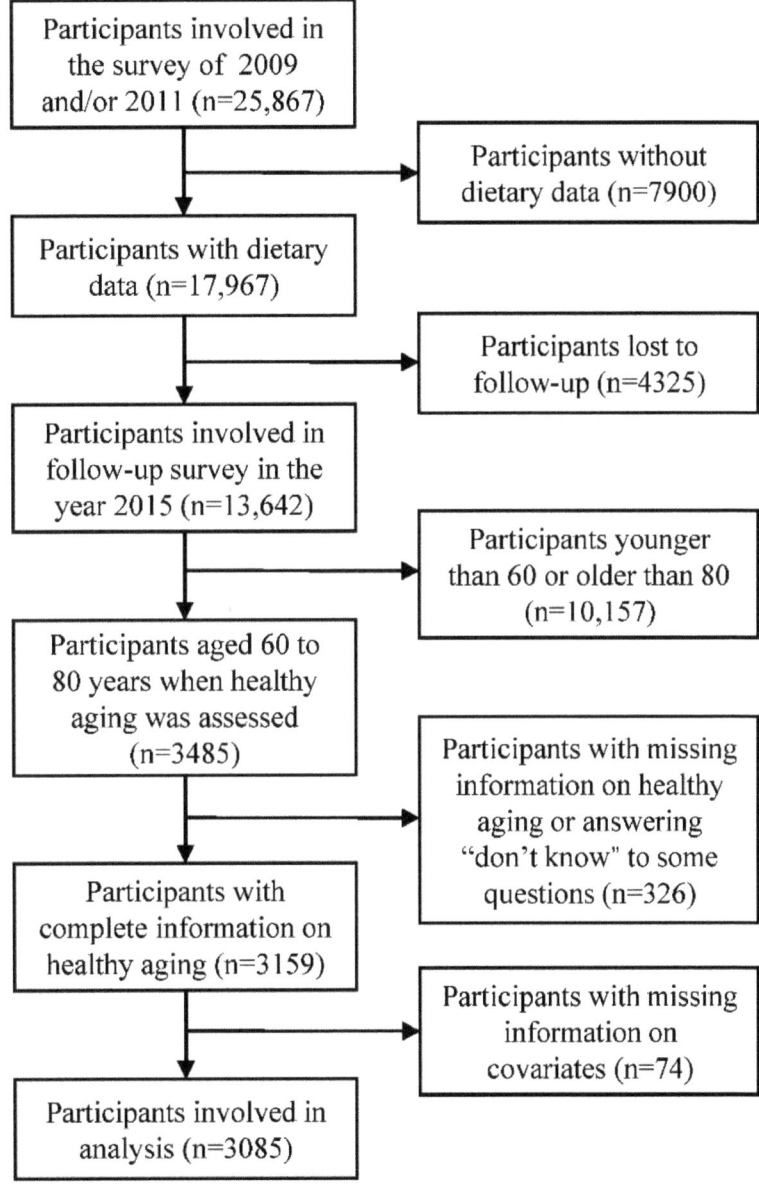

Figure 1. Flow chart of sample selection.

2.3. Healthy Aging Score

According to the definition established by Young et al., healthy aging includes three domains: physiological, psychological, and sociological [13]. As the CHNS only covered questions on two of the three domains, the healthy aging score (HAS) in this study was calculated based on physiological and psychological aspects.

The physiological aspect included two indices: physical functional limitation and comorbidity. Physical functional limitation was defined as the number of basic tasks that participants reported difficulty in performing, including lifting a 5 kg bag, squatting down, standing up, sitting continuously, and walking a kilometer. Comorbidity was defined as the number of chronic conditions, including hypertension, diabetes, myocardial infarction, stroke, apoplexy, and asthma. Both previously diagnosed hypertension and systolic blood pressure ≥ 140 mmHg and/or diastolic blood pressure ≥ 90 mmHg in the survey were regarded as hypertension. Other medical histories were based on self-reports.

The psychological aspect includes two indices: cognitive function and psychological stress. A subset of tests from the Telephone Interview for Cognitive Status-modified was used to estimate the cognitive function of adults aged 55 years and above in the CHNS [28], including immediate and delayed free-recall test (10 words), the Serial 7s test, and counting backward from 20. Responses to the four questions were summed to give a score ranging from 0 to 27, with a higher score indicating better cognitive function. Psychological stress was estimated by the Perceived Stress Scale (PSS), which has been previously validated in Chinese populations [29]. The PSS uses 14 questions to measure the stress that participants have felt during the last month, e.g., "In the last month, how often have you felt that you were unable to control the important things in your life?". The answers were recorded on a Likert response scale, consisting of "never", "almost never", "sometimes", "fairly often", "very often", and "don't know". In the analysis, "don't know" was replaced by "sometimes", the neutral midpoint of the Likert scale [30]. The total PSS score was then calculated according to the standard methods [31]. PSS scores ranged from 0 to 56, with a higher score indicating that participants felt more stress.

The HAS was calculated by summing the scores of the four indices mentioned above. Before summation, each index was converted to a continuous distribution between 0 and 1 by dividing the full score of each. The value of cognitive function was reversed before summation. Finally, we obtained a HAS ranging from 0 to 4, with a lower score indicating healthier aging.

2.4. Self-Reported Life Quality

Self-reported life quality was surveyed in the year 2015. Participants were asked "How do you rate the quality of your life at present?" (very good, good, fair, bad, very bad, and don't know). Participants who chose "don't know" were excluded. We grouped the participants' life quality into good (very good/good), fair, and bad (bad/very bad) for further analysis.

2.5. Covariates

Information on covariates of interest was obtained from the baseline survey, including sociodemographic characteristics (age, gender, region of residence, residency, education, household income, and marriage status), lifestyle behaviors (smoking and alcohol use), and anthropometric measurements (weight and height).

Per capita household income was grouped into tertiles and labeled as low, middle, and high at each wave of the survey. Missing values for income were imputed by the medians of each site at each wave of the survey. Body mass index (BMI) was calculated as weight/(height)^2.

2.6. Statistics

Results were presented as means and standard deviations for normally distributed variables; otherwise, medians and interquartile ranges (IQR) were presented. Categorical variables were presented as percentages. ANOVA and Chi-square tests were performed to compare the differences across DDS tertiles for normally distributed continuous variables and categorical variables, respectively.

The association between DDS tertiles and HAS was investigated with linear regression models; association between DDS tertiles and healthy aging components (physical functional limitation, comorbidity, cognitive function, and psychological stress) were investigated by ordinal logistic regression models. Physical functional limitation and comorbidity were grouped into categorical variables according to participants' number of limitations or comorbidities (0, 1–2, or ≥ 3). Cognitive function and psychological stress scores were grouped into tertiles from low to high. Multivariate models were adjusted for age (years), gender (men or women), BMI (kg/m^2), region of residence (southern or northern China), residency (rural or urban), education (primary school and below or middle school and above), income (low, middle, or high), marriage status (married or others (divorced, widowed, separated, or never married)), smoking (current smoker or not), and alcohol use (≥ 1 or <1 time per week).

We further investigated food group consumption in relation to HAS. Data on food consumption were converted into categorical variables, then linear regression models were created. For food groups with a relatively low proportion of consumers (milk and dairy products, aquatic products, and fruits), the daily average food consumption was grouped into non-consumer, low (below the median in consumers), and high (above the median in consumers). Other food groups were grouped into tertiles and labeled as low, middle, and high. The covariates mentioned above were also adjusted in the analysis.

Multinomial logistic regression models were created to investigate the association of HAS with self-reported life quality (fair, good, or poor).

Subgroup analyses of the association between DDS tertiles and healthy aging were conducted according to age (≤ 60 or >60 years), gender (man or women), region of residence (southern or northern China), BMI (<24 or ≥ 24 kg/m^2), smoking (current smoker or not), and alcohol use (≥ 1 or <1 time per week). Interaction was tested by likelihood ratio tests, which compared the model with and without interaction terms between DDS tertiles and the baseline stratifying variables. Sensitivity analysis was conducted by excluding participants who answered "don't know" to at least one of the questions in the assessment of psychological stress.

Tests for linear trends across categories were conducted by assigning the medians of each category and treating the variable as continuous in a separate regression model. All the statistics were analyzed using R 4.0.5 (R Core Team, Vienna, Austria). Additional packages were used for ordinal logistic regression (MASS [32]), multinomial logistic regression (nnet [32]), and likelihood ratio test (lmtest [33]). All p values were two-sided, and statistical significance was defined as $p < 0.05$.

3. Results

3.1. Baseline Characteristics

The baseline characteristics of participants across DDS tertiles are shown in Table 1. Participants with a higher DDS had a higher BMI, had higher proportions of people living in southern China and urban areas, had higher levels of education and per capita household income, were more likely to be married, and had a lower proportion of smokers.

Table 1. Baseline characteristics of the participants across dietary diversity score tertiles.

Variables	Dietary Diversity Score [a]			p
	T1	T2	T3	
Number of participants	991	1076	1018	
Age (year)	62.1(5.6)	61.6(5.5)	61.9(5.6)	0.088
Body mass index (kg/m^2)	23.3(3.8)	23.9(3.4)	24.4(3.2)	<0.001
Gender				0.166
Men	44.1	48.2	46.7	
Women	55.9	51.8	53.3	
Region of residence				<0.001
Southern China	60.9	69.1	63.0	
Northern China	39.1	30.9	37.0	
Residency				<0.001
Rural	84.2	65.1	36.1	
Urban	15.8	34.9	63.9	
Education				<0.001
Primary school and below	80.7	61.9	35.1	
Middle school and above	19.3	38.1	64.9	
Per capita household income				<0.001
Low	54.0	32.4	11.8	
Middle	31.1	37.7	25.3	
High	14.9	29.9	62.9	
Marriage status				<0.001
Married	83.9	88.4	90.2	
Others	16.1	11.6	9.8	
Smoking				0.001
Current smoker	30.1	28.0	23.1	
Non-smoker	69.9	72.0	76.9	
Alcohol use (times/week)				0.474
<1	79.8	78.0	77.8	
≥1	20.2	22.0	22.2	

[a] Dietary diversity scores were grouped into tertiles from low to high (T1: 1.7–3.3, T2: 3.5–4.3, and T3: 4.4–8.0). Continuous variables are presented as means and standard deviations; categorical variables are presented as percentages. Continuous variables were compared across dietary diversity score tertiles by ANOVA; categorical variables were compared by Chi-square tests.

3.2. Dietary Diversity Score and Healthy Aging

The average HAS of the participants was 1.26 ± 0.50. The DDS was inversely associated with HAS after the adjustment of covariates (a lower HAS indicated healthier aging). Higher DDS was associated with better cognitive function, fewer physical functional limitations, and less psychological stress. The association between DDS and the number of comorbidities was insignificant (Table 2).

Table 2. Association of dietary diversity score with healthy aging.

Variables		Dietary Diversity Score [a]		p-Trend
	T1	T2	T3	
Healthy aging score [b]				
Crude	Ref	−0.12(−0.16, −0.08)	−0.26(−0.31, −0.22)	<0.001
Model 1	Ref	−0.06(−0.10, −0.02)	−0.15(−0.20, −0.11)	<0.001
Model 2	Ref	−0.06(−0.10, −0.02)	−0.16(−0.20, −0.11)	<0.001
Physical functional limitation [c]				
Crude	Ref	0.77(0.65, 0.90)	0.58(0.49, 0.68)	<0.001
Model 1	Ref	0.87(0.73, 1.04)	0.64(0.52, 0.79)	<0.001
Model 2	Ref	0.86(0.73, 1.03)	0.64(0.52, 0.78)	<0.001
Comorbidity [c]				
Crude	Ref	1.07(0.90, 1.27)	1.26(1.06, 1.50)	0.010
Model 1	Ref	1.09(0.91, 1.31)	1.19(0.97, 1.47)	0.101
Model 2	Ref	1.01(0.84, 1.22)	1.09(0.88, 1.35)	0.441
Cognitive function [c]				
Crude	Ref	1.58(1.34, 1.85)	2.88(2.44, 3.39)	<0.001
Model 1	Ref	1.25(1.05, 1.48)	1.80(1.48, 2.19)	<0.001
Model 2	Ref	1.23(1.04, 1.46)	1.77(1.46, 2.15)	<0.001
Psychological stress [c]				
Crude	Ref	0.56(0.48, 0.66)	0.42(0.36, 0.50)	<0.001
Model 1	Ref	0.63(0.53, 0.74)	0.59(0.48, 0.71)	<0.001
Model 2	Ref	0.63(0.53, 0.75)	0.59(0.49, 0.72)	<0.001

Ref, reference. [a] Dietary diversity scores were grouped into tertiles from low to high (T1: 1.7–3.3, T2: 3.5–4.3, and T3: 4.4–8.0). [b] Linear regression models were created to estimate the association of dietary diversity score with healthy aging score; values are β (95% confidence intervals) unless specified. [c] Ordinal logistic regression models were created to estimate the association of dietary diversity score with physical functional limitation, comorbidity, cognitive function, and psychological stress; values are odds ratios (95% confidence intervals) unless specified. Comorbidity and physical functional limitations were classified into categorical variables according to the number of comorbidities or functional limitations (0, 1–2, or ≥3). Scores for cognitive function and psychological stress are grouped into tertiles from low to high. Multivariate models were adjusted for: model 1: age, gender, region of residence, residency, education, income, and marriage status; model 2: additionally included body mass index, smoking, and alcohol use.

Significant interactions were observed between DDS tertiles and gender, region of residence, smoking status, and alcohol use in relation to HAS (Figure 2). The association of DDS tertiles with cognitive function was modified by age and region of residence, while the association of DDS tertiles with psychological stress was modified by BMI and region of residence (Figure 2).

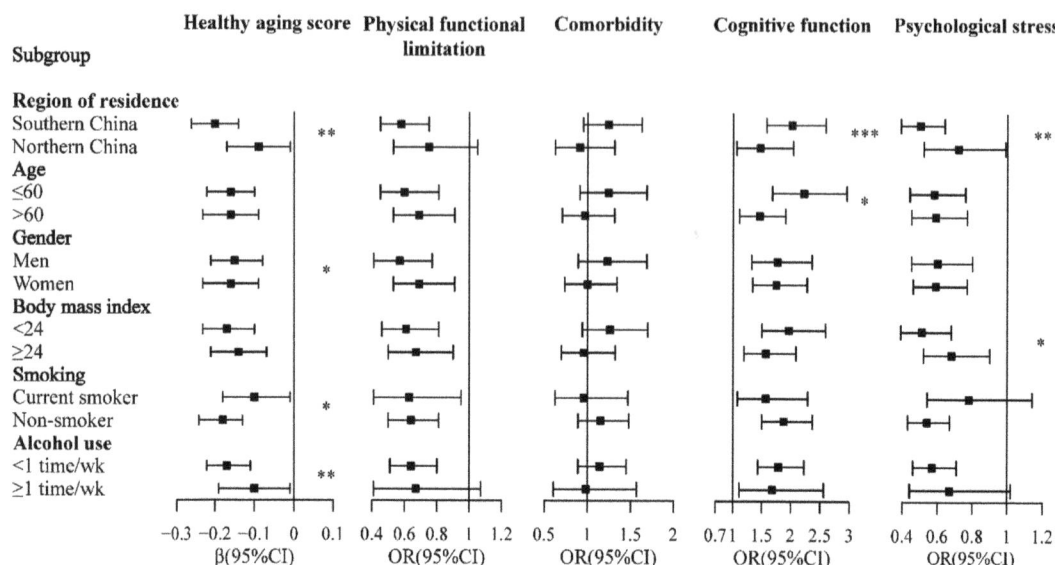

Figure 2. Subgroup analysis of the association between dietary diversity score tertiles and healthy aging. Dietary diversity scores were grouped into tertiles from low to high (T1: 1.7–3.3, T2: 3.5–4.3, and T3: 4.4–8.0). Squares and horizontal lines showed the results of T3 vs. T1. * $p < 0.05$, ** $p < 0.01$, *** $p < 0.001$. OR, odds ratio; CI, confidence interval. Association of DDS tertiles with healthy aging score (lower score indicated healthier aging) was estimated by a linear regression model. Association of DDS tertiles with physical functional limitation, comorbidity, cognitive function, and psychological stress was estimated by an ordinal logistic regression model. Comorbidity and physical functional limitations were classified into categorical variables according to the number of comorbidities or functional limitations (0, 1–2, or ≥3). Cognition and PSS were grouped into tertiles from low to high. Multivariate models were adjusted for age, gender, region of residence, residency, education, income, marriage status, body mass index, smoking, and alcohol use. Analyses within subgroups were adjusted for all other covariates.

In the sensitivity analysis, the association of DDS with HAS and psychological stress did not change appreciably after excluding participants who answered "don't know" in the assessment of psychological stress (Table S1).

3.3. Food Group Consumption and Healthy Aging

The consumption of meat and poultry, aquatic products, and fruits was inversely associated with HAS. Compared with non-consumers, a low consumption of milk and dairy products was associated with a lower HAS. Participants in the highest tertile of staple foods consumption had a higher HAS than those in the lowest tertile. The association of the consumption of eggs and HAS became insignificant after the adjustment of covariates. There was no significant association between HAS and the consumption of vegetables and the consumption of soybeans and nuts (Table 3).

Table 3. Association between food consumption and healthy aging score.

Food Groups	Number of Participants	Median (IQR)	Crude β (95%CI)	Crude p-Trend	Adjusted β (95%CI)	Adjusted p-Trend
Staple foods				<0.001		0.060
Low	1028	130.8 (33.2)	Ref		Ref	
Middle	1028	178.2 (20.5)	0.05 (0.01, 0.10)		0 (−0.04, 0.04)	
High	1029	228.2 (41.5)	0.12 (0.08, 0.16)		0.04 (0, 0.08)	
Soybeans and nuts				0.180		0.995
Low	1028	0 (2.2)	Ref		Ref	
Middle	1028	8.4 (4.1)	−0.05 (−0.09, −0.01)		−0.03 (−0.07, 0.01)	
High	1029	21.2 (13.5)	−0.03 (−0.08, 0.01)		0 (−0.04, 0.04)	
Vegetables				0.585		0.167
Low	1028	95.8 (33.5)	Ref		Ref	
Middle	1028	149.6 (26.2)	0 (−0.05, 0.04)		−0.01 (−0.05, 0.02)	
High	1029	225.0 (70.2)	−0.01 (−0.06, 0.03)		−0.03 (−0.07, 0.01)	
Fruits				<0.001		<0.001
Non-consumer	1482	0	Ref		Ref	
Low	802	31.2 (20.2)	−0.10 (−0.14, −0.06)		−0.05 (−0.09, −0.01)	
High	801	88.1 (54.0)	−0.13 (−0.18, −0.09)		−0.09 (−0.13, −0.05)	
Meat and poultry				<0.001		0.047
Low	1028	16.1 (24.0)	Ref		Ref	
Middle	1028	42.7 (12.2)	−0.08 (−0.13, −0.04)		−0.04 (−0.08, 0)	
High	1029	76.9 (30.6)	−0.13 (−0.17, −0.08)		−0.04 (−0.09, 0)	
Aquatic products				<0.001		<0.001
Non-consumer	1436	0	Ref		Ref	
Low	824	13.8 (8.9)	−0.12 (−0.16, −0.07)		−0.05 (−0.09, −0.01)	
High	825	38.0 (21.7)	−0.17 (−0.21, −0.13)		−0.10 (−0.14, −0.06)	
Eggs				0.006		0.113
Low	1028	0 (5.1)	Ref		Ref	
Middle	1028	14.6 (5.7)	−0.02 (−0.06, 0.02)		0.01 (−0.03, 0.05)	
High	1029	30.7 (15.3)	−0.06 (−0.10, −0.02)		−0.03 (−0.07, 0.01)	
Milk and dairy products				<0.001		0.054
Non-consumer	2493	0	Ref		Ref	
Low	296	45.9 (30.3)	−0.13 (−0.19, −0.06)		−0.08 (−0.14, −0.02)	
High	296	126.2 (65.4)	−0.13 (−0.19, −0.07)		−0.05 (−0.11, 0.01)	

IQR, interquartile range; CI, confidence interval; Ref, reference. Consumption of fruits, aquatic products, and milk and dairy products were grouped into non-consumer, low (below the median in consumers), and high (above the median in consumers). Other food groups were grouped into tertiles and labeled as low, middle, and high. Linear regression models were created to estimate the association of food consumption with healthy aging score (a lower score indicates healthier aging). Multivariate models were adjusted for age, gender, region of residence, residency, education, income, marriage status, body mass index, smoking, and alcohol use.

3.4. Healthy Aging Score and Self-Reported Life Quality

The association of HAS with self-reported life quality is shown in Table 4. HAS was inversely associated with good self-reported life quality and positively associated with bad life quality.

Table 4. Healthy aging score and self-reported life quality [a].

Self-Reported Life Quality	Number of Participants	Crude		Adjusted	
		OR (95%CI)	p	OR (95%CI)	p
Fair	1148	Ref		Ref	
Good	1763	0.38 (0.32, 0.44)	<0.001	0.38 (0.32, 0.45)	<0.001
Poor	168	4.15 (3.05, 5.66)	<0.001	4.41 (3.12, 6.25)	<0.001

OR, odds ratio; CI, confidence interval; Ref, reference. [a] 3079 participants were included in analysis. Multinomial logistic regression models were created to estimate the association of healthy aging score (a lower score indicates healthier aging) with self-reported life quality. Multivariate models were adjusted for age, gender, region of residence, residency, education, income, and marriage status.

4. Discussion

Our study revealed that the consumption of some food groups may impact the aging process and that a more diverse diet contributed to a healthier aging process in older adults. Moreover, healthy aging was associated with good self-reported life quality. To the best of our knowledge, the present study is the first to explore the association of DDS with overall healthy aging. The results confirm that the adoption of a diverse diet may provide a cost-effective intervention to promote healthy aging.

Our study found that higher DDS was associated with overall healthy aging in elderly Chinese people. The analyses of DDS in relation to healthy aging components showed that a higher DDS was associated with better cognitive function and fewer physical functional limitations and psychological stress, which was consistent with results from the literature. Prospective studies have proven that an increase in DDS is associated with reduced risk of cognitive impairment in elderly Chinese and Japanese people [34,35], and previous studies have also indicted that having a higher dietary diversity is associated with better physical function in elderly Japanese people [36]. We assumed that several pathways might contribute to the association between DDS and healthy aging. First, the aging process is characterized by a loss of muscle mass and strength [37], increasing the risks of functional impairment [38], disability [39], and frailty [40]. Sufficient protein intake is good for preserving good muscle function in older people [41,42]. Our previous work showed that higher DDS was associated with a higher intake of protein in Chinese adults [21], which may slow down the loss of muscle mass caused by aging. The analysis of food group consumption and healthy aging supported this assumption, which showed that higher intakes of meat and aquatic products, both good sources of high-quality protein, were inversely associated with HAS. Second, older people usually experience a degeneration in their physical and mental capability, including a decrease in mobility, degeneration of the digestive system, and decline in income, causing them to be at higher risks of malnutrition [43–45]. Higher DDS was reported to be inversely associated with the risk of nutrient inadequacy [46,47], which may prevent health problems related to insufficient nutrient intake. Third, inflammation and oxidative stress are thought to be one of the major causes of aging, accelerating the loss of muscle and bone mass and the degeneration of the function of the central nervous system [48–51]. As vegetables and fruits are good sources of antioxidants, a higher DDS may promote healthier aging by reducing inflammation and oxidative stress [52]. Last but not least, it is suggested that age-related gut microbiota dysbiosis can trigger the innate immune response and chronic low-grade inflammation, leading to frailty and unhealthy aging [53,54]. A diverse diet was reported to promote a healthier gut microbiota [55], which may further promote healthy aging [56].

Specifically, psychological stress is an important aspect of wellbeing, and stress has been reported to play an important role in the development of depression [57], which is an increasing social concern in elderly Chinese people [58]. Previous studies have reported that psychological stress may be a risk factor for chronic diseases (e.g., diabetes and cardiovascular diseases) [59,60]. As China is experiencing a fast transition in technology, economy, and lifestyle, older people may face more stress from these changes [61,62]. The impact of diet on psychological stress is relatively difficult to investigate, as the association is bidirectional [63]. However, it has been proven by clinical trials that the Mediterranean diet is protective against depression and psychological problems [64,65]. Our prospective study found that higher DDS was associated with lower PSS scores in elderly Chinese people. The beneficial effect of higher DDS on psychological stress may be related to the elevated intake of antioxidants from a diverse diet [66]. Moreover, recent findings on the gut–brain axis have suggested that maintaining a healthy microbiota might be important for mental health [63,67], thus a higher DDS might also contribute to better mental health through a healthier gut microbiota.

Regarding food groups, the present study found that participants in the highest tertile of staple foods consumption had higher HAS than those in the lowest tertile while there was no significant difference between participants in the lowest and middle tertiles. Staple foods were the major source of carbohydrates in the Chinese diet. Evidence in the literature has suggested that high carbohydrate intake might have negative effects on mental health. Prospective studies have reported that dietary patterns characterized by high intake of protein and fat and low intake of carbohydrate were associated with lower risks of cognitive impairment and dementia [68,69]. Some other studies have reported that a low-carbohydrate diet was associated with lower risks of depression in Iranian women [70] and patients with diabetes [71]. Moreover, we propose that another possible reason for this association may be that individuals with a high consumption of staples foods have a lower score for DDS in the study population.

In the subgroup analyses, we observed that the association of DDS with HAS was less pronounced in individuals who were current smokers or who drank alcohol ≥1 time per week compared to their counterparts. Smoking generates radicals and increases inflammation, causing lipid peroxidation and the oxidation of proteins [51,72,73]. It has been recognized as one of the most important risk factors for respiratory diseases, cardiovascular diseases, and cancers, which are the major causes of disability and mortality [74,75]. Alcohol use is another leading risk factor for disease burden and health loss [76], increasing the risk of hypertension [77], liver cancer [78], and gastrointestinal cancer [79]. Thus, smoking and alcohol use might attenuate the positive association between DDS and healthy aging. Moreover, our study found that the association between DDS and healthy aging was more pronounced among individuals living in southern China than those living in northern areas. This may be because the northern and southern populations of China have some differences in terms of lifestyle, diet, and the environment. According to previous studies, the northern dietary pattern is more likely to contribute to the development of overweight and obesity [80], and the northern population is more likely to have clustered cardiovascular risk factors than the southern population [81].

In addition, the present study found that higher HAS was negatively associated with self-reported good life quality and positively associated with bad life quality. This is reasonable, as a higher HAS means more physical functional limitation, comorbidity, psychological stress, and poor cognitive function. The results suggest that improving dietary diversity may be regarded as one of the strategies to promote healthy aging and to improve the life quality of elderly people.

When constructing a DDS, the food groups included were different across studies, partly due to the study population and purpose [18,82,83]. In the literature, the five-food-group DDS according to the USDA Food Guide Pyramid or a modified version of the score have been used relatively more frequently [82,83]. In the present study, we calculated the DDS based on the dietary guidelines for Chinese populations [20], which additionally includes some food groups which play important roles in the Chinese diet.

The present study had several potential limitations. First, although the present study was based on a prospective setting, participants' baseline information regarding outcomes was not taken into consideration, as most of these indices were not included in the baseline survey. This may impact the causal inference in this study. Second, the definition of healthy aging and the indices included in the estimation of healthy aging were different across studies. We calculated the healthy aging score based on the data available, which may impact comparison with other studies. In the present study, the HAS was constructed based on participants' physiological and psychological conditions, and the sociological aspect was not included. Thus, the association of dietary diversity and healthy aging was not comprehensively investigated. However, as physiological and mental capacities were regarded as the intrinsic capacity of individuals according to the WHO report [12], this work could contribute to our knowledge on dietary intake and healthy aging. Further studies in regard to sociological aspects of aging are still needed to provide a more comprehensive picture.

5. Conclusions

In summary, we found that the consumption of some food groups may impact the aging process and adherence to a more diverse diet was associated with a healthier aging process in elderly people. Higher DDS was associated with better cognitive function, fewer physical functional limitations, and less psychological stress. This study confirmed that the adoption of a diverse diet may provide a cost-effective intervention for the promotion of healthy aging.

Supplementary Materials: The following are available online at https://www.mdpi.com/article/10.3390/nu13061787/s1, Table S1: Sensitivity analysis of the association between dietary diversity score and healthy aging.

Author Contributions: Conceptualization, J.Z. and A.Z.; methodology, J.Z.; formal analysis, J.Z.; writing—original draft preparation, J.Z.; writing—review and editing, A.Z.; supervision, A.Z. Both authors have read and agreed to the published version of the manuscript.

Funding: This research received no external funding.

Institutional Review Board Statement: The CHNS was approved by institutional review boards at the University of North Carolina at Chapel Hill and the National Institute of Nutrition and Food Safety, Chinese Center for Disease Control and Prevention. The ethics of data use of this study were approved by the institution review board of Tsinghua University (No. 20210072).

Informed Consent Statement: All the participants gave written informed consent before they participated in the survey.

Data Availability Statement: The raw data supporting the conclusions of this article can be found here: https://www.cpc.unc.edu/projects/china/ (accessed on 23 May 2019).

Acknowledgments: This research uses data from CHNS. We are grateful to research grant funding from the National Institute for Health (NIH), the Eunice Kennedy Shriver National Institute of Child Health and Human Development (NICHD) for R01 HD30880, National Institute on Aging (NIA) for R01 AG065357, National Institute of Diabetes and Digestive and Kidney Diseases (NIDDK) for R01DK104371 and R01HL108427, the NIH Fogarty grant D43 TW009077 since 1989, the China-Japan Friendship Hospital, Ministry of Health for support for CHNS 2009, Chinese National Human Genome Center at Shanghai since 2009, and Beijing Municipal Center for Disease Prevention and Control since 2011. We thank the National Institute for Nutrition and Health, China Center for Disease Control and Prevention, Beijing Municipal Center for Disease Control and Prevention, and the Chinese National Human Genome Center at Shanghai.

Conflicts of Interest: The authors declare no conflict of interest.

References

1. United Nations, Department of Economic and Social Affairs, Population Division (2020). World Population Ageing 2019 (ST/ESA/SER.A/444). Available online: https://www.un.org/en/development/desa/population/publications/pdf/ageing/WorldPopulationAgeing2019-Report.pdf (accessed on 4 October 2020).
2. National Bureau of Statistics. Main Data of the Seventh National Census of China. Available online: http://www.stats.gov.cn/tjsj/zxfb/202105/t20210510_1817176.html (accessed on 20 May 2021).
3. Fang, E.F.; Xie, C.; Schenkel, J.A.; Wu, C.; Long, Q.; Cui, H.; Aman, Y.; Frank, J.; Liao, J.; Zou, H.; et al. A research agenda for ageing in China in the 21st century (2nd edition): Focusing on basic and translational research, long-term care, policy and social networks. *Ageing Res. Rev.* **2020**, *64*, 101174. [CrossRef] [PubMed]

4. Chen, H.; Qian, Y.; Dong, Y.; Yang, Z.; Guo, L.; Liu, J.; Shen, Q.; Wang, L. Patterns and changes in life expectancy in China, 1990-2016. *PLoS ONE* **2020**, *15*, e0231367. [CrossRef]
5. Kontis, V.; Bennett, J.E.; Mathers, C.D.; Li, G.; Foreman, K.; Ezzati, M. Future life expectancy in 35 industrialised countries: Projections with a Bayesian model ensemble. *Lancet* **2017**, *389*, 1323–1335. [CrossRef]
6. Salomon, J.A.; Wang, H.; Freeman, M.K.; Vos, T.; Flaxman, A.D.; Lopez, A.D.; Murray, C.J. Healthy life expectancy for 187 countries, 1990–2010: A systematic analysis for the Global Burden Disease Study 2010. *Lancet* **2012**, *380*, 2144–2162. [CrossRef]
7. Zhou, M.G.; Li, Y.C.; Wang, H.D.; Zeng, X.Y.; Wang, L.J.; Liu, S.W.; Liu, Y.N.; Liang, X.F. Analysis on life expectancy and healthy life expectancy in China, 1990-2015. *Chin. J. Epidemiol.* **2016**, *37*, 1439–1443. [CrossRef]
8. Havighurst, R.J. Successful Aging1. *Gerontol.* **1961**, *1*, 8–13. [CrossRef]
9. Aronson, L. Healthy Aging Across the Stages of Old Age. *Clin. Geriatr. Med.* **2020**, *36*, 549–558. [CrossRef]
10. Anton, S.D.; Woods, A.J.; Ashizawa, T.; Barb, D.; Buford, T.W.; Carter, C.S.; Clark, D.J.; Cohen, R.A.; Corbett, D.B.; Cruz-Almeida, Y.; et al. Successful aging: Advancing the science of physical independence in older adults. *Ageing Res. Rev.* **2015**, *24*, 304–327. [CrossRef] [PubMed]
11. Fallon, C.K.; Karlawish, J. Is the WHO Definition of Health Aging Well? Frameworks for "Health" After Three Score and Ten. *Am. J. Public Health* **2019**, *109*, 1104–1106. [CrossRef]
12. World Health Organization. World Report on Ageing and Health 2015. Available online: https://www.who.int/ageing/events/world-report-2015-launch/en/ (accessed on 10 September 2020).
13. Young, Y.; Frick, K.D.; Phelan, E.A. Can Successful Aging and Chronic Illness Coexist in the Same Individual? A Multidimensional Concept of Successful Aging. *J. Am. Med Dir. Assoc.* **2009**, *10*, 87–92. [CrossRef]
14. Young, Y.; Fan, M.-Y.; Parrish, J.M.; Frick, K.D. Validation of a Novel Successful Aging Construct. *J. Am. Med Dir. Assoc.* **2009**, *10*, 314–322. [CrossRef]
15. Black, M.; Bowman, M. Nutrition and Healthy Aging. *Clin. Geriatr. Med.* **2020**, *36*, 655–669. [CrossRef]
16. Ademowo, O.S.; Dias, H.K.I.; Pararasa, C.; Griffiths, H.R. Chapter 6—Nutritional Hormesis in a Modern Environment. In *The Science of Hormesis in Health and Longevity*; Rattan, S.I.S., Kyriazis, M., Eds.; Academic Press: London, UK, 2019; pp. 75–86. ISBN 978-0-12-814253-0.
17. Milte, C.M.; McNaughton, S.A. Dietary patterns and successful ageing: A systematic review. *Eur. J. Nutr.* **2016**, *55*, 423–450. [CrossRef] [PubMed]
18. United Nations, Food and Agriculture Organization, Nutrition and Consumer Protection Division. Guidelines for Measuring Household and Individual Dietary Diversity. Available online: http://www.fao.org/publications/card/en/c/5aacbe39-068f-513b-b17d-1d92959654ea/ (accessed on 19 November 2019).
19. World Health Organization. Healthy Diet. Available online: https://www.who.int/news-room/fact-sheets/detail/healthy-diet (accessed on 22 April 2021).
20. Chinese Nutrition Society. *Dietary Guidelines for Chinese (2016)*; People's Medical Publishing House Co., Ltd.: Beijing, China, 2016; ISBN 978-7-117-22214-3.
21. Zhang, J.; Zhao, A.; Wu, W.; Yang, C.; Ren, Z.; Wang, M.; Wang, P.; Zhang, Y. Dietary Diversity Is Associated With Memory Status in Chinese Adults: A Prospective Study. *Front. Aging Neurosci.* **2020**, *12*, 580760. [CrossRef]
22. Tao, L.; Xie, Z.; Huang, T. Dietary Diversity and All-Cause Mortality among Chinese Adults Aged 65 or Older: A Community-Based Cohort Study. *Asia Pac J Clin Nutr.* **2020**, *29*, 152–160. [CrossRef] [PubMed]
23. Otsuka, R.; Tange, C.; Nishita, Y.; Kato, Y.; Tomida, M.; Imai, T.; Ando, F.; Shimokata, H. Dietary Diversity and All-Cause and Cause-Specific Mortality in Japanese Community-Dwelling Older Adults. *Nutrients* **2020**, *12*, 1052. [CrossRef] [PubMed]
24. Popkin, B.M.; Du, S.; Zhai, F.; Zhang, B. Cohort Profile: The China Health and Nutrition Survey–monitoring and understanding socio-economic and health change in China, 1989-2011. *Int. J. Epidemiol.* **2009**, *39*, 1435–1440. [CrossRef]
25. Zhai, F.; Guo, X.; Popkin, B.M.; Ma, L.; Wang, Q.; Yu, W.; Jin, S.; Ge, K. Evaluation of the 24-Hour Individual Recall Method in China. *Food Nutr. Bull.* **1996**, *17*, 1–17. [CrossRef]
26. Yang, Y.; Wang, G.; Pan, X. *China Food Composition (Book 1)*, 2nd ed.; Peking University Medical Press: Beijing, China, 2009.
27. Yang, Y. *China Food Composition (Book 2)*; Peking University Medical Press: Beijing, China, 2004.
28. Qin, B.; Adair, L.S.; Plassman, B.L.; Batis, C.; Edwards, L.J.; Popkin, B.M.; Mendez, M.A. Dietary Patterns and Cognitive Decline Among Chinese Older Adults. *Epidemiology* **2015**, *26*, 758–768. [CrossRef] [PubMed]
29. Leung, D.Y.; Lam, T.-H.; Chan, S.S. Three versions of Perceived Stress Scale: Validation in a sample of Chinese cardiac patients who smoke. *BMC Public Health* **2010**, *10*, 513–517. [CrossRef]
30. Downey, R.G.; King, C.V. Missing Data in Likert Ratings: A Comparison of Replacement Methods. *J. Gen. Psychol.* **1998**, *125*, 175–191. [CrossRef] [PubMed]
31. Cohen, S.; Kamarck, T.; Mermelstein, R. A global measure of perceived stress. *J. Health Soc. Behav.* **1983**, *24*, 385–396. [CrossRef] [PubMed]
32. Venables, W.; Ripley, B. *Modern Applied Statistics New York*; Fourth, S., Ed.; Springer: New York, NY, USA, 2002; ISBN 978-0-387-21706-2.
33. Zeileis, A.; Hothorn, T. Diagnostic Checking in Regression Relationships. R News 2002, 2, 7–10. Available online: https://cran.r-project.org/web/packages/lmtest/vignettes/lmtest-intro.pdf (accessed on 15 March 2021).

34. Zheng, J.; Zhou, R.; Li, F.; Chen, L.; Wu, K.; Huang, J.; Liu, H.; Huang, Z.; Xu, L.; Yuan, Z.; et al. Association between dietary diversity and cognitive impairment among the oldest-old: Findings from a nationwide cohort study. *Clin. Nutr.* **2021**, *40*, 1452–1462. [CrossRef]
35. Otsuka, R.; Nishita, Y.; Tange, C.; Tomida, M.; Kato, Y.; Nakamoto, M.; Imai, T.; Ando, F.; Shimokata, H. Dietary diversity decreases the risk of cognitive decline among Japanese older adults. *Geriatr. Gerontol. Int.* **2016**, *17*, 937–944. [CrossRef]
36. Yokoyama, Y.; Nishi, M.; Murayama, H.; Amano, H.; Taniguchi, Y.; Nofuji, Y.; Narita, M.; Matsuo, E.; Seino, S.; Kawano, Y.; et al. Association of dietary variety with body composition and physical function in community-dwelling elderly Japanese. *J. Nutr. Heal. Aging* **2015**, *20*, 691–696. [CrossRef] [PubMed]
37. Goodpaster, B.H.; Park, S.W.; Harris, T.B.; Kritchevsky, S.B.; Nevitt, M.; Schwartz, A.V.; Simonsick, E.M.; Tylavsky, F.A.; Visser, M.; Newman, A.B.; et al. The Loss of Skeletal Muscle Strength, Mass, and Quality in Older Adults: The Health, Aging and Body Composition Study. *Journals Gerontol. Ser. A Boil. Sci. Med Sci.* **2006**, *61*, 1059–1064. [CrossRef] [PubMed]
38. Visser, M.; Kritchevsky, S.B.; Goodpaster, B.H.; Newman, A.B.; Nevitt, M.; Stamm, E.; Harris, T.B. Leg Muscle Mass and Composition in Relation to Lower Extremity Performance in Men and Women Aged 70 to 79: The Health, Aging and Body Composition Study. *J. Am. Geriatr. Soc.* **2002**, *50*, 897–904. [CrossRef]
39. Rantanen, T. Muscle strength, disability and mortality. *Scand. J. Med. Sci. Sports* **2003**, *13*, 3–8. [CrossRef]
40. Evans, W.J.; Paolisso, G.; Abbatecola, A.M.; Corsonello, A.; Bustacchini, S.; Strollo, F.; Lattanzio, F. Frailty and muscle metabolism dysregulation in the elderly. *Biogerontology* **2010**, *11*, 527–536. [CrossRef]
41. Houston, D.K.; Nicklas, B.J.; Ding, J.; Harris, T.B.; Tylavsky, F.A.; Newman, A.B.; Lee, J.S.; Sahyoun, N.R.; Visser, M.; Kritchevsky, S.B.; et al. Dietary protein intake is associated with lean mass change in older, community-dwelling adults: The Health, Aging, and Body Composition (Health ABC) Study. *Am. J. Clin. Nutr.* **2008**, *87*, 150–155. [CrossRef]
42. McGrath, R.; Stastny, S.; Casperson, S.; Jahns, L.; Roemmich, J.; Hackney, K.J. Daily Protein Intake and Distribution of Daily Protein Consumed Decreases Odds for Functional Disability in Older Americans. *J. Aging Health* **2020**, *32*, 1075–1083. [CrossRef] [PubMed]
43. Fávaro-Moreira, N.C.; Krausch-Hofmann, S.; Matthys, C.; Vereecken, C.; Vanhauwaert, E.; Declercq, A.; Bekkering, G.E.; Duyck, J. Risk Factors for Malnutrition in Older Adults: A Systematic Review of the Literature Based on Longitudinal Data. *Adv. Nutr.* **2016**, *7*, 507–522. [CrossRef] [PubMed]
44. Donini, L.M.; Scardella, P.; Piombo, L.; Neri, B.; Asprino, R.; Proietti, A.R.; Carcaterra, S.; Cava, E.; Cataldi, S.; Cucinotta, D.; et al. Malnutrition in elderly: Social and economic determinants. *J. Nutr. Health Aging* **2013**, *17*, 9–15. [CrossRef] [PubMed]
45. Agarwal, E.; Miller, M.; Yaxley, A.; Isenring, E. Malnutrition in the elderly: A narrative review. *Maturitas* **2013**, *76*, 296–302. [CrossRef] [PubMed]
46. Cano-Ibáñez, N.; Gea, A.; Martínez-González, M.A.; Salas-Salvadó, J.; Corella, D.; Zomeño, M.D.; Romaguera, D.; Vioque, J.; Aros, F.; Warnberg, J.; et al. Dietary Diversity and Nutritional Adequacy among an Older Spanish Population with Metabolic Syndrome in the PREDIMED-Plus Study: A Cross-Sectional Analysis. *Nutrients* **2019**, *11*, 958. [CrossRef] [PubMed]
47. Oldewage-Theron, W.H.; Kruger, R. Food Variety and Dietary Diversity as Indicators of the Dietary Adequacy and Health Status of an Elderly Population in Sharpeville, South Africa. *J. Nutr. Elder.* **2008**, *27*, 101–133. [CrossRef]
48. Meng, S.J.; Yu, L.J. Oxidative Stress, Molecular Inflammation and Sarcopenia. *Int. J. Mol. Sci.* **2010**, *11*, 1509–1526. [CrossRef] [PubMed]
49. Domazetovic, V. Oxidative stress in bone remodeling: Role of antioxidants. *Clin. Cases Miner. Bone Metab.* **2017**, *14*, 209–216. [CrossRef]
50. Mulero, J.; Zafrilla, P.; Martinez-Cacha, A. Oxidative stress, frailty and cognitive decline. *J. Nutr. Health Aging* **2011**, *15*, 756–760. [CrossRef]
51. Sui, S.X.; Williams, L.J.; Holloway-Kew, K.L.; Hyde, N.K.; Pasco, J.A. Skeletal Muscle Health and Cognitive Function: A Narrative Review. *Int. J. Mol. Sci.* **2020**, *22*, 255. [CrossRef]
52. Welch, A.A. Nutritional Influences on Age-Related Skeletal Muscle Loss. *Proc. Nutr. Soc.* **2014**, *73*, 16–33. [CrossRef]
53. Kim, S.; Jazwinski, S.M. The Gut Microbiota and Healthy Aging: A Mini-Review. *Gerontology* **2018**, *64*, 513–520. [CrossRef] [PubMed]
54. Mello, A.M.; Paroni, G.; Daragjati, J.; Pilotto, A. Gastrointestinal Microbiota and Their Contribution to Healthy Aging. *Dig. Dis.* **2016**, *34*, 194–201. [CrossRef]
55. Heiman, M.L.; Greenway, F.L. A healthy gastrointestinal microbiome is dependent on dietary diversity. *Mol. Metab.* **2016**, *5*, 317–320. [CrossRef]
56. Sanchez-Morate, E.; Gimeno-Mallench, L.; Stromsnes, K.; Sanz-Ros, J.; Román-Domínguez, A.; Parejo-Pedrajas, S.; Inglés, M.; Olaso, G.; Gambini, J.; Mas-Bargues, C. Relationship between Diet, Microbiota, and Healthy Aging. *Biomed.* **2020**, *8*, 287. [CrossRef]
57. Richter-Levin, G.; Xu, L. How could stress lead to major depressive disorder? *IBRO Rep.* **2018**, *4*, 38–43. [CrossRef]
58. Lim, L.L.; Chang, W.; Yu, X.; Chiu, H.; Chong, M.-Y.; Kua, E.-H. Depression in Chinese elderly populations. *Asia-Pacific Psychiatry* **2011**, *3*, 46–53. [CrossRef]
59. Novak, M.; Björck, L.; Giang, K.W.; Heden-Ståhl, C.; Wilhelmsen, L.; Rosengren, A. Perceived stress and incidence of Type 2 diabetes: A 35-year follow-up study of middle-aged Swedish men. *Diabet. Med.* **2012**, *30*, e8–e16. [CrossRef] [PubMed]
60. Steptoe, A.; Kivimäki, M. Stress and cardiovascular disease. *Nat. Rev. Cardiol.* **2012**, *9*, 360–370. [CrossRef]

61. Bakkeli, N. Older Adults' Mental Health in China: Examining the Relationship Between Income Inequality and Subjective Wellbeing Using Panel Data Analysis. *J. Happiness Stud.* **2020**, *21*, 1349–1383. [CrossRef]
62. Chen, S.; Geldsetzer, P.; Bärnighausen, T. The causal effect of retirement on stress in older adults in China: A regression discontinuity study. *SSM Popul. Health* **2020**, *10*, 100462. [CrossRef] [PubMed]
63. Bremner, J.D.; Moazzami, K.; Wittbrodt, M.T.; Nye, J.A.; Lima, B.B.; Gillespie, C.F.; Rapaport, M.H.; Pearce, B.D.; Shah, A.J.; Vaccarino, V. Diet, Stress and Mental Health. *Nutrients* **2020**, *12*, 2428. [CrossRef] [PubMed]
64. Wade, A.T.; Davis, C.R.; Dyer, K.A.; Hodgson, J.M.; Woodman, R.J.; Keage, H.A.D.; Murphy, K.J. A Mediterranean diet supplemented with dairy foods improves mood and processing speed in an Australian sample: Results from the MedDairy randomized controlled trial. *Nutr. Neurosci.* **2020**, *23*, 646–658. [CrossRef]
65. Parletta, N.; Zarnowiecki, D.; Cho, J.; Wilson, A.; Bogomolova, S.; Villani, A.; Itsiopoulos, C.; Niyonsenga, T.; Blunden, S.; Meyer, B.; et al. A Mediterranean-style dietary intervention supplemented with fish oil improves diet quality and mental health in people with depression: A randomized controlled trial (HELFIMED). *Nutr. Neurosci.* **2019**, *22*, 474–487. [CrossRef] [PubMed]
66. Abshirini, M.; Siassi, F.; Koohdani, F.; Qorbani, M.; Mozaffari, H.; Aslani, Z.; Soleymani, M.; Entezarian, M.; Sotoudeh, G. Dietary total antioxidant capacity is inversely associated with depression, anxiety and some oxidative stress biomarkers in postmenopausal women: A cross-sectional study. *Ann. Gen. Psychiatry* **2019**, *18*, 3. [CrossRef]
67. Clapp, M.; Aurora, N.; Herrera, L.; Bhatia, M.; Wilen, E.; Wakefield, S. Gut Microbiota's Effect on Mental Health: The Gut-Brain Axis. *Clin. Pr.* **2017**, *7*, 131–136. [CrossRef]
68. Roberts, R.O.; Roberts, L.A.; Geda, Y.E.; Cha, R.H.; Pankratz, V.S.; O'Connor, H.M.; Knopman, D.S.; Petersen, R.C. Relative Intake of Macronutrients Impacts Risk of Mild Cognitive Impairment or Dementia. *J. Alzheimer's Dis.* **2012**, *32*, 329–339. [CrossRef]
69. Shang, X.; Hill, E.; Li, Y.; He, M. Energy and macronutrient intakes at breakfast and cognitive declines in community-dwelling older adults: A 9-year follow-up cohort study. *Am. J. Clin. Nutr.* **2021**, *113*, 1093–1103. [CrossRef]
70. Sangsefidi, Z.S.; Salehi-Abarghouei, A.; Sangsefidi, Z.S.; Mirzaei, M.; Hosseinzadeh, M. The relation between low carbohydrate diet score and psychological disorders among Iranian adults. *Nutr. Metab.* **2021**, *18*, 1–9. [CrossRef]
71. Daneshzad, E.; Keshavarz, S.; Qorbani, M.; Larijani, B.; Azadbakht, L. Association between a low-carbohydrate diet and sleep status, depression, anxiety, and stress score. *J. Sci. Food Agric.* **2020**, *100*, 2946–2952. [CrossRef]
72. Ozguner, F.; Koyu, A.; Cesur, G. Active smoking causes oxidative stress and decreases blood melatonin levels. *Toxicol. Ind. Health* **2005**, *21*, 21–26. [CrossRef] [PubMed]
73. Doggui, R.; Elsawy, W.; Conti, A.A.; Baldacchino, A. Association between chronic psychoactive substances use and systemic inflammation: A systematic review and meta-analysis. *Neurosci. Biobehav. Rev.* **2021**, *125*, 208–220. [CrossRef] [PubMed]
74. West, R. Tobacco smoking: Health impact, prevalence, correlates and interventions. *Psychol. Health* **2017**, *32*, 1018–1036. [CrossRef] [PubMed]
75. Ren, Y.; Zhang, M.; Luo, X.; Zhao, J.; Yin, L.; Pang, C.; Feng, T.; Wang, S.; Wang, B.; Zhang, H.; et al. Secular trend of the leading causes of death in China from 2003 to 2013. *Afr. Health Sci.* **2017**, *17*, 532–537. [CrossRef]
76. Griswold, M.G.; Fullman, N.; Hawley, C.; Arian, N.; Zimsen, S.R.M.; Tymeson, H.D.; Venkateswaran, V.; Tapp, A.D.; Forouzanfar, M.H.; Salama, J.S.; et al. Alcohol use and burden for 195 countries and territories, 1990–2016: A systematic analysis for the Global Burden of Disease Study 2016. *Lancet* **2018**, *392*, 1015–1035. [CrossRef]
77. Jung, M.-H.; Shin, E.-S.; Ihm, S.-H.; Jung, J.-G.; Lee, H.-Y.; Kim, C.-H. The effect of alcohol dose on the development of hypertension in Asian and Western men: Systematic review and meta-analysis. *Korean J. Intern. Med.* **2020**, *35*, 906–916. [CrossRef]
78. Park, H.; Shin, S.K.; Joo, I.; Song, D.S.; Jang, J.W.; Park, J.-W. Systematic Review with Meta-Analysis: Low-Level Alcohol Consumption and the Risk of Liver Cancer. *Gut Liver* **2020**, *14*, 792–807. [CrossRef]
79. Scherübl, H. Alcohol Use and Gastrointestinal Cancer Risk. *Visc. Med.* **2020**, *36*, 175–181. [CrossRef]
80. Tang, D.; Bu, T.; Feng, Q.; Liu, Y.; Dong, X. Differences in Overweight and Obesity between the North and South of China. *Am. J. Health Behav.* **2020**, *44*, 780–793. [CrossRef]
81. Wu, J.; Cheng, X.; Qiu, L.; Xu, T.; Zhu, G.; Han, J.; Xia, L.; Qin, X.; Cheng, Q.; Liu, Q. Prevalence and Clustering of Major Cardiovascular Risk Factors in China. *Medicine* **2016**, *95*, e2712. [CrossRef]
82. SalehiAbargouei, A.; Akbari, F.; Bellissimo, N.; Azadbakht, L. Dietary diversity score and obesity: A systematic review and meta-analysis of observational studies. *Eur. J. Clin. Nutr.* **2016**, *70*, 1–9. [CrossRef] [PubMed]
83. Qorbani, M.; Mahdavi-Gorabi, A.; Khatibi, N.; Ejtahed, H.-S.; Khazdouz, M.; Djalalinia, S.; Sahebkar, A.; Esmaeili-Abdar, M.; Hasani, M. Dietary diversity score and cardio-metabolic risk factors: An updated systematic review and meta-analysis. *Eat. Weight. Disord. Stud. Anorex. Bulim. Obes.* **2021**, 1–16. [CrossRef]

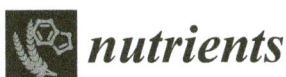

Article

Caloric Restriction Prevents Metabolic Dysfunction and the Changes in Hypothalamic Neuropeptides Associated with Obesity Independently of Dietary Fat Content in Rats

Marina Martín [1], Amaia Rodríguez [2,3], Javier Gómez-Ambrosi [2,3], Beatriz Ramírez [2,3], Sara Becerril [2,3], Victoria Catalán [2,3], Miguel López [3,4], Carlos Diéguez [3,4], Gema Frühbeck [2,3,5] and María A. Burrell [1,3,*]

1. Department of Pathology, Anatomy and Physiology, University of Navarra, IdiSNA, 31008 Pamplona, Spain; mmartinr.1@unav.es
2. Metabolic Research Laboratory, Clínica Universidad de Navarra, IdiSNA, 31008 Pamplona, Spain; arodmur@unav.es (A.R.); jagomez@unav.es (J.G.-A.); bearamirez@unav.es (B.R.); sbecman@unav.es (S.B.); vcatalan@unav.es (V.C.); gfruhbeck@unav.es (G.F.)
3. CIBER Fisiopatología de la Obesidad y Nutrición (CIBEROBN), Instituto de Salud Carlos III, 28029 Madrid, Spain; m.lopez@usc.es (M.L.); carlos.dieguez@usc.es (C.D.)
4. Department of Physiology, CIMUS, University of Santiago de Compostela-Instituto de Investigación Sanitaria, 15782 Santiago de Compostela, Spain
5. Department of Endocrinology and Nutrition, Clínica Universidad de Navarra, 31008 Pamplona, Spain
* Correspondence: mburrell@unav.es; Tel.: +34-948-425600 (ext. 806247)

Citation: Martín, M.; Rodríguez, A.; Gómez-Ambrosi, J.; Ramírez, B.; Becerril, S.; Catalán, V.; López, M.; Diéguez, C.; Frühbeck, G.; Burrell, M.A. Caloric Restriction Prevents Metabolic Dysfunction and the Changes in Hypothalamic Neuropeptides Associated with Obesity Independently of Dietary Fat Content in Rats. *Nutrients* 2021, 13, 2128. https://doi.org/10.3390/nu13072128

Academic Editors: Emiliana Giacomello, Luana Toniolo and Marcellino Monda

Received: 14 May 2021
Accepted: 15 June 2021
Published: 22 June 2021

Publisher's Note: MDPI stays neutral with regard to jurisdictional claims in published maps and institutional affiliations.

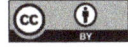

Copyright: © 2021 by the authors. Licensee MDPI, Basel, Switzerland. This article is an open access article distributed under the terms and conditions of the Creative Commons Attribution (CC BY) license (https://creativecommons.org/licenses/by/4.0/).

Abstract: Energy restriction is a first therapy in the treatment of obesity, but the underlying biological mechanisms have not been completely clarified. We analyzed the effects of restriction of high-fat diet (HFD) on weight loss, circulating gut hormone levels and expression of hypothalamic neuropeptides. Ten-week-old male Wistar rats (n = 40) were randomly distributed into four groups: two fed ad libitum a normal diet (ND) (N group) or a HFD (H group) and two subjected to a 25% caloric restriction of ND (NR group) or HFD (HR group) for 9 weeks. A 25% restriction of HFD over 9 weeks leads to a 36% weight loss with regard to the group fed HFD ad libitum accompanied by normal values in adiposity index and food efficiency ratio (FER). This restriction also carried the normalization of NPY, AgRP and POMC hypothalamic mRNA expression, without changes in CART. Caloric restriction did not succeed in improving glucose homeostasis but reduced HFD-induced hyperinsulinemia. In conclusion, 25% restriction of HFD reduced adiposity and improved metabolism in experimental obesity, without changes in glycemia. Restriction of the HFD triggered the normalization of hypothalamic NPY, AgRP and POMC expression, as well as ghrelin and leptin levels.

Keywords: food restriction; gut hormones; hypothalamic neuropeptides and obesity

1. Introduction

Obesity constitutes a persistent major health concern linked to increased morbidity and mortality [1]. Dietary intervention is still considered the cornerstone for the treatment of obesity and its associated metabolic alterations [2]. Many patients with obesity can achieve short-term weight reduction through diet alone, but successful long-term weight maintenance is much more difficult. The rise in obesity rates over the past 30 years has been related to increases in the portion size of energy-dense and highly palatable inexpensive food. Therefore, a reduction in portion size seems a logical alternative as a first therapeutic approach before progressing to a normal diet. Dietary interventions should be personalized, adapted to food preferences and enable flexible approaches to reduce calorie intake in order to strengthen motivation and adherence of patients with obesity [3]. In this regard, several control studies have shown that low-carbohydrate, high-fat diets (HFD) in patients with obesity and diabetes induce short-term favorable effects on weight loss, blood glucose and insulin [4]. Caloric restriction alleviates multiple complications of obesity and aging, including insulin resistance, dyslipidemia, hypertension, atherosclerosis and systemic inflammation [5,6]. However, it is not clear whether weight loss caused by a restricted HFD is accompanied by modifications in signals involved in the regulation of body weight and energy homeostasis.

Body weight is regulated by complex homeostatic mechanisms that include interactions between peripheral organs and the central nervous system [7]. In the hypothalamus, the arcuate nucleus (ARC) constitutes one of the main regulatory feeding centers. ARC neurons containing the orexigenic peptides neuropeptide Y (NPY) and agouti-related peptide (AgRP) and the anorexigenic factors proopiomelanocortin (POMC) and cocaine- and amphetamine-regulated transcript (CART) receive and integrate information about the metabolic state [8,9]. This integration occurs via receptors for hormones such as leptin, glucagon-like peptide 1 (GLP-1), peptide YY (PYY) and ghrelin [10], and also sensing the circulating levels of nutrients, such as glucose and fatty acids [11].

The hypothesis of the present study was that caloric restriction in rats fed a HFD might produce metabolic benefits. Therefore, we analyzed if body weight reduction derived from a restricted HFD is linked to modifications in glucose homeostasis, adipocyte size, gut hormone levels and hypothalamic neuropeptide expression.

2. Materials and Methods

2.1. Experimental Animals and Study Design

Ten-week-old male Wistar rats ($n = 40$) (breeding house of the University of Navarra) with a mean body weight of 308 ± 11 g were caged individually in a room under controlled temperature (22 ± 2 °C), relative humidity ($50 \pm 10\%$), ventilation (at least 15 complete changes of air/h) and a 12:12 h light–dark cycle (lights on at 8:00 a.m.). To analyze the effect of diet-induced obesity and caloric restriction, rats were divided into four dietary groups for 9 weeks ($n = 10$/group): rats fed ad libitum a ND (N group) (12.1 kJ: 4% fat, 82% carbohydrate and 14% protein, diet 2014S, Teklad Global Diets, Harlan, Barcelona, Spain) or a HFD (H group) (23.0 kJ/g: 59% fat, 27% carbohydrate and 14% protein, diet F3282; Bio-Serv, Frenchtown, NJ, USA) and rats fed a ND (NR group) or a HFD (HR group) with a caloric restriction of 25%. After 8 h fasting, rats were sacrificed by decapitation. Blood samples were immediately collected, and sera were obtained by cold centrifugation (4 °C) at $700 \times g$ for 15 min and stored at -20 °C. The perirenal, subcutaneous and epididymal white adipose tissue (WAT) depots were harvested, weighed and a small fragment of the fat tissues was fixed in 4% formaldehyde. The brain was also dissected out and frozen for study of the expression of hypothalamic neuropeptides. All experimental procedures were performed in accordance with the European Guidelines for the care and use of Laboratory Animals (directive 2010/63/EU) and were approved by the Ethical Committee for Animal Experimentation of the University of Navarra (049/10).

2.2. Body Weight, Body Composition and Food Efficiency Ratio

Body weight was recorded twice a week and food intake was monitored daily. The adiposity index was calculated as the sum of the weight of perirenal, subcutaneous and epididymal WAT depots in absolute (g) or relative (g/body weight) values. The food efficiency ratio (FER) was determined as body weight gained per week divided by total energy (kcal) consumed over this period.

2.3. Blood Measurements

Serum glucose concentrations were determined with a sensitive-automatic glucose sensor (Ascensia Elite, Bayer, Barcelona, Spain). Fasting serum leptin, PYY, GLP-1 and insulin concentrations were measured using a MILLIPLEX™ MAP rat gut hormone panel kit (RGT-88K Millipore Corporation, Billerica, MA, USA) in accordance with the manufacturer's recommendations. Total ghrelin serum levels were assessed using a commercial ELISA kit (EZRGRT-91K, Millipore). Intra- and inter-assay coefficients of variation for measurements of total ghrelin were <5%.

2.4. Histological Analyses

Subcutaneous WAT samples were fixed in 4% formaldehyde, embedded in paraffin. Five μm-sections were stained with hematoxylin–eosin. Three fields per section from each animal were imaged with the 20× objective, and diameters from, at least, 100 adipocytes/section were determined with the Adiposoft software (version 1.13) plugin within ImageJ software (MATLAB).

2.5. In Situ Hybridization for Hypothalamic Neuropeptides

Cryostat coronal brain sections (16 μm) were obtained and stored at −80 °C until hybridization. In situ hybridization was carried out as earlier described [12]. Sections were probed with specific oligonucleotides for AgRP, CART, NPY and POMC (Table 1). These probes were 3′-end labeled with 35S-αdATP (Perkin Elmer, Waltham, MA, USA) using terminal deoxynucleotidyl transferase (New England Biolabs; Ipswich, MA, USA). The incubation of the sections with an excess of the unlabeled probes allowed to confirm the specificity of the probes. The frozen sections were treated with 4% paraformaldehyde in 0.1 mol/L phosphate buffer (pH 7.40) at room temperature (RT) for 30 min and then dehydrated using 70, 80, 90, 95% and absolute ethanol (5 min each). The hybridization was performed overnight at 37 °C in a moist chamber. Hybridization solution contained 0.5×10^6 cpm (AgRP, CART and POMC) or 1×10^6 (NPY) cpm per slide of the labeled probe, 4× saline-sodium citrate buffer (SSC), 50% deionized formamide, 1× Denhardt's solution, 10% dextran sulfate and 10 μg/mL sheared, single-stranded salmon sperm DNA (all of them, Sigma-Aldrich; St. Louis, MO, USA). Then, the sections were washed in 1× SSC at RT, four times in 1× SSC at 42 °C (30 min per wash), one time in 1× SSC at RT for 1 h and then rinsed in water and ethanol. Finally, the sections were air-dried and exposed to Hyperfilm β-Max (KODAK; Rochester, NY, USA) at RT. All the slides were exposed under the same conditions and developed in developer/replenisher (Developer G150, AGFA HealthCare: Mortsel, Belgium) and Fixator (Manual Fixing G354; AGFA HealthCare: Mortsel, Belgium). Sections were scanned, and the hybridization signal was measured by densitometry using ImageJ-1.33 software (NIH; Bethesda, MD, USA). The optical density (OD) of the hybridization signal was quantified and corrected by the OD of its adjacent background value. A rectangle was outlined, always with the same dimensions, enclosing the hybridization signal over each nucleus and over adjacent brain areas of each section [12]. Sixteen to twenty sections for each animal (4–5 slides with 4 sections per slide) were used, and the mean was used as densitometry value for each animal.

Table 1. List of in situ hybridization oligonucleotides.

Gene	GenBank ID	Sequence (5′-3′)
Agrp	NM_033650.1	CGACGCGGAGAACGAGACTCGCGGTTCTGTGGATCTAGCACCTCTGCC
Cart	NM_017110	CCGAAGGAGGCTGTCACCCCTTCACA
Npy	NM_012614.2	AGATGAGATGTGGGGGGAAACTAGGAAAAGTCAGGAGAGCAAGTTTCATT
Pomc	NM_139326	TCCATAGACGTGTGGAGCTG

Agrp, agouti-related neuropeptide; *Cart*, cocaine- and amphetamine-regulated transcript prepropeptide; *Npy*, neuropeptide Y; *Pomc*, proopiomelanocortin.

2.6. Statistical Analysis

Data are shown as mean ± SEM. Differences between groups were analyzed by a two-way ANOVA (diet × caloric restriction) or a one-way ANOVA followed by the least significant difference (LSD) post hoc test, if an interaction was detected. The statistical analyses were performed using the SPSS v. 15.0 software (SPSS Inc., Chicago, IL, USA).

3. Results
3.1. Caloric Restriction Improved the Obese Phenotype even in Rats Fed a HFD

As shown in Figure 1A, all experimental groups exhibited similar body weight during the first 3–4 days of the experiment. Significant differences were identified from day 3 onwards. As expected, the H group showed the highest body weight (507 ± 18 g) at the end of the experiment, nearly doubling the initial one, while the NR group exhibited the lowest body mass (329 ± 4 g). Particularly relevant was the evolution of the HR group, which presented similar body weight to that of the N group throughout the experimental period ($p = 0.165$), being even lower at the end of the study.

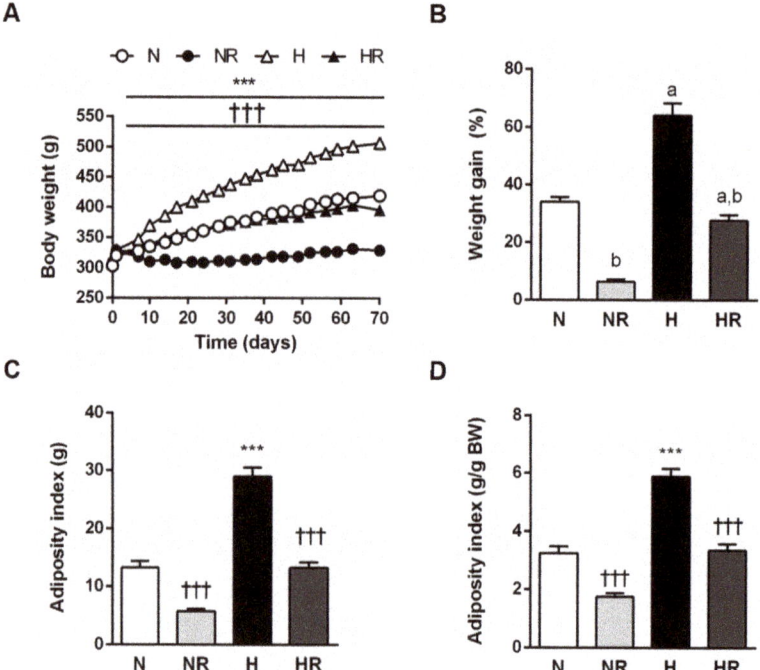

Figure 1. Growth curves of body weight (**A**), percentage of weight gain (**B**) and whole-body adiposity in absolute (**C**) and relative (**D**) values of the four experimental groups during the 9 weeks of dietary interventions. ^{a} $p < 0.05$ effect of diet; ^{b} $p < 0.05$ effect of caloric restriction. *** $p < 0.001$ vs. the same group fed a ND; ††† $p < 0.001$ vs. the same group fed ad libitum.

The percentage of body weight increase in each group during the 9 weeks of the experiment is illustrated in Figure 1B. As expected, groups fed a HFD showed a higher weight gain than those fed a normal diet ($p < 0.0001$) (Figure 1B) and higher relative and absolute adiposity indices (Figure 1C,D). Groups fed ad libitum experienced a more pronounced percentage of body weight increase than the corresponding groups subjected to caloric restriction ($p < 0.0001$). The comparison between N and HR groups was again noteworthy, since the percentage of body weight increase ($p = 0.124$) as well as absolute ($p = 0.988$) (Figure 1C) and relative ($p = 0.721$) (Figure 1D) adiposity index values were similar in both groups.

The histological observation of subcutaneous WAT samples of the four groups revealed evident differences in adipocyte size (Figure 2). As expected, the H group presented the highest percentage of large adipocytes (diameter > 150 μm) (Figure 2C), while the NR group showed the highest percentage of small adipocytes (diameter < 150 μm) (Figure 2B). The WAT of the HR group exhibited hypertrophic adipocytes (diameter ≥ 250 µm) interspersed among a majority population of small adipocytes (diameter ≤ 50 µm) (Figure 2D).

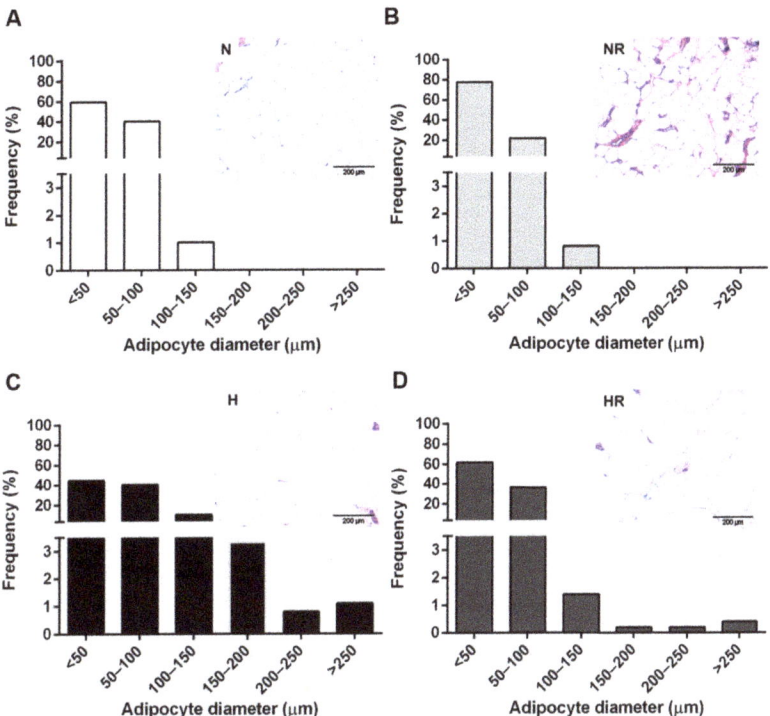

Figure 2. Adipocyte diameter distribution of subcutaneous WAT obtained from rats fed a normal diet (ND) (**A**) or a high-fat diet (HFD) ad libitum (**C**) or subjected to a 25% caloric restriction of ND (**B**) or HFD (**D**) for 9 weeks. Representative histological sections of subcutaneous WAT stained with hematoxylin–eosin are shown at the top of the histograms.

3.2. Caloric Restriction Reduced Food Efficiency Independently of the Type of Diet

Since the ND and the HFD provide a different energy content, food intake is illustrated both as total grams of food consumed and the corresponding kilocalories ingested (Figure 3). The evolution of food intake in grams relative to body weight (Figure 3A,C) revealed higher food consumption in groups fed a normal diet with or without caloric restriction ($p < 0.0001$). However, groups fed a HFD ingested more calories ($p < 0.0001$) (Figure 3B,D) and exhibited a higher FER ($p < 0.0001$) (Figure 3C) than those fed a normal diet. No significant differences were observed in the total energy content of food ingested by N and HR groups ($p = 0.916$), nor in the FER values ($p = 0.193$).

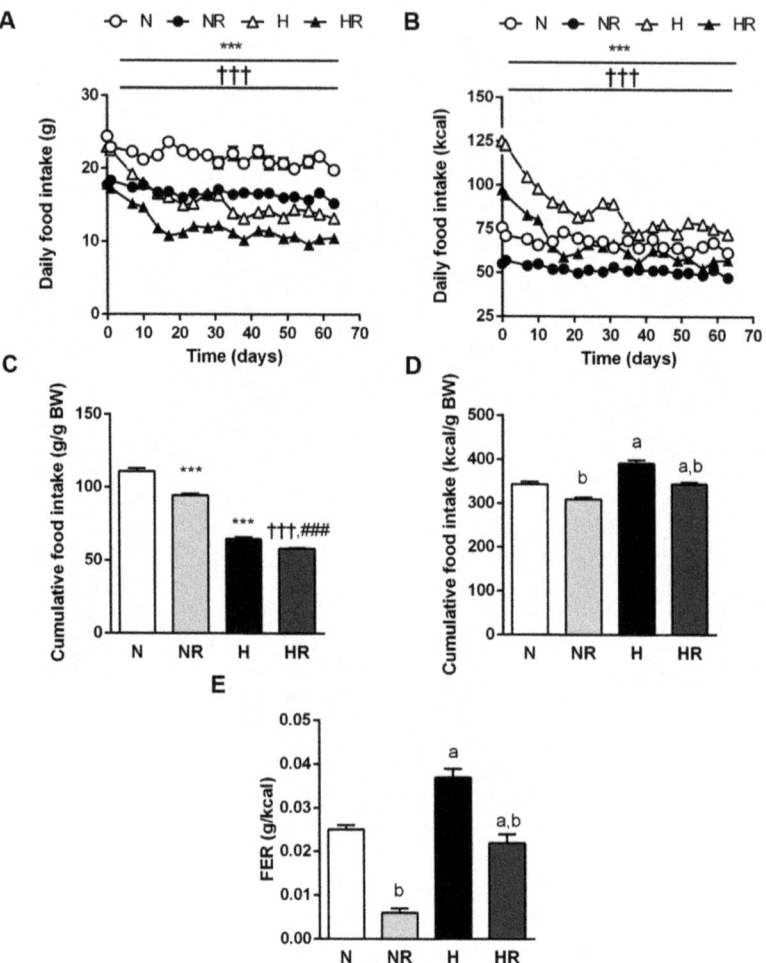

Figure 3. Curves of daily food intake in grams (**A**) and kilocalories (**B**) of the experimental animals ($n = 10$ per group). Bar graphs represent cumulative food intake relative to body weight in grams (**C**) and in kilocalories (**D**) as well as food efficiency ratio (FER) (**E**) during dietary interventions. [a] $p < 0.05$ effect of diet; [b] $p < 0.05$ effect of caloric restriction. *** $p < 0.001$ vs. the same group fed a ND; ††† $p < 0.001$ vs. the same group fed ad libitum; ### $p < 0.001$ vs. N.

3.3. Caloric Restriction Ameliorated Metabolic Profile even in Rats Fed a HFD

The general characteristics of the metabolic profile of experimental animals during the dietary interventions are summarized in Figure 4. Consumption of a HFD increased both glucose ($p < 0.0001$) and insulin ($p < 0.0001$) concentrations, while restriction diminished only insulin circulating levels ($p < 0.0001$) (Figure 4A,B). The N and HR groups had similar insulinemia ($p = 0.614$), but glycemia was higher in the HR group ($p < 0.01$) (Figure 4A,B).

In accordance with the adiposity index data, leptinemia was augmented in the HFD and ad libitum fed groups ($p < 0.001$) (Figure 4C). Furthermore, as expected, consumption of HFD decreased ghrelin levels ($p < 0.0001$), while restriction increased them ($p < 0.05$) (Figure 4D). In the case of circulating GLP-1, no changes were observed between the four groups (Figure 4E). PYY serum concentrations were decreased in groups fed a HFD ($p < 0.05$) (Figure 4F). Interestingly, the N and HR groups showed similar leptinemia

(p = 0.266) (Figure 4C) and ghrelinemia (p = 0.196) (Figure 4D), but different serum PYY levels, which were higher in the N group (p < 0.05) (Figure 4F).

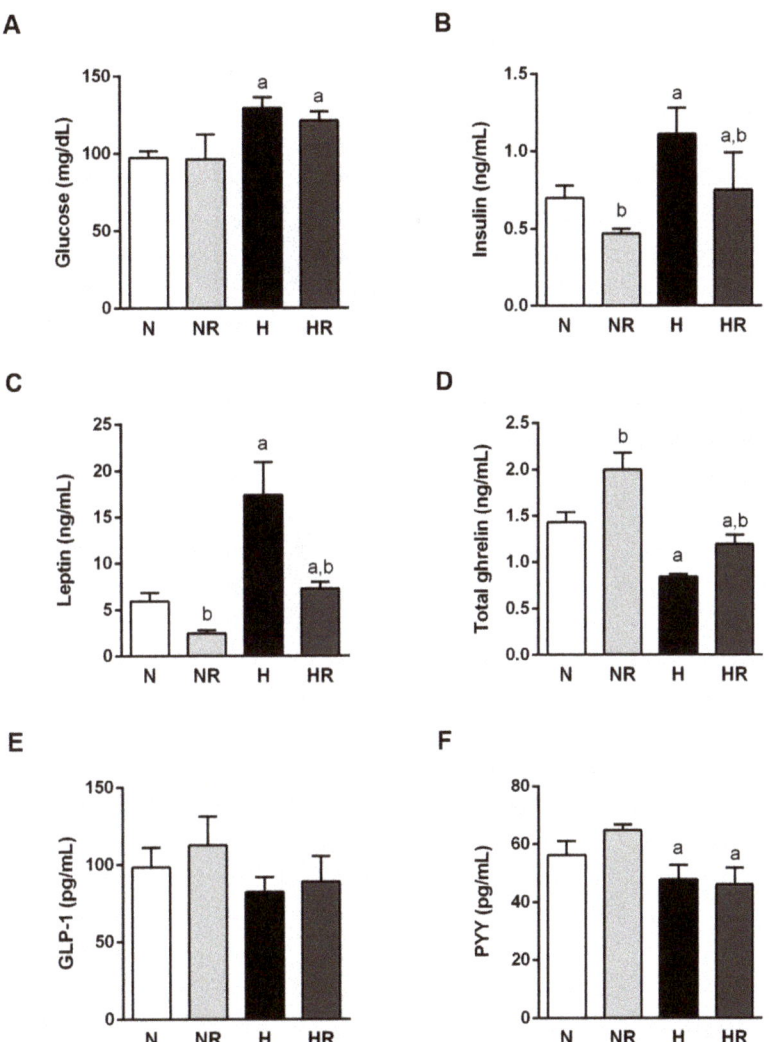

Figure 4. Fasting serum glucose (**A**), insulin (**B**), leptin (**C**), total ghrelin (**D**), GLP-1 (**E**) and PYY (**F**) levels of the four experimental groups. [a] p < 0.05 effect of diet; [b] p < 0.05 effect of caloric restriction.

3.4. Caloric Restriction Ameliorated Metabolic Profile even in Rats Fed a HFD

Expression of the hypothalamic neuropeptides controlling appetite, NPY, AgRP, POMC and CART was measured by in situ hybridization (Figure 5). Type of diet and restriction affected the orexigenic neuropeptides NPY and AgRP in a different manner. The effect of restriction on NPY expression depended on the type of diet (Figure 5A), so that restriction of the normal diet caused a decrease in NPY (p < 0.01). By contrast, restriction of the HFD increased NPY (p < 0.01). AgRP was decreased in the groups fed the HFD (p < 0.05) and increased in the groups fed the restricted diet, although there was only a marginal effect (p = 0.055) on both normal diet and HFD (Figure 5B). Interestingly, N and HR presented comparable expression of NPY, AgRP and POMC but not of CART. CART expression was lower in the groups fed the HFD ($p < 0.05$) and ad libitum ($p < 0.0001$) (Figure 5D).

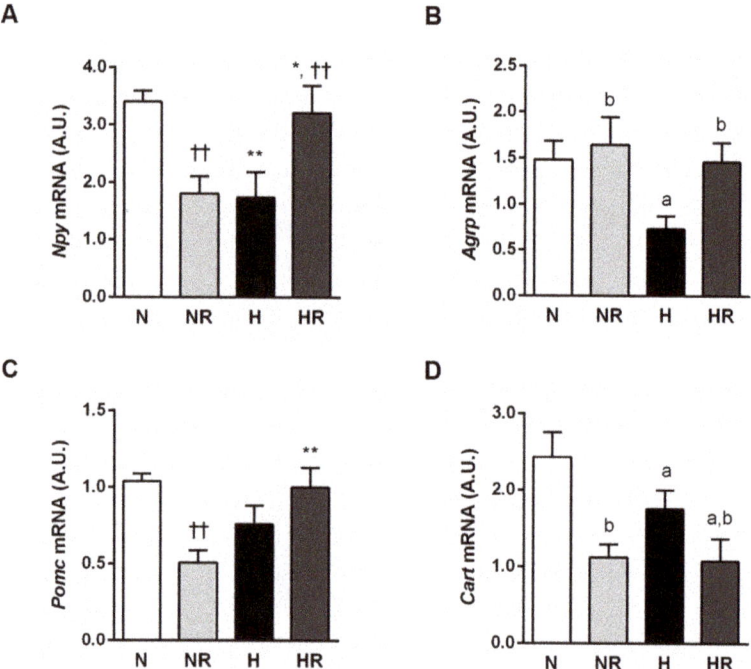

Figure 5. Hypothalamic gene expression of neuropeptides NPY (A), AgRP (B), POMC (C) and CART (D) in the arcuate nucleus of the four experimental groups. [a] $p < 0.05$ effect of diet; [b] $p < 0.05$ effect of caloric restriction. * $p < 0.05$; ** $p < 0.01$ vs. the same group fed a ND; †† $p < 0.01$ vs. the same group fed ad libitum.

4. Discussion

The significant global burden of overweight and obesity requires lifestyle strategies facilitating successful long-term body weight management. Dietary weight loss programs are mainly based on a decrease in fat or carbohydrate content in food, along with an important reduction in meal size [13]. Although this reduction often results in initial weight loss, patients with obesity often fail to maintain the treatment [14]. Numerous studies support the beneficial effects of food restriction, but only some of them have analyzed the results of restricting a HFD [15–17]. Moreover, the findings available are difficult to compare because these studies differ in numerous parameters (species/humans, duration of the experimental period or percentage of intake restriction). The present study demonstrates that a 25% restriction of a HFD for 9 weeks led to a similar body weight evolution and adiposity index than ad libitum intake of a normal diet. Other authors have concluded that animals fed a HFD with caloric content similar to the control group entail increased adiposity in the absence of significant changes in body weight [18] and that body composition is not normalized unless dietary fat is reduced [19]. However, our results regarding food intake clearly demonstrate that eating diets with the same caloric content but different fat amount leads to normalization of body weight and whole-body adiposity. Thus, dietary fat content is not the unique determinant of body fat when caloric intake is not excessive.

The intake of diets with a high fat content exerts deleterious effects on metabolism, especially on the glucose homeostasis. Previous studies indicate that energy restriction decreases plasma glucose and improves glucose tolerance and insulin sensitivity [20,21], even when restricting a HFD [22]. Our data revealed that the intake of a restricted HFD results in normal insulin values but higher glycemia, suggesting the persistence of insulin resistance, which is related to the type of diet rather than to the amount of weight loss or the body fat content.

The amelioration of glucose homeostasis is usually associated with modifications in adipose tissue morphology [23]. Adipocyte hyperplasia and hypertrophy are independent of body weight but correlate with insulin sensitivity [23–25]. Consistently, we observed evident differences in adipocyte size between groups fed the normal diet ad libitum and the restricted HFD. The HR group presented a heterogeneous population of adipocytes containing very large and very small adipocytes. These observations agree with other authors reporting that individuals with obesity whose fat depots are constituted predominantly by few large adipocytes exhibit higher glucose intolerance than those subjects with the same degree of obesity but with many small adipocytes [24]. Thus, increased adipocyte size can be considered an independent marker of insulin resistance and hyperleptinemia [26]. The underlying mechanisms responsible for the dimension of fat cells are complex and appear to be related to the dynamics of adipocyte storage and removal rate in different locations and metabolic situations [23,27,28]. Data from our study suggest that not only the distribution but also the morphology of WAT have to be considered when assessing glucose homeostasis and obesity.

The deregulation of glucose homeostasis caused by the intake of a HFD could also lead to modifications of some regulatory peptides, such as GLP-1 or PYY. In addition to improving glycemia [29], GLP-1 reduces appetite, thereby supporting its use in the treatment of obesity and its comorbidities [30,31]. In the present study, serum GLP-1 concentrations remained unaltered, which is in accordance with previous observations [32]. However, other authors suggest that over 11 weeks of intake modifications result in a progressive change in the concentration of circulating GLP-1 [33]. Therefore, it seems plausible that the duration of our dietary intervention is not enough to detect significant modifications in GLP-1. On the other hand, different studies have shown the relevance of PYY in the etiology of obesity and type 2 diabetes [34–36]. PYY acts in the hypothalamus to activate melanocortin neurons that affect insulin sensitivity [37]. Our data are in agreement with this observation, since HFD intake led to a significant decrease in PYY concentrations. When comparing the N and HR groups, PYY serum levels were lower in the HR group. The hypothesis that glycemic control would be improved with restricted HFD was not supported by the study findings. It seems that the hormonal profile that improves insulin secretion includes the elevation of both PYY and GLP-1 levels [38].

Ghrelin and leptin constitute crucial factors for the control of body composition and glucose homeostasis. Many studies have determined that the presence of specific macronutrients in the lumen of the gastrointestinal tract influences serum concentrations of different gastrointestinal hormones [39–41]. Global analysis of the influence of the type of diet and restriction yielded significant differences in ghrelin and leptin circulating levels. It is noteworthy that no significant differences were found when comparing the N and HR groups. Considering the parallel evolution in body weight and energy intake of both groups, it can be concluded that modifications in ghrelin and leptin are mainly influenced by body composition. In the case of leptin, this correlation is clear since WAT is the main source of leptin [42]. Reports of modifications in circulating ghrelin after feeding diets with different macronutrients are highly variable [43–45]. Although early ghrelin studies indicated its key role in the control of food intake [46–48], based on the present study, a direct correlation between ghrelin secretion and body composition can also be put forward. New insights indicate that induced ablation of ghrelin cells in adult mice does not decrease food intake and body weight, so ghrelin may not be so determinant in appetite control and body weight [49]. Thus, the ghrelin system may have evolved to play a role in protecting against starvation and hypoglycemia [50] as it seems to occur in the NR group.

To directly evaluate the metabolic effects of restricting a HFD in the ARC, we measured the expression of hypothalamic neuropeptides. The prototypic first-order neuronal targets of leptin, insulin and ghrelin action are the catabolic POMC/CART and the anabolic NPY/AgRP neurons. These neurons trigger opposing effects on energy balance and are reciprocally regulated by changes in energy stores. Adaptive responses to perturbations in body fat mass involve changes in the activity of NPY/AgRP and POMC/CART neurons in the ARC. Feeding a HFD produces a decrease in the expression of hypothalamic NPY and AgRP [7,51]. By contrast, restriction increases the expression of NPY/AgRP [52] and decreases the POMC/CART [53]. Our data are only partially in agreement with these general premises. First of all, the abnormal lower expression of NPY in the NR group could be explained by the fact that ghrelin induces orexigenic effects in free feeding conditions but has no effect in animals under negative energy balance conditions such as being chronically food-restricted [54]. The N and HR groups showed a similar expression of NPY, AgRP and POMC. This finding is not surprising given that both groups presented similar body weight, adiposity index, total intake of calories and FER. Nevertheless, the lower expression of CART in the HR group compared to the N group does not follow this trend. Some authors reported that CART affects several biological processes in both lipid and glucose homeostasis. Depending on the hormonal context, CART has insulin-like or insulin-antagonistic effects [55,56]. Consequently, lower CART expression in the HR group might be related to the deregulation of glucose homeostasis observed in this group. In line with our observations, several studies have reported incongruous correlations of hypothalamic expression of orexigenic factors NPY and AgRP as well as anorexigenic peptides POMC and CART under conditions of caloric restriction and/or obesogenic environment [57,58]. Interestingly, molecular profiling of hypothalamic neurons at a single-cell resolution has revealed molecularly distinct clusters of AgRP- and POMC-expressing neurons with potential divergent metabolic functions, hormonal regulation and response to dietary changes [59–62]. Due to the complexity of the regulation of these hypothalamic centers, further studies are required to unravel the mechanism through which different diets affect the expression of hypothalamic neuropeptides.

5. Conclusions

In conclusion, restricted HFD intake leads to a decrease in body weight, adiposity, FER, circulating ghrelin and leptin levels similar to those produced by a normal diet ad libitum. Furthermore, restricting HFD also normalizes the expression of NPY, AgRP and POMC in the ARC but does not improve glucose homeostasis. Altered levels of circulating PYY and CART mRNA expression in the ARC could be involved in glycemic deregulation. Restriction of a HFD may be used as an initial therapy in overweight and obese patients in order to achieve important improvements in energy status before progressing to a normal diet. The development of first step dietary interventions not involving a dramatic change in the habitual diet of overweight or obese people could represent an interesting alternative in the initial stages of obesity treatment. Further studies are required to investigate this possibility.

Author Contributions: Conceptualization, M.M., J.G.-A., M.A.B. and G.F.; methodology, M.M., A.R., J.G.-A., B.R., S.B., V.C., M.L., C.D. and M.A.B.; formal analysis, M.M., A.R., J.G.-A., B.R., S.B., V.C., M.L., C.D. and M.A.B.; writing—original draft preparation, M.M. and M.A.B.; writing—review and editing, M.M., A.R., J.G.-A., B.R., S.B., V.C., M.L., C.D., G.F. and M.A.B.; supervision, M.M. and M.A.B.; funding acquisition, A.R., M.L. and G.F. All authors have read and agreed to the published version of the manuscript.

Funding: This work was supported by Ministerio de Economía y Competitividad (SAF2015-71026R) and Fondo de Investigación Sanitaria-FEDER (PI19/00785 and PI19/00990). CIBEROBN is an initiative of the Instituto de Salud Carlos III, Spain.

Institutional Review Board Statement: All experimental procedures conformed to the European Guidelines for the care and use of Laboratory Animals (directive 2010/63/EU) and were approved by the Ethical Committee for Animal Experimentation of the University of Navarra (049/10).

Data Availability Statement: The data presented in this study are available on request from the corresponding author. The data are not publicly available due to privacy restrictions.

Acknowledgments: The authors gratefully acknowledge all the staff of the breeding house of the University of Navarra, in particular Elena Ciordia, Juan Percaz and Eneko Etxetxikia. We also express our gratitude to Javier García for his expert help with the histological studies.

Conflicts of Interest: The authors declare no conflict of interest.

References

1. Afshin, A.; Forouzanfar, M.H.; Reitsma, M.B.; Sur, P.; Estep, K.; Lee, A.; Marczak, L.; Mokdad, A.H.; Moradi-Lakeh, M.; Naghavi, M.; et al. Health effects of overweight and obesity in 195 Countries over 25 years. *N. Engl. J. Med.* **2017**, *377*, 13–27.
2. Bray, G.A.; Frühbeck, G.; Ryan, D.H.; Wilding, J.P. Management of obesity. *Lancet* **2016**, *387*, 1947–1956. [CrossRef]
3. Ezquerro, S.; Rodríguez, A.; Portincasa, P.; Frühbeck, G. Effects of diets on adipose tissue. *Curr. Med. Chem.* **2019**, *26*, 3593–3612. [CrossRef] [PubMed]
4. Brouns, F. Overweight and diabetes prevention: Is a low-carbohydrate-high-fat diet recommendable? *Eur. J. Nutr.* **2018**, *57*, 1301–1312. [CrossRef] [PubMed]
5. Kraus, W.E.; Bhapkar, M.; Huffman, K.M.; Pieper, C.F.; Das, S.K.; Redman, L.M.; Villareal, D.T.; Rochon, J.; Roberts, S.B.; Ravussin, E.; et al. 2 years of calorie restriction and cardiometabolic risk (CALERIE): Exploratory outcomes of a multicentre, phase 2, randomised controlled trial. *Lancet Diabetes Endocrinol.* **2019**, *7*, 673–683. [CrossRef]
6. López-Otín, C.; Galluzzi, L.; Freije, J.M.P.; Madeo, F.; Kroemer, G. Metabolic control of longevity. *Cell* **2016**, *166*, 802–821. [CrossRef]
7. Theilade, S.; Christensen, M.B.; Vilsbøll, T.; Knop, F.K. An overview of obesity mechanisms in humans: Endocrine regulation of food intake, eating behaviour and common determinants of body weight. *Diabetes Obes. Metab.* **2021**, *23* (Suppl. 1), 17–35. [CrossRef] [PubMed]
8. Beutler, L.R.; Chen, Y.; Ahn, J.S.; Lin, Y.C.; Essner, R.A.; Knight, Z.A. Dynamics of gut-brain communication underlying hunger. *Neuron* **2017**, *96*, 461–475.e5. [CrossRef] [PubMed]
9. Parker, J.A.; Bloom, S.R. Hypothalamic neuropeptides and the regulation of appetite. *Neuropharmacology* **2012**, *63*, 18–30. [CrossRef]
10. Al Massadi, O.; López, M.; Tschöp, M.; Diéguez, C.; Nogueiras, R. Current understanding of the hypothalamic ghrelin pathways inducing appetite and adiposity. *Trends Neurosci.* **2017**, *40*, 167–180. [CrossRef]
11. López, M.; Nogueiras, R.; Tena-Sempere, M.; Diéguez, C. Hypothalamic AMPK: A canonical regulator of whole-body energy balance. *Nat. Rev. Endocrinol.* **2016**, *12*, 421–432. [CrossRef]
12. Martínez-Sánchez, N.; Seoane-Collazo, P.; Contreras, C.; Varela, L.; Villarroya, J.; Rial-Pensado, E.; Buque, X.; Aurrekoetxea, I.; Delgado, T.C.; Vázquez-Martínez, R.; et al. Hypothalamic AMPK-ER Stress-JNK1 axis mediates the central actions of thyroid hormones on energy balance. *Cell Metab.* **2017**, *26*, 212–229.e12. [CrossRef]
13. Thom, G.; Lean, M. Is there an optimal diet for weight management and metabolic health? *Gastroenterology* **2017**, *152*, 1739–1751. [CrossRef] [PubMed]
14. Dulloo, A.G.; Montani, J.P. Pathways from dieting to weight regain, to obesity and to the metabolic syndrome: An overview Introduction. *Obes. Rev.* **2015**, *16*, 1–6. [CrossRef]
15. Briggs, D.I.; Lockie, S.H.; Wu, Q.; Lemus, M.B.; Stark, R.; Andrews, Z.B. Calorie-restricted weight loss reverses high-fat diet-induced ghrelin resistance, which contributes to rebound weight gain in a ghrelin-dependent manner. *Endocrinology* **2013**, *154*, 709–717. [CrossRef]
16. Lewis, H.B.; Ahern, A.L.; Solis-Trapala, I.; Walker, C.G.; Reimann, F.; Gribble, F.M.; Jebb, S.A. Effect of reducing portion size at a compulsory meal on later energy intake, gut hormones, and appetite in overweight adults. *Obesity* **2015**, *23*, 1362–1370. [CrossRef]
17. Hall, K.D.; Bemis, T.; Brychta, R.; Chen, K.Y.; Courville, A.; Crayner, E.J.; Goodwin, S.; Guo, J.; Howard, L.; Knuth, N.D.; et al. Calorie for calorie, dietary fat restriction results in more body fat loss than carbohydrate restriction in people with obesity. *Cell Metab.* **2015**, *22*, 427–436. [CrossRef] [PubMed]
18. Boozer, C.N.; Schoenbach, G.; Atkinson, R.L. Dietary fat and adiposity: A dose-response relationship in adult male rats fed isocalorically. *Am. J. Physiol.* **1995**, *268*, E546–E550. [CrossRef]
19. Boozer, C.N.; Brasseur, A.; Atkinson, R.L. Dietary fat affects weight loss and adiposity during energy restriction in rats. *Am. J. Clin. Nutr.* **1993**, *58*, 846–852. [CrossRef] [PubMed]
20. Park, S.Y.; Choi, G.H.; Choi, H.I.; Ryu, J.; Jung, C.Y.; Lee, W. Calorie restriction improves whole-body glucose disposal and insulin resistance in association with the increased adipocyte-specific GLUT4 expression in Otsuka Long-Evans Tokushima fatty rats. *Arch. Biochem. Biophys.* **2005**, *436*, 276–284. [CrossRef] [PubMed]
21. Kalupahana, N.S.; Voy, B.H.; Saxton, A.M.; Moustaid-Moussa, N. Energy-restricted high-fat diets only partially improve markers of systemic and adipose tissue inflammation. *Obesity* **2011**, *19*, 245–254. [CrossRef] [PubMed]

22. Eriksson-Hogling, D.; Andersson, D.P.; Backdahl, J.; Hoffstedt, J.; Rössner, S.; Thorell, A.; Arner, E.; Arner, P.; Rydén, M. Adipose tissue morphology predicts improved insulin sensitivity following moderate or pronounced weight loss. *Int. J. Obes.* **2015**, *39*, 893–898. [CrossRef]
23. Heinonen, S.; Saarinen, L.; Naukkarinen, J.; Rodriguez, A.; Fruhbeck, G.; Hakkarainen, A.; Lundbom, J.; Lundbom, N.; Vuolteenaho, K.; Moilanen, E.; et al. Adipocyte morphology and implications for metabolic derangements in acquired obesity. *Int.˚J. Obes.* **2014**, *38*, 1423–1431. [CrossRef] [PubMed]
24. Arner, E.; Westermark, P.O.; Spalding, K.L.; Britton, T.; Rydén, M.; Frisén, J.; Bernard, S.; Arner, P. Adipocyte turnover: Relevance to human adipose tissue morphology. *Diabetes* **2010**, *59*, 105–109. [CrossRef] [PubMed]
25. Dahlman, I.; Ryden, M.; Arner, P. Family history of diabetes is associated with enhanced adipose lipolysis: Evidence for the implication of epigenetic factors. *Diabetes Metab.* **2018**, *44*, 155–159. [CrossRef] [PubMed]
26. Lundgren, M.; Svensson, M.; Lindmark, S.; Renström, F.; Ruge, T.; Eriksson, J.W. Fat cell enlargement is an independent marker of insulin resistance and 'hyperleptinaemia'. *Diabetologia* **2007**, *50*, 625–633. [CrossRef]
27. Arner, P.; Bernard, S.; Appelsved, L.; Fu, K.Y.; Andersson, D.P.; Salehpour, M.; Thorell, A.; Ryden, M.; Spalding, K.L. Adipose lipid turnover and long-term changes in body weight. *Nat. Med.* **2019**, *25*, 1385–1389. [CrossRef]
28. Spalding, K.L.; Arner, E.; Westermark, P.O.; Bernard, S.; Buchholz, B.A.; Bergmann, O.; Blomqvist, L.; Hoffstedt, J.; Naslund, E.; Britton, T.; et al. Dynamics of fat cell turnover in humans. *Nature* **2008**, *453*, 783–787. [CrossRef]
29. Sharma, D.; Verma, S.; Vaidya, S.; Kalia, K.; Tiwari, V. Recent updates on GLP-1 agonists: Current advancements & challenges. *Biomed. Pharmacother.* **2018**, *108*, 952–962.
30. Beiroa, D.; Imbernon, M.; Gallego, R.; Senra, A.; Herranz, D.; Villarroya, F.; Serrano, M.; Ferno, J.; Salvador, J.; Escalada, J.; et al. GLP-1 agonism stimulates brown adipose tissue thermogenesis and browning through hypothalamic AMPK. *Diabetes* **2014**, *63*, 3346–3358. [CrossRef]
31. Parker, J.A.; McCullough, K.A.; Field, B.C.T.; Minnion, J.S.; Martin, N.M.; Ghatei, M.A.; Bloom, S.R. Glucagon and GLP-1 inhibit food intake and increase c-fos expression in similar appetite regulating centres in the brainstem and amygdala. *Int. J. Obes.* **2013**, *37*, 1391–1398. [CrossRef]
32. Méndez-Giménez, L.; Becerril, S.; Camões, S.P.; da Silva, I.V.; Rodrigues, C.; Moncada, R.; Valentí, V.; Catalán, V.; Gómez-Ambrosi, J.; Miranda, J.P.; et al. Role of aquaporin-7 in ghrelin- and GLP-1-induced improvement of pancreatic beta-cell function after sleeve gastrectomy in obese rats. *Int. J. Obes.* **2017**, *41*, 1394–1402. [CrossRef] [PubMed]
33. Chandarana, K.; Gelegen, C.; Karra, E.; Choudhury, A.I.; Drew, M.E.; Fauveau, V.; Viollet, B.; Andreelli, F.; Withers, D.J.; Batterham, R.L. Diet and gastrointestinal bypass-induced weight loss: The roles of ghrelin and peptide YY. *Diabetes* **2011**, *60*, 810–818. [CrossRef] [PubMed]
34. Batterham, R.L.; Cowley, M.A.; Small, C.J.; Herzog, H.; Cohen, M.A.; Dakin, C.L.; Wren, A.M.; Brynes, A.E.; Low, M.J.; Ghatei, M.A.; et al. Gut hormone PYY(3-36) physiologically inhibits food intake. *Nature* **2002**, *418*, 650–654. [CrossRef] [PubMed]
35. le Roux, C.W.; Batterham, R.L.; Aylwin, S.J.; Patterson, M.; Borg, C.M.; Wynne, K.J.; Kent, A.; Vincent, R.P.; Gardiner, J.; Ghatei, M.A.; et al. Attenuated peptide YY release in obese subjects is associated with reduced satiety. *Endocrinology* **2006**, *147*, 3–8. [CrossRef]
36. Sam, A.H.; Gunner, D.J.; King, A.; Persaud, S.J.; Brooks, L.; Hostomska, K.; Ford, H.E.; Liu, B.; Ghatei, M.A.; Bloom, S.R.; et al. Selective ablation of peptide YY cells in adult mice reveals their role in beta cell survival. *Gastroenterology* **2012**, *143*, 459–468. [CrossRef]
37. Shen, W.J.; Yao, T.; Kong, X.; Williams, K.W.; Liu, T. Melanocortin neurons: Multiple routes to regulation of metabolism. *Biochim. Biophys. Acta Mol. Basis Dis.* **2017**, *1863*, 2477–2485. [CrossRef]
38. Plum, L.; Ahmed, L.; Febres, G.; Bessler, M.; Inabnet, W.; Kunreuther, E.; McMahon, D.J.; Korner, J. Comparison of glucostatic parameters after hypocaloric diet or bariatric surgery and equivalent weight loss. *Obesity* **2011**, *19*, 2149–2157. [CrossRef]
39. Foster-Schubert, K.E.; Overduin, J.; Prudom, C.E.; Liu, J.; Callahan, H.S.; Gaylinn, B.D.; Thorner, M.O.; Cummings, D.E. Acyl and total ghrelin are suppressed strongly by ingested proteins, weakly by lipids, and biphasically by carbohydrates. *J. Clin. Endocrinol. Metab.* **2008**, *93*, 1971–1979. [CrossRef]
40. Orr, J.; Davy, B. Dietary influences on peripheral hormones regulating energy intake: Potential applications for weight management. *J. Am. Diet. Assoc.* **2005**, *105*, 1115–1124. [CrossRef]
41. Little, T.J.; Feinle-Bisset, C. Effects of dietary fat on appetite and energy intake in health and obesity—Oral and gastrointestinal sensory contributions. *Physiol. Behav.* **2011**, *104*, 613–620. [CrossRef]
42. Becerril, S.; Rodríguez, A.; Catalán, V.; Ramírez, B.; Unamuno, X.; Portincasa, P.; Gómez-Ambrosi, J.; Frühbeck, G. Functional relationship between leptin and nitric oxide in metabolism. *Nutrients* **2019**, *11*, 2129. [CrossRef]
43. Ellis, A.C.; Chandler-Laney, P.; Casazza, K.; Goree, L.L.; McGwin, G.; Gower, B.A. Circulating ghrelin and GLP-1 are not affected by habitual diet. *Regul. Pept.* **2012**, *176*, 1–5. [CrossRef]
44. Al Massadi, O.; Pardo, M.; Roca-Rivada, A.; Castelao, C.; Casanueva, F.F.; Seoane, L.M. Macronutrients act directly on the stomach to regulate gastric ghrelin release. *J. Endocrinol. Investig.* **2010**, *33*, 599–602. [CrossRef]
45. Koliaki, C.; Kokkinos, A.; Tentolouris, N.; Katsilambros, N. The effect of ingested macronutrients on postprandial ghrelin response: A critical review of existing literature data. *Int. J. Pept.* **2010**. [CrossRef]
46. Nakazato, M.; Murakami, N.; Date, Y.; Kojima, M.; Matsuo, H.; Kangawa, K.; Matsukura, S. A role for ghrelin in the central regulation of feeding. *Nature* **2001**, *409*, 194–198. [CrossRef] [PubMed]
47. Wren, A.M.; Seal, L.J.; Cohen, M.A.; Brynes, A.E.; Frost, G.S.; Murphy, K.G.; Dhillo, W.S.; Ghatei, M.A.; Bloom, S.R. Ghrelin enhances appetite and increases food intake in humans. *J. Clin. Endocrinol. Metab.* **2001**, *86*, 5992. [CrossRef] [PubMed]

48. Sleeman, M.W.; Spanswick, D.C. Starving for ghrelin. *Cell Metab.* **2014**, *20*, 1–2. [CrossRef] [PubMed]
49. McFarlane, M.R.; Brown, M.S.; Goldstein, J.L.; Zhao, T.J. Induced ablation of ghrelin cells in adult mice does not decrease food intake, body weight, or response to high-fat diet. *Cell Metab.* **2014**, *20*, 54–60. [CrossRef] [PubMed]
50. Goldstein, J.L.; Zhao, T.J.; Li, R.L.; Sherbet, D.P.; Liang, G.; Brown, M.S. Surviving starvation: Essential role of the ghrelin-growth hormone axis. *Cold Spring Harb. Symp. Quant. Biol.* **2011**, *76*, 121–127. [CrossRef] [PubMed]
51. Widdowson, P.S.; Upton, R.; Henderson, L.; Buckingham, R.; Wilson, S.; Williams, G. Reciprocal regional changes in brain NPY receptor density during dietary restriction and dietary-induced obesity in the rat. *Brain Res.* **1997**, *774*, 1–10. [CrossRef]
52. Yu, Y.; Deng, C.; Huang, X.F. Obese reversal by a chronic energy restricted diet leaves an increased Arc NPY/AgRP, but no alteration in POMC/CART, mRNA expression in diet-induced obese mice. *Behav. Brain Res.* **2009**, *205*, 50–56. [CrossRef]
53. Kristensen, P.; Judge, M.E.; Thim, L.; Ribel, U.; Christjansen, K.N.; Wulff, B.S.; Clausen, J.T.; Jensen, P.B.; Madsen, O.D.; Vrang, N.; et al. Hypothalamic CART is a new anorectic peptide regulated by leptin. *Nature* **1998**, *393*, 72–76. [CrossRef]
54. Alen, F.; Crespo, I.; Ramirez-Lopez, M.T.; Jagerovic, N.; Goya, P.; de Fonseca, F.R.; de Heras, R.G.; Orio, L. Ghrelin-induced orexigenic effect in rats depends on the metabolic status and is counteracted by peripheral CB1 receptor antagonism. *PLoS ONE* **2013**, *8*, e60918. [CrossRef]
55. Banke, E.; Riva, M.; Shcherbina, L.; Wierup, N.; Degerman, E. Cocaine- and amphetamine-regulated transcript is expressed in adipocytes and regulate lipid- and glucose homeostasis. *Regul. Pept.* **2013**, *182*, 35–40. [CrossRef] [PubMed]
56. Nakhate, K.T.; Subhedar, N.K.; Kokare, D.M. Involvement of neuropeptide CART in the central effects of insulin on feeding and body weight. *Pharmacol. Biochem. Behav.* **2019**, *181*, 101–109. [CrossRef] [PubMed]
57. Mariano, I.R.; Yamada, L.A.; Soares Rabassi, R.; Rissi Sabino, V.L.; Bataglini, C.; Azevedo, S.; Garcia, R.F.; Pedrosa, M.M.D. Differential responses of liver and hypothalamus to the nutritional condition during lactation and adult life. *Front. Physiol.* **2020**, *11*, 553. [CrossRef] [PubMed]
58. Patkar, P.P.; Hao, Z.; Mumphrey, M.B.; Townsend, R.L.; Berthoud, H.R.; Shin, A.C. Unlike calorie restriction, Roux-en-Y gastric bypass surgery does not increase hypothalamic AgRP and NPY in mice on a high-fat diet. *Int. J. Obes.* **2019**, *43*, 2143–2150. [CrossRef]
59. Adriaenssens, A.E.; Biggs, E.K.; Darwish, T.; Tadross, J.; Sukthankar, T.; Girish, M.; Polex-Wolf, J.; Lam, B.Y.; Zvetkova, I.; Pan, W.; et al. Glucose-dependent insulinotropic polypeptide receptor-expressing cells in the hypothalamus regulate food Intake. *Cell Metab.* **2019**, *30*, 987–996.e6. [CrossRef] [PubMed]
60. Deng, G.; Morselli, L.L.; Wagner, V.A.; Balapattabi, K.; Sapouckey, S.A.; Knudtson, K.L.; Rahmouni, K.; Cui, H.; Sigmund, C.D.; Kwitek, A.E.; et al. Single-nucleus RNA sequencing of the hypothalamic arcuate nucleus of C57BL/6J mice after prolonged diet-induced obesity. *Hypertension* **2020**, *76*, 589–597. [CrossRef] [PubMed]
61. Lam, B.Y.H.; Cimino, I.; Polex-Wolf, J.; Nicole Kohnke, S.; Rimmington, D.; Iyemere, V.; Heeley, N.; Cossetti, C.; Schulte, R.; Saraiva, L.R.; et al. Heterogeneity of hypothalamic pro-opiomelanocortin-expressing neurons revealed by single-cell RNA sequencing. *Mol. Metab.* **2017**, *6*, 383–392. [CrossRef] [PubMed]
62. Quarta, C.; Claret, M.; Zeltser, L.M.; Williams, K.W.; Yeo, G.S.H.; Tschop, M.H.; Diano, S.; Bruning, J.C.; Cota, D. POMC neuronal heterogeneity in energy balance and beyond: An integrated view. *Nat. Metab.* **2021**, *3*, 299–308. [CrossRef] [PubMed]

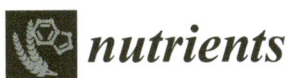

Review

The Potential of Calorie Restriction and Calorie Restriction Mimetics in Delaying Aging: Focus on Experimental Models

Emiliana Giacomello [1],* and Luana Toniolo [2],*

1. Department of Medicine, Surgery and Health Sciences, University of Trieste, 34149 Trieste, Italy
2. Laboratory of Muscle Biophysics, Department of Biomedical Sciences, University of Padova, 35131 Padova, Italy
* Correspondence: egiacomello@units.it (E.G.); luana.toniolo@unipd.it (L.T.)

Citation: Giacomello, E.; Toniolo, L. The Potential of Calorie Restriction and Calorie Restriction Mimetics in Delaying Aging: Focus on Experimental Models. *Nutrients* **2021**, *13*, 2346. https://doi.org/10.3390/nu13072346

Academic Editor: Donald K. Ingram

Received: 11 June 2021
Accepted: 6 July 2021
Published: 9 July 2021

Publisher's Note: MDPI stays neutral with regard to jurisdictional claims in published maps and institutional affiliations.

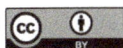

Copyright: © 2021 by the authors. Licensee MDPI, Basel, Switzerland. This article is an open access article distributed under the terms and conditions of the Creative Commons Attribution (CC BY) license (https:// creativecommons.org/licenses/by/ 4.0/).

Abstract: Aging is a biological process determined by multiple cellular mechanisms, such as genomic instability, telomere attrition, epigenetic alterations, loss of proteostasis, deregulated nutrient sensing, mitochondrial dysfunction, cellular senescence, stem cell exhaustion, and altered intercellular communication, that ultimately concur in the functional decline of the individual. The evidence that the old population is steadily increasing and will triplicate in the next 50 years, together with the fact the elderlies are more prone to develop pathologies such as cancer, diabetes, and degenerative disorders, stimulates an important effort in finding specific countermeasures. Calorie restriction (CR) has been demonstrated to modulate nutrient sensing mechanisms, inducing a better metabolic profile, enhanced stress resistance, reduced oxidative stress, and improved inflammatory response. Therefore, CR and CR-mimetics have been suggested as powerful means to slow aging and extend healthy life-span in experimental models and humans. Taking into consideration the difficulties and ethical issues in performing aging research and testing anti-aging interventions in humans, researchers initially need to work with experimental models. The present review reports the major experimental models utilized in the study of CR and CR-mimetics, highlighting their application in the laboratory routine, and their translation to human research.

Keywords: aging; life-span; health-span; calorie restriction; calorie restriction mimetic; resveratrol; experimental models

1. Introduction

The rapid growth of the world's aging population (https://population.un.org/wpp/; reporting the World population prospect of 2019, accessed on March 2021) has motivated a large effort in the investigation of the mechanisms underlying aging, and in the search of possible countermeasures.

Aging is characterized by two connected aspects: the malfunctioning of multiple basic biological processes and the parallel functional decline of the individual. Actually, the alteration of the molecular mechanisms regulating basic processes can increase the risk of developing chronic diseases (e.g., cardiovascular disease, diabetes, cancer, and neurodegeneration), meanwhile the functional decline of the individual contributes to a negative outcome to health-challenging situations.

More recently, it has been suggested that aging is determined by nine biological processes, which are: genomic instability, telomere attrition, epigenetic alterations, loss of proteostasis, deregulated nutrient sensing, mitochondrial dysfunction, cellular senescence, stem cell exhaustion, and altered intercellular communication [1]. Each distinct hallmark of aging has been identified based on the following three characteristics: (1) it is displayed during normal aging; (2) its experimental intensification accelerates aging; and (3) its experimental abatement delays aging [1]. The accumulation of the effects of this damage over time inevitably leads to cell death.

Among the multiple alterations that have a profound impact on aging, the nutrient sensing cell pathways have recently captured much interest thanks to their potential as therapeutic targets in the prevention of age-related diseases, and the extension of the healthy life-span. The nutrient sensing pathways are mainly regrouped in the IGF (insulin-like growth factor)/insulin, the TOR (target of rapamycin), and the AMPK (AMP-Activated Protein Kinase) pathways [2]. It has been extensively shown that, the presence of cellular nutrients induces the stimulation of insulin receptor and IGF-1R generating a phosphorylation cascade that activates AKT (Ak transforming), which induces glucose metabolism through GSK-3β, suppresses a wide range of cellular responses via the FOXO (Forkhead box) transcription factor, and stimulates protein synthesis by activating TORC1 (TOR Complex1), leading to protein synthesis and cell growth. Moreover, IGF-1R dependent signal, activates the Ras/MAPK signaling pathway, which results in cell proliferation. Contrarily, when the cell is deprived of nutrients or in low energetic conditions, AMPK levels increase and inhibit protein synthesis through TORC1, reducing anabolic processes and inducing mitochondrial respiration [2].

Accordingly, data from different experimental models have largely demonstrated that the mutations that induce life-span extension are associated with an altered activity of the above-listed signaling pathways [3].

Interestingly, the extension of the life-span upon inhibition of the nutrient sensing signaling pathways, has also been associated to the physiological condition induced by calorie restriction (CR). Actually, CR, which consists of the reduction in the caloric intake without malnutrition, has been reported as a robust intervention to promote life-span elongation and healthy aging in rodents at the beginning of last century [4], and has been further suggested to have similar effects in humans [5,6]. CR regimens have been shown to induce metabolic adaptations, such as reduced oxidative stress and improved inflammatory response [7,8], that ultimately result in better life- and health-spans. Studies performed on experimental models allowed to attribute the life prolongation effects to the modulation of the IGF-1 [9,10], TOR [11], and AMPK signaling pathways [12], but also to other targets, such as the above mentioned FOXO that stimulates protein synthesis, NfkappaB, which is involved in the inflammatory response, and Nfr2 that is implicated in mitochondrial biogenesis [2,13–15]. Moreover, recent work brought to the identification of the Sir2/SIRT1 NAD-dependent histone deacetylase, which is involved in the chromatin silencing pathway, as the key regulator of life- and health-span extension induced by CR [16–18]. The identification of the regulatory properties of Sirtuins, together with the evidence that this pathway is conserved among different species [16], has provided to this molecular pathway a target role, pharmacologically adjustable, for the amelioration of the health-span, especially in those individuals who cannot afford CR interventions. As a consequence, at present there is a wide field of research focused on the investigation of natural and synthetic compounds (CR-mimetics), aiming at improving life- and health-span in humans [19–21]. Among the most known, the natural polyphenol resveratrol, a potent SIRT1 activator is largely investigated in both experimental models and humans [22–25].

The study of the aging mechanisms and the possible countermeasures to contrast them in humans is challenging due to the long duration of the aging process itself. Longitudinal studies are difficult to perform because they need an important effort, traceability and continuity that, trivially, are very problematic to maintain for a long time. On the other side, cross-sectional studies can be influenced by multiple factors, especially if we consider that in the last century several parameters characterizing the life quality, as the socio-sanitary conditions, the nutritional regimens and psychophysical activities, have undergone dramatic changes. In addition, the heterogeneity of population characteristics can further complicate the analyses.

Mainly for these reasons, but also for ethical issues, the study of aging is conducted on experimental models. Unfortunately, experimental models are not devoid of pitfalls, flaws or obstacles. Multiple factors must be considered when planning experiments to investigate the influence of CR and CR mimetics on the aging process. Although theoretical life-span curves are quite homogeneous in shape across several experimental models, they can be enormously different in length [26], and cannot provide information on the real health condition (health-span) of the experimental model [27]. Furthermore, aging can induce diverse modifications at the tissue or organ level depending on the experimental model used [28,29]. Not least, CR mechanisms underlying life-span extension can differ among species [30,31].

The present review aims at providing an overview of the major experimental models utilized in aging research, highlighting the characteristics that allow their use in the study of CR and CR mimetics, and their translation to human research, with a daily-laboratory routine perspective.

2. Saccharomyces cerevisiae

The first studies on aging in the budding yeast *Saccharomyces cerevisiae* date back to 60 years ago [32], since then its application in aging research has been continuously active. More recently, at the beginning of the 21st century, the use of yeast in aging research saw an important outburst thanks to the discovery of Sirtuins, a class of histone deacetylases involved in life-span regulation.

Saccharomyces cerevisiae is a unicellular eukaryotic organism with 6000 completely sequenced genes [33,34], and with a short life cycle. Yeast cells proliferate in both haploid or diploid state depending on nutrients abundance. With a sufficient nutritional supply, cells proliferate in a diploid state with a cell cycle of 2 h, while they enter meiosis and spore formation upon nutrient withdrawal. Spores can survive from hours to months, and in favorable conditions haploid a and alpha spores can proliferate and mate to form diploid cells. The simple laboratory equipment required, the short generation time, and a well-characterized genome displaying high similarities with mammalian cells, easily modifiable by means of genetic approaches, make *Saccharomyces cerevisiae* an optimal tool to dissect the molecular mechanisms of multiple pathways involved in aging.

The life cycle and senescence in the budding yeast has been defined exploiting two different experimental protocols, which measure two different biological properties. These are the replicative life-span and chronological life-span, respectively [32,35,36]. The first experimental protocol is based on the evidence that the budding capacity of a single mother-cell decreases with time. The second experimental protocol is based on the analysis of the growth to plateau concentration of a population in a liquid medium, and the estimation of percentage of viable or metabolic active cells [34].

Evidences showing that reduction in glucose availability in the growth medium from 2% to 0.01% induced an extension of *Saccharomyces cerevisiae* life-span, have made this organism an excellent model to study the fundamental mechanisms of life prolongation upon CR [17,37]. Interestingly, in 2000, studies from separate groups allowed the identification the Sir-2 NAD-dependent histone deacetylase pathway [17,18,38] as a key regulator of life-span extension. Only subsequently, the Sir2 pathway has been shown to be conserved among species [16].

At date, the signaling pathways regulating the replicative and the chronological life-span are better characterized. In fact, the RAS-PKA and Tor-Sch9 signaling pathways have been demonstrated to be consistent in both the replicative and the chronological life-span, while the effects of the modulation of Sir2 pathway on the chronological life-span are opposite to replicative life-span [17,39]. These evidences provide a further element to orient the researcher in the choice of the most appropriate experimental protocol.

Interestingly, the above-mentioned characteristics make the budding yeast very suitable for high-throughput methodologies, particularly in the screening of anti-aging compounds [40–42]. In this context, the work of Howitz and collaborators [20], reported the discovery of small molecules, such as resveratrol, able to activate Sirtuins and induce life-span extension, tracing the pace to the design and screening of new CR-mimetic compounds.

Although the yeast allows a precise characterization of some molecular pathways involved in aging, its application in the study of CR and CR-mimetics is limited, not only because it cannot provide information at the tissue and organ level, but also because CR mechanisms can differ among species [31]. Indeed, mammals contain seven homologs of the yeast Sir2, which have different cellular localization, different protein interactions and different biological function [30].

3. Caenorhabditis elegans

Since the 1970s the small nematode *Caenorhabditis elegans* is one of the most used organisms in aging research and in the study of genetics of aging [43,44]. Interestingly, it allowed the identification of the insulin/IGF-1 signaling pathway, and afterwards FOXO, as key regulators of the life-span extension [9,10,45]. Only subsequently, the insulin/IGF-1 pathway was found and better characterized in other model animals and humans [46–48].

In normal conditions (20 °C), *C. elegans* develops from an egg and undergoes four larva stages (L1–L4) to become a reproductive adult hermaphrodite worm in three days. The mean life-span of the *C. elegans* is around 15 days, and the maximum life-span around 27 days. In adverse conditions (i.e., temperature or nutrients restriction), worms after the larval stage L2 can enter an alternative developmental state named dauer larvae, which is stress and age-resistant [49,50]. When conditions become more favorable, dauer larvae can convert into a reproductive adult. The adult worm is a simple organism composed by about 1000 cells, that form distinct tissues and organs with a functional similarity to human organs [51,52]. With age progression, *C. elegans* worms reduce their activity, become less coordinate and can eventually stop moving in an age-dependent fashion [53]. Moreover, normal and transgenic *C. elegans* have shown to display some of the aging features as sarcopenia [54], and neurodegeneration [55,56].

From the laboratory routine perspective, *C. elegans* is an interesting experimental model since it is relatively easy to maintain, and the growth medium easily tunable [53]. The *C. elegans* genome is deciphered, easily modifiable, and with good association to human genes [57,58]. The presence of a RNAi library that covers about 80% of the genes allows extensive screens to detect genes involved in the modulation of life-span [59,60]. The life-spans of a population have generally no, or little, fluctuation, allowing the identification of factors that increase or reduce the life-span by 10–15% with statistical significance [60].

C. elegans has been adopted as the prominent model in aging research for several years because it has been found that mutations to genes that regulate the dauer stage correlate with life-span. For instance, the analyses of age-1 and daf-2 mutants, which displayed a longer life-span, led to the identification of the insulin/IGF-1 signaling pathway [9,10]. Subsequently, daf-16 mutants allowed the identification of the FOXO pathway, and revealed the importance of this pathway in improving the resistance to oxidative stress. As a result of these important discoveries, and thanks to the ease to work with mutants and to manipulate its genome, *C. elegans* was exploited to show that CR induced modulation of life-span is strictly correlated with mitochondrial integrity [31,61,62], revealing the central role of mitochondria in the determination of metabolic plasticity.

Interestingly, the availability of the wide array of experimental tools, together with the possibility to control the bacterial food and the presence of specific nutrients, allowed the dissection of the molecular mechanisms involved in the CR dependent life-span extension, showing that different dietary regimens can modulate life-span by independent or overlapping mechanisms [63]. As a result, it is now widely accepted that the effects of CR are caused by the interference with a network of genetic pathways rather than by with a single, linear pathway.

C. elegans was also employed in the first studies on the dissection of the molecular pathways affected by resveratrol [21], confirming AMPK as energy sensor responsible of life-span extension, and guiding the search and screening of new CR-mimetics [64].

Although the use of *C. elegans* in the study of longevity lead to important discoveries, this organism in not free of weaknesses. Being the body organization very simple, and due to the fact that the mechanisms involved in the beneficial action of CR can differ in the different organisms [31], its correlation with humans has to be cautiously evaluated.

4. Drosophila melanogaster

Used for the first time in aging experiments in 1916, demonstrating that its life-span was food and temperature dependent [65], *Drosophila melanogaster* is still considered a suitable model in aging research. Thanks to the feasibility of performing largescale screens for demographic analyses, the fruit fly has a bridging role in the validation of findings discovered in other model organisms [45,66]. As a consequence, *D. melanogaster* is largely exploited in the study of CR mechanisms and in the search of CR-mimetics [21,67].

At 25 °C, *D. melanogaster* has a life-span of approximately 60 days, which can be reduced increasing the temperature, and vice versa, increased by reducing the growth temperature. *D. melanogaster*, as other insects, can enter a reproductive diapause following light cycle and temperature modulation. As reported for *C. elegans*, diapause is connected to a better stress resistance and increased life-span.

D. melanogaster has been described to undergo functional senescence at tissue and organ level [68]. Interestingly, similarly to what has been observed in humans, during aging, flies present the alteration of selected biomarkers as the advanced glycation end products, or carbonylated proteins [69]. At the organ level, age progression induces unbalanced gut homeostasis, altered cardiac and skeletal muscle function, and neurological and neurosecretory modifications [70,71]. More importantly, although it is needless to stress that *D. melanogaster* is far from mirroring the human organism, it is an excellent model to study the genetic complexity of the aging process.

From the laboratory point of view, *D. melanogaster* requires a simple and cost-effective maintenance, and researchers can acquire a very good knowledge on the factors that should be considered when working with the fruit fly [68]. The simplicity of its genome, consisting of 13,000 genes belonging, approximately, to the same mammalian gene families [45], together with the availability of strains with the same genotype, facilitate demographic analyses and the performance of largescale screens [45,66]. Actually, *D. melanogaster* is an excellent model to perform genetic analyses thanks to the availability of mutant and transgenic strains, and the accessibility to temporal, hormone-inducible, and tissue-specific expression of mutated proteins [72]. Not last, a collection of RNAi lines enables the targeting of most transcripts to perform knockdown screens [73].

The above-mentioned characteristics make the fruit fly an experimental model often exploited to delve into the genetics of CR, and into the search and characterization of CR-mimetics [67]. Life-span prolongation upon CR in *D. melanogaster* has been shown to be mediated by five mechanisms: the cotransporter encoded by Indy [74], the insulin/GF-like signaling pathway [75], the Rpd3 deacetylase [76], the dSir2 deacetylase [77], and TOR signaling pathway [78]. The broad knowledge of the CR restriction mechanisms in *D. melanogaster*, together with the relative ease to work with this organism allowed to confirm resveratrol as a CR-mimetic, and to screen interventions with potential effects in life-span extension [79,80].

Although *D. melanogaster* is still far from the human organisms, this experimental model has supplemental advantages compared to yeast and *C. elegans* that justify its employment in the study of CR. It is an obligate aerobe, and it is dioecious, two factors that can have an important impact on aging [81], and on the response to anti-aging measures, making *D. melanogaster* a model organism suitable to perform both genetic manipulation and physiological analyses.

5. Fishes

The fishes include the shortest- and longest-lived vertebrates in nature [82–84]. The heterogeneity in longevity provides a unique possibility for exploring the molecular mechanisms that determine the differences in the rate of aging by applying comparative studies [85,86].

In the view of the laboratory application, the small tropical fish species are considered to have the best potential in aging research, since they display a short life-span, gradual senescence, and development of degenerative processes and tissue lesions in an age dependent way [87,88]. Although the zebrafish (*Danio rerio*) is the most utilized model system in the research laboratories, guppy and killifish have a potential in aging research due to their short life-span [87,89].

Widely employed in developmental studies, the zebrafish is increasingly used in aging research, due to its relative short life-span (2–3 years), and based on the evidence that it shows hallmarks of gradual senescence, such as spinal curvature, muscle degeneration, and reduced physical ability [90–92]. Interestingly, recent research shows that zebrafish can be exploited for the investigation of neurodegenerative pathologies as Alzheimer disease, Parkinson disease [93], but also osteoporosis, sarcopenia [94], and age-dependent trainability [95].

Zebrafish have several advantages for routine research because housing is quite simple, it has a good reproductive capacity, and can provide sufficient amounts of tissues for sampling. Zebrafish have a conserved genome, which is easily modifiable [96]. Moreover, research with zebrafish is greatly supported by the availability of well-established methodological and biological tools, spanning from genetic manipulation [96], live imaging [97], adaptation to high-throughput screenings [98–100]. Moreover, as discussed for *D. melanogaster*, zebrafish can be exploited for demographic studies.

For the above-mentioned reasons, zebrafish have an interesting potential as a model to investigate CR and CR-mimetics. Interestingly, zebrafish feeding conditions can be easily modified upon need, providing the possibility to control the diet to reduce the caloric intake [101,102], or to induce obesity [103], causing genetic modulations similar to those observed in mammals. Likewise, zebrafish is largely used to test CR-mimetics and in the investigation of resveratrol for its CR-mimetic properties [104,105].

The above-mentioned features together with the fact that this is a more complex organism with defined organs and apparatuses, confer to zebrafish a bridging role between more simple organisms and mammals, in the search for anti-aging molecules.

6. Rodents

Rodents are the most common mammalian used in research, and include species with different life-spans, such as mice, rats, naked rat, moles, and others. To date, the mouse and the rat models are the most exploited mammalian models used in aging research, and have enabled important progress in the field of CR and CR-mimetics. Actually, the CR capability to induce life-span elongation was demonstrated for the first time by McCay and collaborators on albino rats [4], and the potential of resveratrol as CR-mimetic was demonstrated in C57BL/6 mice. Despite the awareness of multiple differences with the human aging [28,29], the most used animal model are mice, and, here, we attempt to shortly describe the main advantages and disadvantages of the use of mouse models in the perspective of planning experiments to delve into CR and CR-mimetics potential in attenuating aging.

Mice have about 3 years life-span, with slight changes depending on the strain, with inbred strains being more prone to aging [106,107]. Mice are quite similar to humans in their physiology, cellular functions, and, to a lesser extent, in their anatomy. Mouse aging has been shown to cause changes in many organ systems, in the body composition, in the cognition, and to induce a decline of the physical function [106,107]. The genome of the mouse, with 2.5 Gbp and 40 chromosomes, encodes almost the same number of genes of the human genome, with the 99% of the mouse genes having a human orthologue. Mice are available as inbred strains, therefore they have a genomic homogeneity [45]. To date, there is a large availability of mutant strains and gene-modifying tools that allow to delve into multiple cellular mechanisms. Moreover, the rapid advances in gene editing techniques have made the development of mutant strains less complicated and more rapid compared to the past.

In the context of the aging and CR research, models as the Ames and the Snell dwarf mice have demonstrated to have a longer life-span, ascribable to naturally occurring point mutations to the Prop1 gene [108] and Pou1f1 [109] that, similarly to what demonstrated in yeast, *C. elegans* and *D. melanogaster*, envisage an alteration of the insulin/IGF-1 pathway [110,111]. On the other hand, the availability of strains that display obesity [112], or accelerated aging [113–115], provides a further tool to investigate, in a restricted time-window, the effects of CR regimens and CR-mimetics.

A further advantage in adopting mice as an experimental model in the study of CR is the tuneability of the feeding conditions that allow to simulate obesity or diabetes, but also different nutrition-dependent contexts [112,116]. In this context, C57BL/6 mice fed with a high fat regimen revealed the CR-mimetic properties of resveratrol in mammals, showing that this small polyphenol is able to mimic some molecular aspects of the CR regimens and to improve the health-span in mice by reducing IGF-1 levels, increasing insulin sensitivity, AMPK and PGC-1alpha activity, and mitochondrial activity [24,117]. At the physiological level resveratrol has been showed to induce protection against type II diabetes [23,24], cardiovascular diseases [118,119], and improve the skeletal muscle functions [25,120–122]. Further data on resveratrol have been obtained by exploiting different mouse models, such as naturally aging C57BL/6 mice, diabetic mice [123], senescence-accelerated mice [124], and transgenic strains [125].

This being said, the exploitation of mice in the investigation of CR and CR-mimetics on the whole organism could seem perfect. However, rodents and humans differ both for basic biological process (i.e., regulation of telomere length, the DNA repair mechanisms, and the immune response), and life conditions (i.e., diet composition, physical activity, and life in a restricted state), that, in turn, have a different impact on aging and on the effects of CR and CR-mimetics [126].

7. Nonhuman Primates

Although working with the above-described experimental models certainly has multiple advantages, the differences with human aging prevent the direct translation of findings from model organism to humans. This gap could be overcome by the use of nonhuman primates, which are considered a good translational model because they have similar genetic, physiological, and behavioral characteristics to humans. Nonhuman primates display about 92% of genetic homology with humans, they exhibit age-associated dysfunctions and diseases, and are outbred with a high inter-individual variability similarly to humans [127,128]. The use of nonhuman primates has provided an important contribution in the study of vaccines, in transplant technology, in the study of infectious diseases, aging [129,130], and have been exploited to investigate the effects of CR in longitudinal protocols [131,132].

Nonhuman primates are grouped in two main categories, the Old World and the New World monkeys [130]. The Old World monkeys, which originate from Asia and Africa, have a medium to large size, variable life-spans, and include rhesus monkey, as macaques, that are the most utilized in aging research [129,130]. The New World monkeys, which originate from South America, have a smaller size and a shorter life-span. The most used New World monkeys in research are the marmosets, which live in multigenerational family units, allowing a simple maintenance. The smaller the size (200–450 g), the shorter the life-span, together with observation that these monkey display most of the aging characteristics observed in humans, means that nonhuman primates could represent a good opportunity to reduce costs and time, providing this model with a huge potential in aging research [130,131].

Fifty years after the first work on CR in rodents [4], at the end of the 1980s, CR experiments were applied on rhesus monkeys by different research groups, with the aim to perform longitudinal studies [133,134]. Since then, CR in nonhuman primates has been shown to have anti-aging properties [135,136], decrease the weight, ameliorate glucoregulation [137], reduce inflammation and cardiovascular diseases risk [135], and, in general, to improve the health-span [136]. In line with the necessity to use CR mimetics in patients that cannot afford a calorie restricted regimen, more recently, nonhuman primates have been largely employed in the study of resveratrol. Resveratrol has been demonstrated to improve several physiological parameters in nonhuman primates fed on a regular or modified diet [138–141], providing good chances for the translation to humans.

Although the nonhuman primates represent the most proximate model to humans, their use in the translational study of CR needs careful evaluation. If, on one side, there is an increasing knowledge of the molecular pathways determining longevity, nowadays there is also the awareness that life-span and health-span are modulated by complementary variables, including the macronutrients in the diet, physical activity, gender, and genetic background [126], which can modify the response to CR regimens.

8. Studies in Humans

Aging research in humans is complicated by the long life-span, the large variability among individuals, and multiple factors, such as socio-economic and cultural conditions, that can affect the aging process.

Studies on human aging can exploit the cross-sectional or the longitudinal design, but neither of them are free of flaws, and can lead to different interpretations [142]. Cross-sectional designs, which analyze different age groups at the same time point, are influenced by the dramatic changes occurred in the last 100 years of social, nutritional, and work conditions. Longitudinal studies, which follow the same individuals along time, reveal a high degree of individual variability, which is likely to depend on the social, nutritional, and work conditions changes, but also on the variation of the physio-pathological status experienced throughout the life-span of the individual.

Nowadays, the search for the effects of long-term lifestyle interventions initiated in early adulthood and carried on throughout the entire life captures much attention, due to the evidence that in some tissues and organs, such as the skeletal muscle [28], the functional decline can begin in adulthood. This interest has prompted several observational studies to understand the correlation between nutrition and health-span, and the potential of CR regimens and CR mimetics in improving the health-span of aging people. An example has been provided by Okinawans who are the world's longest-lived population. The prolongation of the life-span of this population has been attributed principally to CR and the presence of CR mimetics in the diet [5,6].

At date, there is also a large number of studies aimed at directly testing CR regimens and CR-mimetics, but there are still some shadows on their efficacy [143,144], because the time and the interval of the intervention, the variability among individuals, and other factors can compromise their effectiveness [145].

Interestingly, also the investigation on humans can exploit an experimental model of accelerated aging. This is the bed rest model, which became very popular after spaceflights as a tool to investigate the effects of microgravity. The bed rest model is based on the evidence that microgravity and long periods of immobilization cause an alteration of mechano-skeletal and vestibulo-neuromuscular stimuli that have detrimental effects on the normal physiology of several organs and apparatuses, such as skeletal muscle, bones, cardiovascular system, and to unbalance several biomarkers [146]. Although bed rest experiments are restricted due to their nature, in recent years they have allowed the collection of an enormous amount of data, which contributed to expanding the knowledge on physiological changes during loss of gravitation, and on the mechanisms of aging.

Interestingly, aiming at simulating the nutritional condition of astronauts, who consume fewer calories, bed rest protocols envisaged the application of CR regimens, that have been shown to modulate several physiological parameters [147,148]. Interestingly, although CR enhances protein catabolism in 2-week inactive individuals [149], it prevents the inflammatory state induced by the inactivity [150].

9. Conclusions

The increase in the world's aging population (https://population.un.org/wpp/; reporting the World population prospect of 2019, accessed on March 2021) has motivated a large effort in the investigation of the mechanisms underlying aging, and in the search of possible countermeasures. The search of strategies to improve the health-span in humans face with the intrinsic complexity of investigating in humans, such as the presence of ethical issues, and the difficulties to perform both longitudinal and cross-sectional studies. Mainly for these reasons, researchers opt in favor of using experimental models. Hence, the researcher has to deal with the evidence that, on one hand there are conserved mechanisms that regulated life-span, on the other, there are important variations in the fine mechanisms underlying aging in different organisms, between related species, and even among distinct individuals, conferring to aging a multifactorial nature [151].

Consequently, the cautious choice of one experimental model compared to another (Table 1), is based on the questions the researcher wants to answer. In the investigation of CR and CR-mimetics, the experimental models used are multiple, generally starting with a simple organism, and subsequently translating to more complex organisms. This approach has been exploited both for the study of several signaling pathways [14,16], and in the search of anti-aging agents [20,22]. Special attention has to be dedicated to the target tissue or organ, because senescence can affect tissue and organs dependently of the experimental model considered. It is important to mention that, the set-up, the availability of dedicated facilities, and the know-how of the laboratory are important in guiding the selection of the experimental model.

It is worthwhile to mention that, nowadays the researcher can afford new methods of analysis and new knowledge to tackle aging mechanisms and anti-aging interventions. These include silico analysis and simulations [152], and system biology studies [153], which can be of fundamental help when planning a research project on aging, and searching for interventions able to ameliorate life-span and health-span [151,154–156].

Table 1. Summary of the most relevant properties of the described model systems.

	Yeast	Worms	Flies	Fishes	Rodents	Non-Human Primates
Life span	Very short	Very short with little fluctuation	Very short	Variable	Variable	Long
Genome	Restricted number of genes, fully characterized genome with a low similarity with human	Restricted number of genes, fully characterized genome with a low similarity with human	Restricted number of genes, fully characterized genome with a medium similarity with human	High number of genes, with a medium-high similarity with human	High number of genes, with a medium-high similarity with human	Similar number of genes, with high similarity with human
Anatomo-physiology	Unicellular	Very simple organism with tissues similar to human, hermaphrodite	Simple organism, with tissues similar to human, aerobe	Organism with defined organs and apparatuses	Mammals, with high similarity except some tissues and organs	Similar physiological and behavioral characteristics
Experimental tools	Easy genetic interventions	Easy genetic interventions, Mutant strains, RNAi libraries, Control of feeding conditions	Easy genetic interventions, Mutant strains, transgenic tunable strains, RNAi libraries, Control of feeding conditions	Easy genetic interventions, Mutant strains, transgenic tunable strains, RNAi libraries, Control of feeding conditions	Inbred strains, Control of feeding and diet conditions	High inter-individual variability similar to humans, Life in multigenerational family units
Major applications in CR research	Studies on mechanisms of CR, Screening of CR-mimetics, High-throughput analyses	Studies on mechanisms of CR, Screening of CR-mimetics, High-throughput analyses	Studies of mechanisms of CR, Screening of CR-mimetics, High-throughput and largescale screens for demographic analyses	Studies of mechanisms of CR, Screening of CR-mimetics, High-throughput and largescale screens for demographic analyses	Application of CR and CR-mimetics treatments in normal and pathological conditions	Longitudinal studies on CR and CR-mimetics
Pitfalls	Unicellular organisms, Restricted gene homologs	Different life cycle compared to mammals, Very simple organs	Different life cycle compared to mammals, Simple organs,	Different life cycle and habitat compared to mammals, Relatively simple organs and apparatuses, Dedicated facility	Different anatomo-physiological and aging properties of some organs and tissues, Dedicated facility	Long-term studies, Ethical concerns, Dedicated facility

Author Contributions: Conceptualization, E.G. and L.T.; writing—original draft preparation, E.G. and L.T.; writing—review and editing, E.G. and L.T. Both authors have read and agreed to the published version of the manuscript.

Funding: This research received no external funding.

Institutional Review Board Statement: Not applicable.

Informed Consent Statement: Not applicable.

Data Availability Statement: The study did not report original data.

Acknowledgments: Not applicable.

Conflicts of Interest: The authors declare no conflict of interest.

References

1. López-Otín, C.; Blasco, M.A.; Partridge, L.; Serrano, M.; Kroemer, G. The hallmarks of aging. *Cell* **2013**, *153*, 1194–1217. [CrossRef]
2. Riera, C.E.; Merkwirth, C.; De Magalhaes Filho, C.D.; Dillin, A. Signaling Networks Determining Life Span. *Annu. Rev. Biochem.* **2016**, *85*. [CrossRef]
3. Fontana, L.; Partridge, L.; Longo, V.D. Extending healthy life span-from yeast to humans. *Science* **2010**, *328*, 321–326. [CrossRef] [PubMed]
4. McCay, C.M.; Maynard, L.A.; Sperling, G.; Barnes, L.L. Retarded Growth, Life Span, Ultimate Body Size and Age Changes in the Albino Rat after Feeding Diets Restricted in Calories. *J. Nutr.* **1939**. [CrossRef]
5. Willcox, D.C.; Willcox, B.J.; Todoriki, H.; Suzuki, M. The okinawan diet: Health implications of a low-calorie, nutrient-dense, antioxidant-rich dietary pattern low in glycemic load. *J. Am. Coll. Nutr.* **2009**, *28*, 500S–516S. [CrossRef] [PubMed]
6. Willcox, D.C.; Willcox, B.J.; Todoriki, H.; Curb, J.D.; Suzuki, M. Caloric restriction and human longevity: What can we learn from the Okinawans? *Biogerontology* **2006**, *7*, 173–177. [CrossRef]
7. Stankovic, M.; Mladenovic, D.; Ninkovic, M.; Vucevic, D.; Tomasevic, T.; Radosavljevic, T. Effects of caloric restriction on oxidative stress parameters. *Gen. Physiol. Biophys.* **2013**. [CrossRef]
8. Ungvari, Z.; Parrado-Fernandez, C.; Csiszar, A.; De Cabo, R. Mechanisms underlying caloric restriction and lifespan regulation: Implications for vascular aging. *Circ. Res.* **2008**, *102*, 519–528. [CrossRef] [PubMed]
9. Kenyon, C.; Chang, J.; Gensch, E.; Rudner, A.; Tabtiang, R. A *C. elegans* mutant that lives twice as long as wild type. *Nature* **1993**, *366*. [CrossRef]
10. Kenyon, C. The first long-lived mutants: Discovery of the insulin/IGF-1 pathway for ageing. *Philos. Trans. R. Soc. B Biol. Sci.* **2011**, *366*, 9–16. [CrossRef] [PubMed]
11. Powers, R.W.; Kaeberlein, M.; Caldwell, S.D.; Kennedy, B.K.; Fields, S. Extension of chronological life span in yeast by decreased TOR pathway signaling. *Genes Dev.* **2006**, *20*. [CrossRef]
12. Cantó, C.; Auwerx, J. Calorie restriction: Is AMPK a key sensor and effector? *Physiology* **2011**, *26*, 214–224. [CrossRef]
13. Pallauf, K.; Giller, K.; Huebbe, P.; Rimbach, G. Nutrition and healthy ageing: Calorie restriction or polyphenol-rich "mediterrAsian" diet? *Oxid. Med. Cell. Longev.* **2013**. [CrossRef] [PubMed]
14. Pan, H.; Finkel, T. Key proteins and pathways that regulate lifespan. *J. Biol. Chem.* **2017**, *292*, 6452–6460. [CrossRef] [PubMed]
15. Ungvari, Z.; Bagi, Z.; Feher, A.; Recchia, F.A.; Sonntag, W.E.; Pearson, K.; De Cabo, R.; Csiszar, A. Resveratrol confers endothelial protection via activation of the antioxidant transcription factor Nrf2. *Am. J. Physiol. Hear. Circ. Physiol.* **2010**, *299*. [CrossRef] [PubMed]
16. Smith, J.S.; Brachmann, C.B.; Celic, I.; Kenna, M.A.; Muhammad, S.; Starai, V.J.; Avalos, J.L.; Escalante-Semerena, J.C.; Grubmeyer, C.; Wolberger, C.; et al. A phylogenetically conserved NAD+-dependent protein deacetylase activity in the Sir2 protein family. *Proc. Natl. Acad. Sci. USA* **2000**. [CrossRef]
17. Lin, S.J.; Defossez, P.A.; Guarente, L. Requirement of NAD and SIR2 for life-span extension by calorie restriction in *Saccharomyces cerevisiae*. *Science* **2000**. [CrossRef]
18. Imai, S.I.; Armstrong, C.M.; Kaeberlein, M.; Guarente, L. Transcriptional silencing and longevity protein Sir2 is an NAD-dependent histone deacetylase. *Nature* **2000**. [CrossRef]
19. Madeo, F.; Carmona-Gutierrez, D.; Hofer, S.J.; Kroemer, G. Caloric Restriction Mimetics against Age-Associated Disease: Targets, Mechanisms, and Therapeutic Potential. *Cell Metab.* **2019**, *29*, 529–610. [CrossRef]
20. Howitz, K.T.; Bitterman, K.J.; Cohen, H.Y.; Lamming, D.W.; Lavu, S.; Wood, J.G.; Zipkin, R.E.; Chung, P.; Kisielewski, A.; Zhang, L.L.; et al. Small molecule activators of sirtuins extend *Saccharomyces cerevisiae* lifespan. *Nature* **2003**. [CrossRef]
21. Wood, J.G.; Regina, B.; Lavu, S.; Hewitz, K.; Helfand, S.L.; Tatar, M.; Sinclair, D. Sirtuin activators mimic caloric restriction and delay ageing in metazoans. *Nature* **2004**. [CrossRef]
22. Timmers, S.; Auwerx, J.; Schrauwen, P. The journey of resveratrol from yeast to human. *Aging (Albany NY)* **2012**, *4*, 146. [CrossRef]
23. Lagouge, M.; Argmann, C.; Gerhart-Hines, Z.; Meziane, H.; Lerin, C.; Daussin, F.; Messadeq, N.; Milne, J.; Lambert, P.; Elliott, P.; et al. Resveratrol Improves Mitochondrial Function and Protects against Metabolic Disease by Activating SIRT1 and PGC-1α. *Cell* **2006**, *127*. [CrossRef]

24. Baur, J.A.; Pearson, K.J.; Price, N.L.; Jamieson, H.A.; Lerin, C.; Kalra, A.; Prabhu, V.V.; Allard, J.S.; Lopez-Lluch, G.; Lewis, K.; et al. Resveratrol improves health and survival of mice on a high-calorie diet. *Nature* **2006**. [CrossRef] [PubMed]
25. Toniolo, L.; Giacomello, E. Resveratrol, aging, and fatigue. *Aging* **2020**. [CrossRef]
26. Mitchell, S.J.; Scheibye-Knudsen, M.; Longo, D.L.; De Cabo, R. Animal models of aging research: Implications for human aging and age-related diseases. *Annu. Rev. Anim. Biosci.* **2015**. [CrossRef] [PubMed]
27. Hamczyk, M.R.; Nevado, R.M.; Barettino, A.; Fuster, V.; Andrés, V. Biological Versus Chronological Aging: JACC Focus Seminar. *J. Am. Coll. Cardiol.* **2020**, *75*, 919–930. [CrossRef]
28. Larsson, L.; Degens, H.; Li, M.; Salviati, L.; Lee, Y.I.; Thompson, W.; Kirkland, J.L.; Sandri, M. Sarcopenia: Aging-related loss of muscle mass and function. *Physiol. Rev.* **2019**. [CrossRef]
29. Burns, T.C.; Li, M.D.; Mehta, S.; Awad, A.J.; Morgan, A.A. Mouse models rarely mimic the transcriptome of human neurodegenerative diseases: A systematic bioinformatics-based critique of preclinical models. *Eur. J. Pharmacol.* **2015**. [CrossRef] [PubMed]
30. Haigis, M.C.; Guarente, L.P. Mammalian sirtuins-Emerging roles in physiology, aging, and calorie restriction. *Genes Dev.* **2006**, *20*, 2913–2921. [CrossRef]
31. Guarente, L. Sirtuins in aging and disease. *Cold Spring Harb. Symp. Quant. Biol.* **2007**, *72*, 483–488. [CrossRef] [PubMed]
32. Mortimer, R.K.; Johnston, J.R. Life span of individual yeast cells. *Nature* **1959**. [CrossRef] [PubMed]
33. Longo, V.D. Mutations in signal transduction proteins increase stress resistance and longevity in yeast, nematodes, fruit flies, and mammalian neuronal cells. *Neurobiol. Aging* **1999**. [CrossRef]
34. Longo, V.D.; Shadel, G.S.; Kaeberlein, M.; Kennedy, B. Replicative and chronological aging in *Saccharomyces cerevisiae*. *Cell Metab.* **2012**, *16*, 18–31. [CrossRef] [PubMed]
35. Kennedy, B.K.; Austriaco, N.R.; Guarente, L. Daughter cells of *Saccharomyces cerevisiae* from old mothers display a reduced life span. *J. Cell Biol.* **1994**. [CrossRef] [PubMed]
36. Fabrizio, P.; Longo, V.D. The chronological life span of *Saccharomyces cerevisiae*. *Aging Cell* **2003**, *2*, 73–81. [CrossRef]
37. Kaeberlein, M.; Andalis, A.A.; Fink, G.R.; Guarente, L. High Osmolarity Extends Life Span in *Saccharomyces cerevisiae* by a Mechanism Related to Calorie Restriction. *Mol. Cell. Biol.* **2002**, *22*. [CrossRef]
38. Landry, J.; Sutton, A.; Tafrov, S.T.; Heller, R.C.; Stebbins, J.; Pillus, L.; Sternglanz, R. The silencing protein SIR2 and its homologs are NAD-dependent protein deacetylases. *Proc. Natl. Acad. Sci. USA* **2000**, *97*. [CrossRef] [PubMed]
39. Fabrizio, P.; Gattazzo, C.; Battistella, L.; Wei, M.; Cheng, C.; McGrew, K.; Longo, V.D. Sir2 blocks extreme life-span extension. *Cell* **2005**. [CrossRef]
40. Sarnoski, E.A.; Liu, P.; Acar, M. A High-Throughput Screen for Yeast Replicative Lifespan Identifies Lifespan-Extending Compounds. *Cell Rep.* **2017**. [CrossRef]
41. Petranovic, D.; Nielsen, J. Can yeast systems biology contribute to the understanding of human disease? *Trends Biotechnol.* **2008**. [CrossRef] [PubMed]
42. Zimmermann, A.; Hofer, S.; Pendl, T.; Kainz, K.; Madeo, F.; Carmona-Gutierrez, D. Yeast as a tool to identify anti-aging compounds. *FEMS Yeast Res.* **2018**. [CrossRef] [PubMed]
43. Kenyon, C.J. The genetics of ageing. *Nature* **2010**, *464*, 504–512. [CrossRef]
44. Mack, H.I.D.; Heimbucher, T.; Murphy, C.T. The nematode *Caenorhabditis elegans* as a model for aging research. *Drug Discov. Today Dis. Model.* **2018**, *27*, 3–13. [CrossRef]
45. Taormina, G.; Ferrante, F.; Vieni, S.; Grassi, N.; Russo, A.; Mirisola, M.G. Longevity: Lesson from model organisms. *Genes* **2019**, *10*, 518. [CrossRef] [PubMed]
46. Partridge, L.; Thornton, J.; Bates, G. The new science of ageing. *Philos. Trans. R. Soc. B Biol. Sci.* **2011**. [CrossRef]
47. Ziv, E.; Hu, D. Genetic variation in insulin/IGF-1 signaling pathways and longevity. *Ageing Res. Rev.* **2011**, *10*, 201–204. [CrossRef]
48. Bonafe, M.; Bonafe, B.; Barbieri, M.; Marchegiani, F.; Olivieri, F.; Ragno, E.; Giampieri, C.; Mugianesi, E.; Centurelli, M.; Franceschi, C.; et al. Polymorphic Variants of Insulin-Like Growth Factor I (IGF-I) Receptor and Phosphoinositide 3-Kinase Genes Affect IGF-I Plasma Levels and Human Longevity: Cues for an Evolutionarily Conserved Mechanism of Life Span Control. *J. Clin. Endocrinol. Metab.* **2003**. [CrossRef]
49. Riddle, D.L.; Albert, P.S. Genetic and environmental regulation of Dauer Larva development. In *C. elegans II*; Riddle, B.T., Meyer, B., Priess, J., Eds.; Cold Spring Harbour Laboratory: Cold Spring Harbour, NY, USA.
50. Karp, X. Working with dauer larvae. *WormBook* **2018**. [CrossRef]
51. McGhee, J.D. The *C. elegans* intestine. *WormBook* **2007**. [CrossRef]
52. Altun, Z.F.; Hall, D.H. WormAtlas Hermaphrodite Handbook-Pericellular Structures. *WormAtlas* **2009**. [CrossRef]
53. Olsen, A.; Vantipalli, M.C.; Lithgow, G.J. Using *Caenorhabditis elegans* as a model for aging and age-related diseases. *Ann. N. Y. Acad. Sci.* **2006**, *1067*, 120–128. [CrossRef] [PubMed]
54. Herndon, L.A.; Schmeissner, P.J.; Dudaronek, J.M.; Brown, P.A.; Listner, K.M.; Sakano, Y.; Paupard, M.C.; Hall, D.H.; Driscoll, M. Stochastic and genetic factors influence tissue-specific decline in ageing *C. elegans*. *Nature* **2002**. [CrossRef] [PubMed]
55. Oeda, T.; Shimohama, S.; Kitagawa, N.; Kohno, R.; Imura, T.; Shibasaki, H.; Ishii, N. Oxidative stress causes abnormal accumulation of familial amyotrophic lateral sclerosis-related mutant SOD1 in transgenic *Caenorhabditis elegans*. *Hum. Mol. Genet.* **2001**. [CrossRef]

56. Papaevgeniou, N.; Chondrogianni, N. The ubiquitin proteasome system in *Caenorhabditis elegans* and its regulation. *Redox Biol.* **2014**, *2*, 333–347. [CrossRef] [PubMed]
57. Wheelan, S.J.; Boguski, M.S.; Duret, L.; Makalowski, W. Human and nematode orthologs-Lessons from the analysis of 1800 human genes and the proteome of *Caenorhabditis elegans*. *Gene* **1999**. [CrossRef]
58. C. elegans Sequencing Consortium. Genome sequence of the nematode *C. elegans*: A platform for investigating biology. *Science* **1998**, *282*, 2012–2018. [CrossRef]
59. Ahringer, J. Reverse genetics. *WormBook* **2006**. [CrossRef]
60. Tissenbaum, H.A. Using *C. elegans* for aging research. *Invertebr. Reprod. Dev.* **2015**. [CrossRef]
61. Walker, G.; Houthoofd, K.; Vanfleteren, J.R.; Gems, D. Dietary restriction in *C. elegans*: From rate-of-living effects to nutrient sensing pathways. *Mech. Ageing Dev.* **2005**. [CrossRef]
62. Anson, R.M.; Hansford, R.G. Mitochondrial influence on aging rate in *Caenorhabditis elegans*. *Aging Cell* **2004**, *3*, 29–34. [CrossRef] [PubMed]
63. Greer, E.L.; Brunet, A. Different dietary restriction regimens extend lifespan by both independent and overlapping genetic pathways in *C. elegans*. *Aging Cell* **2009**. [CrossRef]
64. Calvert, S.; Tacutu, R.; Sharifi, S.; Teixeira, R.; Ghosh, P.; de Magalhães, J.P. A network pharmacology approach reveals new candidate caloric restriction mimetics in *C. elegans*. *Aging Cell* **2016**. [CrossRef]
65. Loeb, J.; Northrop, J.H. Is There a Temperature Coefficient for the Duration of Life? *Proc. Natl. Acad. Sci. USA* **1916**. [CrossRef]
66. Tsurumi, A.; Li, W.X. Aging mechanisms—A perspective mostly from Drosophila. *Genet. Genomics Next* **2020**. [CrossRef]
67. Partridge, L.; Piper, M.D.W.; Mair, W. Dietary restriction in Drosophila. *Mech. Ageing Dev.* **2005**. [CrossRef]
68. He, Y.; Jasper, H. Studying aging in Drosophila. *Methods* **2014**. [CrossRef]
69. Jacobson, J.; Lambert, A.J.; Portero-Otín, M.; Pamplona, R.; Magwere, T.; Miwa, S.; Driege, Y.; Brand, M.D.; Partridge, L. Biomarkers of aging in Drosophila. *Aging Cell* **2010**. [CrossRef] [PubMed]
70. Toivonen, J.M.; Partridge, L. Endocrine regulation of aging and reproduction in Drosophila. *Mol. Cell. Endocrinol.* **2009**. [CrossRef] [PubMed]
71. Tatar, M. The neuroendocrine regulation of Drosophila aging. *Exp. Gerontol.* **2004**, *39*, 1745–1750. [CrossRef]
72. McGuire, S.E.; Mao, Z.; Davis, R.L. Spatiotemporal gene expression targeting with the TARGET and gene-switch systems in Drosophila. *Sci. STKE* **2004**. [CrossRef] [PubMed]
73. Perkins, L.A.; Holderbaum, L.; Tao, R.; Hu, Y.; Sopko, R.; McCall, K.; Yang-Zhou, D.; Flockhart, I.; Binari, R.; Shim, H.S.; et al. The transgenic RNAi project at Harvard medical school: Resources and validation. *Genetics* **2015**. [CrossRef] [PubMed]
74. Rogina, B.; Reenan, R.A.; Nilsen, S.P.; Helfand, S.L. Extended life-span conferred by cotransporter gene mutations in Drosophila. *Science* **2000**, *290*. [CrossRef] [PubMed]
75. Clancy, D.J.; Gems, D.; Harshman, L.G.; Oldham, S.; Stocker, H.; Hafen, E.; Leevers, S.J.; Partridge, L. Extension of life-span by loss of CHICO, a Drosophila insulin receptor substrate protein. *Science* **2001**, *292*. [CrossRef]
76. Woods, J.K.; Rogina, B. The effects of Rpd3 on fly metabolism, health, and longevity. *Exp. Gerontol.* **2016**, *86*. [CrossRef]
77. Rogina, B.; Helfand, S.L. Sir2 mediates longevity in the fly through a pathway related to calorie restriction. *Proc. Natl. Acad. Sci. USA* **2004**, *101*. [CrossRef]
78. Colombani, J.; Raisin, S.; Pantalacci, S.; Radimerski, T.; Montagne, J.; Léopold, P. A nutrient sensor mechanism controls Drosophila growth. *Cell* **2003**, *114*. [CrossRef]
79. Moretti, C.H.; Schiffer, T.A.; Montenegro, M.F.; Larsen, F.J.; Tsarouhas, V.; Carlström, M.; Samakovlis, C.; Weitzberg, E.; Lundberg, J.O. Dietary nitrite extends lifespan and prevents age-related locomotor decline in the fruit fly. *Free Radic. Biol. Med.* **2020**, *160*. [CrossRef]
80. Bauer, J.H.; Goupil, S.; Garber, G.B.; Helfand, S.L. An accelerated assay for the identification of lifespan-extending interventions in *Drosophila melanogaster*. *Proc. Natl. Acad. Sci. USA* **2004**, *101*. [CrossRef]
81. Magwere, T.; Chapman, T.; Partridge, L. Sex Differences in the Effect of Dietary Restriction on Life Span and Mortality Rates in Female and Male *Drosophila melanogaster*. *J. Gerontol. Ser. A Biol. Sci. Med. Sci.* **2004**, *59*. [CrossRef]
82. Finch, C.E. *Longevity, Senescence, and the Genome*; University of Chicago Press: Chicago, IL, USA, 1990; Volume 67.
83. Finch, C.E.; Austad, S.N. History and prospects: Symposium on organisms with slow aging. *Exp. Gerontol.* **2001**, *36*, 593–597. [CrossRef]
84. Singh, P.P.; Demmitt, B.A.; Nath, R.D.; Brunet, A. The Genetics of Aging: A Vertebrate Perspective. *Cell* **2019**, *177*, 200–220. [CrossRef] [PubMed]
85. Trifonova, O.P.; Maslov, D.L.; Mikhailov, A.N.; Zolotarev, K.V.; Nakhod, K.V.; Nakhod, V.I.; Belyaeva, N.F.; Mikhailova, M.V.; Lokhov, P.G.; Archakov, A.I. Comparative analysis of the blood plasma metabolome of negligible, gradual and rapidly ageing fishes. *Fishes* **2018**. [CrossRef]
86. Maslov, D.L.; Trifonova, O.P.; Mikhailov, A.N.; Zolotarev, K.V.; Nakhod, K.V.; Nakhod, V.I.; Belyaeva, N.F.; Mikhailova, M.V.; Lokhov, P.G.; Archakov, A.I. Comparative analysis of skeletal muscle metabolites of fish with various rates of aging. *Fishes* **2019**. [CrossRef]
87. Gerhard, G.S. Small laboratory fish as models for aging research. *Ageing Res. Rev.* **2007**, *6*, 64–72. [CrossRef] [PubMed]
88. Patnaik, B.K.; Mahapatro, N.; Jena, B.S. Ageing in fishes. *Gerontology* **1994**, *40*, 113–132. [CrossRef] [PubMed]

89. Kim, Y.; Nam, H.G.; Valenzano, D.R. The short-lived African turquoise killifish: An emerging experimental model for ageing. *DMM Dis. Model. Mech.* **2016**, *9*, 115–129. [CrossRef]
90. Ulloa, P.E.; Iturra, P.; Neira, R.; Araneda, C. Zebrafish as a model organism for nutrition and growth: Towards comparative studies of nutritional genomics applied to aquacultured fishes. *Rev. Fish Biol. Fish.* **2011**, *21*, 649–666. [CrossRef]
91. Shive, H.R. Zebrafish Models for Human Cancer. *Vet. Pathol.* **2013**, *50*, 468–482. [CrossRef] [PubMed]
92. Gerhard, G.S. Comparative aspects of zebrafish (*Danio rerio*) as a model for aging research. *Exp. Gerontol.* **2003**. [CrossRef] [PubMed]
93. Bandmann, O.; Burton, E.A. Genetic zebrafish models of neurodegenerative diseases. *Neurobiol. Dis.* **2010**, *40*, 58–65. [CrossRef]
94. Daya, A.; Donaka, R.; Karasik, D. Zebrafish models of sarcopenia. *DMM Dis. Model. Mech.* **2020**, *13*, dmm0426890. [CrossRef] [PubMed]
95. Gilbert, M.J.H.; Zerulla, T.C.; Tierney, K.B. Zebrafish (*Danio rerio*) as a model for the study of aging and exercise: Physical ability and trainability decrease with age. *Exp. Gerontol.* **2013**. [CrossRef]
96. Mullins, M.C.; Nüsslein-Volhard, C. Mutational approaches to studying embryonic pattern formation in the zebrafish. *Curr. Opin. Genet. Dev.* **1993**. [CrossRef]
97. Keller, P.J. In vivo imaging of zebrafish embryogenesis. *Methods* **2013**. [CrossRef] [PubMed]
98. Spaink, H.P.; Cui, C.; Wiweger, M.I.; Jansen, H.J.; Veneman, W.J.; Marín-Juez, R.; De Sonneville, J.; Ordas, A.; Torraca, V.; van der Ent, W.; et al. Robotic injection of zebrafish embryos for high-throughput screening in disease models. *Methods* **2013**. [CrossRef] [PubMed]
99. Lessman, C.A. The developing zebrafish (*Danio rerio*): A vertebrate model for high-throughput screening of chemical libraries. *Birth Defects Res. Part C Embryo Today Rev.* **2011**, *93*, 268–280. [CrossRef]
100. Bugel, S.M.; Tanguay, R.L.; Planchart, A. Zebrafish: A Marvel of High-Throughput Biology for 21st Century Toxicology. *Curr. Environ. Health Rep.* **2014**, *1*, 341–352. [CrossRef]
101. Gerhard, G.S.; Cheng, K.C. A call to fins! Zebrafish as a gerontological model. *Aging Cell* **2002**, *1*, 104–111. [CrossRef] [PubMed]
102. Novak, C.M.; Jiang, X.; Wang, C.; Teske, J.A.; Kotz, C.M.; Levine, J.A. Caloric restriction and physical activity in zebrafish (*Danio rerio*). *Neurosci. Lett.* **2005**, *383*. [CrossRef]
103. Oka, T.; Nishimura, Y.; Zang, L.; Hirano, M.; Shimada, Y.; Wang, Z.; Umemoto, N.; Kuroyanagi, J.; Nishimura, N.; Tanaka, T. Diet-induced obesity in zebrafish shares common pathophysiological pathways with mammalian obesity. *BMC Physiol.* **2010**, *10*. [CrossRef] [PubMed]
104. Luo, Q.; Liu, S.; Xie, L.; Yu, Y.; Zhou, L.; Feng, Y.; Cai, D. Resveratrol ameliorates glucocorticoid-induced bone damage in a zebrafish model. *Front. Pharmacol.* **2019**, *10*. [CrossRef]
105. Ran, G.; Ying, L.; Li, L.; Yan, Q.; Yi, W.; Ying, C.; Wu, H.; Ye, X. Resveratrol ameliorates diet-induced dysregulation of lipid metabolism in zebrafish (*Danio rerio*). *PLoS ONE* **2017**, *12*. [CrossRef] [PubMed]
106. Ackert-Bicknell, C.L.; Anderson, L.C.; Sheehan, S.; Hill, W.G.; Chang, B.; Churchill, G.A.; Chesler, E.J.; Korstanje, R.; Peters, L.L. Aging Research Using Mouse Models. *Curr. Protoc. Mouse Biol.* **2015**. [CrossRef]
107. Flurkey, K.; Currer, J.M.; Harrison, D.E. Mouse Models in Aging Research. In *The Mouse in Biomedical Research*; Elsevier Inc.: Amsterdam, The Netherlands, 2007; Volume 3, pp. 637–672. ISBN 9780123694546.
108. Dollé, M.E.T.; Snyder, W.K.; Vijg, J. Genotyping the Prop-1 mutation in Ames dwarf mice. *Mech. Ageing Dev.* **2001**. [CrossRef]
109. Snell, G.D. Dwarf, a new mendelian recessive character of the house mouse. *Proc. Natl. Acad. Sci. USA* **1929**. [CrossRef]
110. Hsieh, C.C.; DeFord, J.H.; Flurkey, K.; Harrison, D.E.; Papaconstantinou, J. Effects of the Pit1 mutation on the insulin signaling pathway: Implications on the longevity of the long-lived Snell dwarf mouse. *Mech. Ageing Dev.* **2002**. [CrossRef]
111. Hsieh, C.C.; DeFord, J.H.; Flurkey, K.; Harrison, D.E.; Papaconstantinou, J. Implications for the insulin signaling pathway in Snell dwarf mouse longevity: A similarity with the *C. elegans* longevity paradigm. *Mech. Ageing Dev.* **2002**. [CrossRef]
112. Koya, D.; Kanasaki, K. Biology of obesity: Lessons from animal models of obesity. *J. Biomed. Biotechnol.* **2011**, *2011*, 1–11.
113. Takeda, T.; Hosokawa, M.; Higuchi, K. Senescence-Accelerated Mouse (SAM): A novel murine model of senescence. *Exp. Gerontol.* **1997**, *32*, 105–109. [CrossRef]
114. Takeda, T.; Hosokawa, M.; Takeshita, S.; Irino, M.; Higuchi, K.; Matsushita, T.; Tomita, Y.; Yasuhira, K.; Hamamoto, H.; Shimizu, K.; et al. A new murine model of accelerated senescence. *Mech. Ageing Dev.* **1981**. [CrossRef]
115. Gurkar, A.U.; Niedernhofer, L.J. Comparison of mice with accelerated aging caused by distinct mechanisms. *Exp. Gerontol.* **2015**. [CrossRef]
116. Collins, S.; Martin, T.L.; Surwit, R.S.; Robidoux, J. Genetic vulnerability to diet-induced obesity in the C57BL/6J mouse: Physiological and molecular characteristics. *Physiol. Behav.* **2004**, *81*. [CrossRef] [PubMed]
117. Pearson, K.J.; Baur, J.A.; Lewis, K.N.; Peshkin, L.; Price, N.L.; Labinskyy, N.; Swindell, W.R.; Kamara, D.; Minor, R.K.; Perez, E.; et al. Resveratrol Delays Age-Related Deterioration and Mimics Transcriptional Aspects of Dietary Restriction without Extending Life Span. *Cell Metab.* **2008**, *8*. [CrossRef] [PubMed]
118. Dolinsky, V.W.; Dyck, J.R.B. Calorie restriction and resveratrol in cardiovascular health and disease. *Biochim. Biophys. Acta-Mol. Basis Dis.* **2011**, *1812*, 1477–1489. [CrossRef] [PubMed]
119. Sung, M.M.; Byrne, N.J.; Robertson, I.M.; Kim, T.T.; Samokhvalov, V.; Levasseur, J.; Soltys, C.L.; Fung, D.; Tyreman, N.; Denou, E.; et al. Resveratrol improves exercise performance and skeletal muscle oxidative capacity in heart failure. *Am. J. Physiol. Hear. Circ. Physiol.* **2017**, *312*. [CrossRef] [PubMed]

120. Rodríguez-Bies, E.; Tung, B.T.; Navas, P.; López-Lluch, G. Resveratrol primes the effects of physical activity in old mice. *Br. J. Nutr.* **2016**. [CrossRef]
121. Toniolo, L.; Formoso, L.; Torelli, L.; Crea, E.; Bergamo, A.; Sava, G.; Giacomello, E. Long-term resveratrol treatment improves the capillarization in the skeletal muscles of ageing C57BL/6J mice. *Int. J. Food Sci. Nutr.* **2021**. [CrossRef]
122. Toniolo, L.; Fusco, P.; Formoso, L.; Mazzi, A.; Canato, M.; Reggiani, C.; Giacomello, E. Resveratrol treatment reduces the appearance of tubular aggregates and improves the resistance to fatigue in aging mice skeletal muscles. *Exp. Gerontol.* **2018**. [CrossRef]
123. Lee, Y.E.; Kim, J.W.; Lee, E.M.; Ahn, Y.B.; Song, K.H.; Yoon, K.H.; Kim, H.W.; Park, C.W.; Li, G.; Liu, Z.; et al. Chronic Resveratrol Treatment Protects Pancreatic Islets against Oxidative Stress in db/db Mice. *PLoS ONE* **2012**, *7*. [CrossRef]
124. Bai, C.H.; Alizargar, J.; Peng, C.Y.; Wu, J.P. Combination of exercise training and resveratrol attenuates obese sarcopenia in skeletal muscle atrophy. *Chin. J. Physiol.* **2020**, *63*. [CrossRef]
125. Knutson, M.D.; Leeuwenburgh, C. Resveratrol and novel potent activators of SIRT1: Effects on aging and age-related diseases. *Nutr. Rev.* **2008**, *66*, 591–596. [CrossRef] [PubMed]
126. Vaughan, K.L.; Kaiser, T.; Peaden, R.; Anson, R.M.; De Cabo, R.; Mattison, J.A. Caloric restriction study design limitations in rodent and nonhuman primate studies. *Journals Gerontol. Ser. A Biol. Sci. Med. Sci.* **2018**, *73*. [CrossRef] [PubMed]
127. Phillips, K.A.; Bales, K.L.; Capitanio, J.P.; Conley, A.; Czoty, P.W.; 't Hart, B.A.; Hopkins, W.D.; Hu, S.L.; Miller, L.A.; Nader, M.A.; et al. Why primate models matter. *Am. J. Primatol.* **2014**, *76*, 801–827. [CrossRef]
128. Lane, M.A.; Ingram, D.K.; Roth, G.S. Calorie restriction in nonhuman primates: Effects on diabetes and cardiovascular disease risk. *Toxicol. Sci.* **1999**, *52*. [CrossRef]
129. Colman, R.J. Non-human primates as a model for aging. *Biochim. Biophys. Acta Mol. Basis Dis.* **2018**, *1864*, 2733–2741. [CrossRef]
130. Mattison, J.A.; Vaughan, K.L. An overview of nonhuman primates in aging research. *Exp. Gerontol.* **2017**, *94*. [CrossRef]
131. Colman, R.J.; Anderson, R.M. Nonhuman primate calorie restriction. *Antioxidants Redox Signal.* **2011**, *14*, 229–239. [CrossRef]
132. Roth, G.S.; Ingram, D.K.; Lane, M.A. Calorie restriction in primates: Will it work and how will we know? *J. Am. Geriatr. Soc.* **1999**, *47*. [CrossRef] [PubMed]
133. Kemnitz, J.W.; Weindruch, R.; Roecker, E.B.; Crawford, K.; Kaufman, P.L.; Ershler, W.B. Dietary restriction of adult male rhesus monkeys: Design, methodology, and preliminary findings from the first year of study. *J. Gerontol.* **1993**, *48*. [CrossRef]
134. Ingram, D.K.; Cutler, R.G.; Weindruch, R.; Renquist, D.M.; Knapka, J.J.; April, M.; Belcher, C.T.; Clark, M.A.; Hatcherson, C.D.; Marriott, B.M.; et al. Dietary restriction and aging: The initiation of a primate study. *J. Gerontol.* **1990**, *45*. [CrossRef] [PubMed]
135. Mattison, J.A.; Roth, G.S.; Mark Beasley, T.; Tilmont, E.M.; Handy, A.M.; Herbert, R.L.; Longo, D.L.; Allison, D.B.; Young, J.E.; Bryant, M.; et al. Impact of caloric restriction on health and survival in rhesus monkeys from the NIA study. *Nature* **2012**, *489*. [CrossRef] [PubMed]
136. Colman, R.J.; Anderson, R.M.; Johnson, S.C.; Kastman, E.K.; Kosmatka, K.J.; Beasley, T.M.; Allison, D.B.; Cruzen, C.; Simmons, H.A.; Kemnitz, J.W.; et al. Caloric restriction delays disease onset and mortality in rhesus monkeys. *Science* **2009**, *325*. [CrossRef] [PubMed]
137. Kemnitz, J.W.; Roecker, E.B.; Weindruch, R.; Elson, D.F.; Baum, S.T.; Bergman, R.N. Dietary restriction increases insulin sensitivity and lowers blood glucose in rhesus monkeys. *Am. J. Physiol. Endocrinol. Metab.* **1994**, *266*. [CrossRef]
138. Mattison, J.A.; Wang, M.; Bernier, M.; Zhang, J.; Park, S.S.; Maudsley, S.; An, S.S.; Santhanam, L.; Martin, B.; Faulkner, S.; et al. Resveratrol prevents high fat/sucrose diet-induced central arterial wall inflammation and stiffening in nonhuman primates. *Cell Metab.* **2014**, *20*. [CrossRef] [PubMed]
139. Marchal, J.; Blanc, S.; Epelbaum, J.; Aujard, F.; Pifferi, F. Effects of chronic calorie restriction or dietary resveratrol supplementation on insulin sensitivity markers in a primate, microcebus murinus. *PLoS ONE* **2012**, *7*. [CrossRef] [PubMed]
140. Dal-Pan, A.; Blanc, S.; Aujard, F. Resveratrol suppresses body mass gain in a seasonal non-human primate model of obesity. *BMC Physiol.* **2010**, *10*. [CrossRef]
141. Hyatt, J.P.K.; Nguyen, L.; Hall, A.E.; Huber, A.M.; Kocan, J.C.; Mattison, J.A.; de Cabo, R.; LaRocque, J.R.; Talmadge, R.J. Muscle-specific myosin heavy chain shifts in response to a long-term high fat/high sugar diet and resveratrol treatment in nonhuman primates. *Front. Physiol.* **2016**, *7*. [CrossRef]
142. Metter, E.J.; Lynch, N.; Conwit, R.; Lindle, R.; Tobin, J.; Hurley, B. Muscle quality and age: Cross-sectional and longitudinal comparisons. *J. Gerontol. Ser. A Biol. Sci. Med. Sci.* **1999**, *54*. [CrossRef]
143. Cava, E.; Fontana, L. Will calorie restriction work in humans? *Aging (Albany NY)* **2013**, *5*. [CrossRef]
144. Wahl, D.; Bernier, M.; Simpson, S.J.; De Cabo, R.; Le Couteur, D.G. Future directions of resveratrol research. *Nutr. Health Aging* **2018**, *4*, 287–290. [CrossRef]
145. Ingram, D.K.; Zhu, M.; Mamczarz, J.; Zou, S.; Lane, M.A.; Roth, G.S.; deCabo, R. Calorie restriction mimetics: An emerging research field. *Aging Cell* **2006**, *5*, 97–108. [CrossRef] [PubMed]
146. Kehler, D.S.; Theou, O.; Rockwood, K. Bed rest and accelerated aging in relation to the musculoskeletal and cardiovascular systems and frailty biomarkers: A review. *Exp. Gerontol.* **2019**, *124*, 110643. [CrossRef]
147. Florian, J.P.; Baisch, F.J.; Heer, M.; Pawelczyk, J.A. Caloric restriction diminishes the pressor response to static exercise. *Extrem. Physiol. Med.* **2016**, *5*. [CrossRef]
148. Florian, J.P.; Baisch, F.J.; Heer, M.; Pawelczyk, J.A. Caloric restriction decreases orthostatic tolerance independently from 6° head-down bedrest. *PLoS ONE* **2015**, *10*. [CrossRef] [PubMed]

149. Biolo, G.; Ciocchi, B.; Stulle, M.; Bosutti, A.; Barazzoni, R.; Zanetti, M.; Antonione, R.; Lebenstedt, M.; Platen, P.; Heer, M.; et al. Calorie restriction accelerates the catabolism of lean body mass during 2 wk of bed rest. *Am. J. Clin. Nutr.* **2007**, *86*. [CrossRef] [PubMed]
150. Bosutti, A.; Malaponte, G.; Zanetti, M.; Castellino, P.; Heer, M.; Guarnieri, G.; Biolo, G. Calorie restriction modulates inactivity-induced changes in the inflammatory markers C-reactive protein and pentraxin-3. *J. Clin. Endocrinol. Metab.* **2008**, *93*. [CrossRef]
151. Cohen, A.A. Aging across the tree of life: The importance of a comparative perspective for the use of animal models in aging. *Biochim. Biophys. Acta Mol. Basis Dis.* **2018**, *1864*, 2680–2689. [CrossRef] [PubMed]
152. Freund, A. Untangling Aging Using Dynamic, Organism-Level Phenotypic Networks. *Cell Syst.* **2019**, *8*, 172–181. [CrossRef]
153. Lacroix, S.; Lauria, M.; Scott-Boyer, M.P.; Marchetti, L.; Priami, C.; Caberlotto, L. Systems biology approaches to study the molecular effects of caloric restriction and polyphenols on aging processes. *Genes Nutr.* **2015**, *10*. [CrossRef] [PubMed]
154. Kepp, O.; Chen, G.; Carmona-Gutierrez, D.; Madeo, F.; Kroemer, G. A discovery platform for the identification of caloric restriction mimetics with broad health-improving effects. *Autophagy* **2020**, *16*, 188–189. [CrossRef] [PubMed]
155. Fortney, K.; Morgen, E.K.; Kotlyar, M.; Jurisica, I. In silico drug screen in mouse liver identifies candidate calorie restriction mimetics. *Rejuvenation Res.* **2012**, *15*. [CrossRef] [PubMed]
156. Zhao, G.; Guo, S.; Somel, M.; Khaitovich, P. Evolution of human longevity uncoupled from caloric restriction mechanisms. *PLoS ONE* **2014**, *9*. [CrossRef] [PubMed]

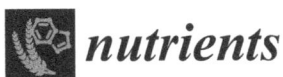

Review

Potential Role of Probiotics for Inflammaging: A Narrative Review

Nikolina Jukic Peladic [1], Giuseppina Dell'Aquila [2,*], Barbara Carrieri [2], Marcello Maggio [3,4], Antonio Cherubini [2,†] and Paolo Orlandoni [1,†]

1. Clinical Nutrition, IRCCS INRCA Ancona, 60127 Ancona, Italy; n.jukicpeladic@inrca.it (N.J.P.); p.orlandoni@inrca.it (P.O.)
2. Geriatria, Accettazione Geriatrica e Centro di Ricerca per L'invecchiamento, IRCCS INRCA, 60127 Ancona, Italy; carrieribarbara@gmail.com (B.C.); a.cherubini@inrca.it (A.C.)
3. Department of Medicine and Surgery, University Medical School of Parma, 43121 Parma, Italy; marcellogiuseppe.maggio@unipr.it
4. Geriatric Clinic Unit, University-Hospital of Parma, 43121 Parma, Italy
* Correspondence: g.dellaquila@inrca.it
† These authors contributed equally to this work.

Abstract: Background and aims: Inflammaging, a chronic, low-grade inflammation (LGI), is one of the mechanisms of adaptation of an organism to aging. Alterations in the composition of gut microbiota and gut permeability are among the main sources of LGI. They may be modulated by supplementation with live microorganisms, i.e. probiotics. This narrative review was performed with the aim to critically examine the current evidence from randomized clinical trials (RCTs) on the effects of probiotics on pro-inflammatory and anti-inflammatory cytokines and C-reactive protein (CRP) in healthy older subjects. Methodology: RCTs on the effects of probiotics on inflammatory parameters in subjects older than 65 years published in English and Italian from 1990 to October 2020 were searched in PubMed. Studies that were not RCTs, those using probiotics together with prebiotics (synbiotics), and studies performed in subjects with acute or chronic diseases were excluded. The findings of RCTs were reported in accordance with the Preferred Reporting Items for Systematic Reviews and Meta-Analyses (PRISMA). Results: A total of nine RCTs met the eligibility criteria and were included in this narrative review. Four articles reported that probiotic supplementation significantly affected inflammatory parameters, respectively, by reducing TGF-β1 concentrations, IL-8, increasing IL-5 and Il-10, and IFN-γ and IL-12. Conclusions: Based on this narrative review, probiotic supplementation showed a limited effect on inflammatory markers in healthy individuals older than 65 years. Besides being few, the studies analyzed have methodological limitations, are heterogeneous, and provide results which are incomparable.

Keywords: inflammaging; probiotics; aging; healthy older subjects

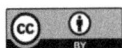

1. Introduction

Independent of variations in fertility, mortality, and migrations, the number of older subjects in the world will continue to increase [1]. Global population aging is the main demographic phenomenon of the twenty-first century, and it is going to have a profound impact on our societies. Therefore, achieving a more thorough understanding of aging and age-related chronic diseases has become the main objective of gerontological and geriatric research. According to accumulating scientific data, aging and age-related diseases share some common biological mechanisms [2,3]. One of the most relevant processes is chronic, low-grade inflammation (LGI), the so-called inflammaging. Pro-inflammatory factors increase in older subjects as a consequence of prolonged stimulation of innate immune system by different agents and of a progressive increase in senescent cells that produce inflammatory molecules [4]. Studies performed on centenarians found that in these long-lived subjects, the constant alert state in which the immune cells are kept by low-grade inflammation is also present, but it is counterbalanced by an effective anti-inflammatory response (anti-inflammaging) [5–7]. The imbalance between pro- and anti-inflammatory factors is one of mechanisms at the basis of several age-associated diseases such as type 2 diabetes, Alzheimer's disease, Parkinson's disease, cardiovascular diseases, osteoarthritis, sarcopenia, major depression, and many types of cancer [8–11]. On these premises, current research is pursuing the identification of factors that could modulate inflammation by acting on its sources, among which there are also alterations in the composition of gut microbiota and gut permeability [12]. Aging, diet, and pharmacotherapy can cause the imbalance of the structure and function of the gut intestinal microbial communities (dysbiosis), leading to increased gut permeability and a higher translocation of substances from gut lumen into the circulation, thus increasing chronic low-grade inflammation [13–18]. The improvement in gut microbiota composition by supplementation with live microorganisms—probiotics—has been advocated as a promising strategy to ameliorate dysbiosis [19,20]. It has been found that, when administered in adequate amounts, probiotics may enhance and/or modulate the functionality of existing microbial communities, influence systemic and mucosal immune function, and improve intestinal barrier function [21–24]. In a recent review, Mohr et al. evaluated the effect of probiotic supplementation on circulating immune and inflammatory markers in healthy adults (aged 18–65 years). The authors concluded that probiotics had a limited effect on immune and inflammatory markers [25]. The aim of the present narrative review was to critically examine the current evidence from randomized clinical trials concerning the ability of various probiotics to affect pro-inflammatory and anti-inflammatory cytokines as well as C-reactive protein (CRP) in healthy older subjects (aged older than 65 years).

2. Materials and Methods

A literature search was performed with the aim to identify and retrieve randomized clinical trials (RCTs) on the effects of probiotics on inflammatory parameters in older subjects (age older than 65 years). Studies that were not RCTs, those using probiotics together with prebiotics (symbiotics), and studies performed in subjects with acute or chronic diseases were excluded. The authors searched in PubMed studies published from 1990 to October 2020. Only articles published in the English and Italian languages were considered. The words used in the search were different combinations of the following terms: "probiotics", "probiotic supplements", "low grade inflammation", "systemic immunity", "immunosenescence", "immunomodulation", "immune response", "immune function", "cytokines", "older", "elderly", and "geriatrics". Reference lists of all included articles and of recent reviews and meta-analyses were searched for additional literature [26–28]. Two authors (NJP and GD) independently evaluated the list of articles and selected the most relevant of them, excluding duplicates. The senior authors (AC and PO) resolved disagreements. A total of 9 RCTs on the influence of probiotics on LGI were identified and analyzed by the authors. The characteristics and main results of each trial are summarized in Table 1. In the absence of specific guidelines for the presentation of the results of the narrative reviews, reporting of findings was conducted, as much as possible, in accordance with the Preferred Reporting Items for Systematic Reviews and Meta-Analyses (PRISMA) [29].

3. Results

Overall, nine randomized controlled trials assessing the efficacy of supplementation with probiotics on modulating the inflammatory parameters in healthy older subjects were identified. The studies identified were extremely heterogeneous with respect to study settings, methodologies used, and bacterial strains administered; thus, the main elements and findings of each study are presented in the text below separately, while the principal characteristics of each study are summarized in Table 1.

Table 1. Randomized controlled trials assessing the efficacy of supplementation with probiotics on modulating inflammatory parameters.

Reference	Study Sample (Age, n. of Subjects Enrolled)	Inclusion Criteria	Probiotic and Placebo Characteristics and Dosage	Duration of Administration and Follow Up	Effect on Inflammatory Markers
De Simone et al. (1992)	Institutionalized older. Mean age 76 years; $n = 25$ subjects enrolled ($n = 15$ intervention vs. $n = 10$ control).	Written informed consent from participants, older than 70 years, no overt diseases according to anamnesis and no fever, pain, cough, dysuria, modification of bowel habits etc.	2 capsules × 4 times/day, containing combined B. bifidum (10^9 CFU) and L. acidophilus (10^9 CFU) vs. 2 capsules × 4 times a day of placebo, containing saccarose and gelatin	4-week intervention	No effect on plasma TNF-α
Guillemart et al. (2010)	Free-living older. Mean age 76 years (range 69–95); $n = 1072$ subjects enrolled in the study.	Both gender, ≥70 years, free living, AGGIR score between 5 and 6, vaccination ag. influenza virus at least 14 d before inclusion, MMSA score ≥24, BMI between 17 and 25 kg/m², compliance with a dietary restriction (no fermented dairy products with other probiotics, yoghurts and medication containing probiotics, vitamins, minerals and other nutrients) during 2 previous weeks and throughout the study, written informed consent.	2 bottles, 100 g each/day, of fermented diary drink containing at least 10^{10} CFU/100 g of the probiotic strain L. Casei DN-114001 vs. non fermented diary drink	12-week intervention + 4-week follow up	No effect on blood CRP, IL-1, IL-6, IFNα, IFNβ, IFNγ, IL-8, IL-10, IL-12 or TNF-α < βγ
Mañé et al. (2011)	Institutionalized older. Mean age 70 years (range 65–84); $n = 60$ subjects enrolled; $n = 20$ placebo, $n = 20$ low dose probiotic, $n = 20$ high dose probiotic.	Written informed consent, older than 65 years.	20 g of powdered skilled milk containing 5×10^8 CFU/day of L. plantarum CECT7315/7316 (low probiotic dose) or 5×10^9 CFU/day of L. plantarum CECT7315/7316 (high probiotic dose) or 20 g of powdered skilled milk (placebo)	12-week intervention + 12 week follow up	TGF-β decreased (value not given) independent from probiotic dosage
Moro-García et al. (2013)	Free-living older. Mean age 70 years (range 65–90); $n = 61$ subjects enrolled.	Older than 65 years, treatment in determined Spanish health centers, written informed consent.	3 capsules/day containing at least 3×10^7 L. delbrueckii subs bulgaricus 8481 vs. placebo capsules with corn starch	24-week intervention	Plasma IL-8 decreased (value not given), hBD-2 increased (value not given); no effect on IFN-γ, IL-1β, IL-2, IL-4, IL-5, IL-6, IL-10, IL-12p70, TNF-α
Dong et al. (2013)	Free-living older. Range 55–74 years; $n = 30$ subjects enrolled; $n = 16$ intervention group vs. $n = 14$ placebo.	Age 55–80 years, BMI 19–30 kg/m², good general health, written informed consent.	2 × 65 mL/day probiotic drink containing 6.5 × 10^9 CFU/bottle L. casei Shirota vs. 130 mL of skimmed milk/day	4-week intervention + 4 weeks of washout	No effect on blood CRP, IL-10/Il-12 ratio increased for LPS-stimulated PBMC
Valentini et al. (2015)	Free living healthy older. Mean age 70.1 ± 3.9 years; $n = 69$ enrolled ($n = 35$ intervention vs. $n = 34$ controls).	Healthy individuals aged 65–85 years, BMI 22–30 kg/m² and Eastern Cooperative Oncology Group Performance Status (ECOG) 0–2, able to use a computer and with access to the internet, by themselves or with help.	RISTOMED personalized diet and 2 capsules/day containing 112 billion lyophilized bacteria consisting of B. infantis DSM 24737, B. longum DSM 24736, B. breve DSM 24732, L. acidophilus DSM 24735, L. delbrückii ssp. bulgaricus DSM 24734, L. paracasei DSM 24733, L. plantarum DSM 24730, and S. thermophilus DSM 24731 vs. RISTOMED personalized diet	8-week intervention (56 ± 2 days)	No effect on hsCRP
Nyangale et al. (2015)	Free-living older 65–80 years, $n = 17$ subjects probiotic period 1, placebo period 2, $n = 17$ subjects placebo period 1, probiotic period 2.	Age 65–80 years, written informed consent.	1 capsule/day containing 10^9 CFU of Bacillus coagulans GBI-36, 6086 (BC30) per day vs. capsules containing microcrystalline cellulose	2 treatment periods consisting of 4-week intervention separated by 3-week washout period	No effect on IL-10, TNF-α or CRP
Spaiser et al. (2015)	Free-living healthy older, range 65–80 years; $n = 42$ subjects enrolled.	Written informed consent	2 capsules/day containing a powder mixture of L. gasseri KS-13, B. bifidum G9-1, B. longum MM2 for a total of 3 × 10^9 viable cells / day vs. capsules containing potato starch and silicon dioxide	3-week intervention and 1-week post intervention for each period of crossover + 5-week washout between the intervention periods	IFN-γ increased after period 1 in intervention and after period 2 in both groups, IFN-γ increased after period 2 in both groups, IL-5 and IL-10 increased with probiotic interventions during both periods

Table 1. Cont.

Reference	Study Sample (Age, n. of Subjects Enrolled)	Inclusion Criteria	Probiotic and Placebo Characteristics and Dosage	Duration of Administration and Follow Up	Effect on Inflammatory Markers
Lee et al. (2017)	Free-living older. Mean age placebo 65.7 ± 0.56 years, probiotic, 65.7 ± 0.50 years; n = 200 subjects enrolled.	Non diabetic (fasting serum glucose concentration < 126 mg/dL), age > 60 years, white blood cell levels between $4 \times 10^3/\mu L$ and $10 \times 10^3/\mu L$, written informed consent.	1 bottle (120 mL)/day of yogurt containing L. paracasei (L. casei 431®) at 12.0×10^8 CFU/day, B. lactis (BB-12®) at 12.0×10^8 CFU/day and 0.0175% heat-treated L. plantarum (nF1) per day vs. 120 mL of milk	12-week intervention	IL-12 and IFN-γ increased, no effect on CRP

CFU, colony forming unit; TNF, tumor necrosis factor; CRP, C-reactive protein; hCRP, high sensitivity C-reactive protein; IL, interleukin; IFN, interferon; TGF, transforming growth factor; hBD-1, human beta defensin; C5a, complement factor 5a, LPS, lipolysaccharide; PBMC, peripheral blood mononuclear cell.

The first study meeting the inclusion criteria for this review dates back to the year 1992. In that year, De Simone et al. performed a randomized controlled trial to investigate the effect of supplementation of *Bifidobacterium bifidum* (BB) and *Lactobacillus acidophilus* (LA), contained in capsules of a specific, commercially available product, on the immune system in a group of older volunteers with no overt diseases [30]. The study was carried out on a small sample of subjects whose blood values were perfectly comparable at baseline. Fifteen subjects were assigned to the intervention group (mean age 76 ± 8 years), ten to the control group (mean age 75 ± 11 years). The authors found that a 4 week period treatment with BB and LA was not sufficient to affect TNF-α levels, which moved from 1.33 ± 5.1 pg/mL at T1 (enrollment) to 1.5 ± 5.1 pg/mg at T2 ($p > 0.05$) in the intervention group, and did not change at all in the placebo group (0 pg/mL both at T1 and T2). Almost 20 years later another group of authors led by Guillemard performed a multi-centric, double blind, controlled, parallel follow-up study in 1072 free living older volunteers to assess whether the consumption of a fermented dairy product containing *Lactobacillus casei* DN-114001 may affect the resistance of the older to common infection diseases [31]. Subjects from the intention to treat population, whose baseline characteristics were well balanced, were randomly assigned to consume 200 g/day of a sweetened, flavored fermented diary product containing at least 10^{10} CFU/100 g of *L. casei* DN-114001 (intervention) or the same quantity of placebo (sweetened, flavored, non-fermented diary product), for a consistently longer period than in the study by De Simone et al. After the three-month intervention, the authors performed blood examinations in a subpopulation of 125 subjects who were randomly selected from the overall sample (63 randomized to fermented product, 62 to control) to assess the changes in biological and immunological parameters following the intake of *L. casei* DN-114001. They tested numerous biological and immunological parameters—CRP, IL-1, IL-6, IFNα, IFNβ, IFNγ, TNF-α, IL-12, IL-10, and IL-8—but, despite a quite long period of administration, they found that none of the parameters tested were modified. A study with similar objectives was carried out a year later by Mañe et al. (2011). The authors investigated the effects of the administration of probiotics *Lactobacillus plantarum*, CECT 7315 and CECT 7316, mixed at a 1:1 ratio, on the systemic immunity in 60 institutionalized healthy older subjects. The parameters tested were TGF-β1, IL-1, and IL-10 [32]. In their study, the authors randomly assigned 20 subjects to high probiotic dose mixture (5×10^9 CFU/day), 20 subjects to low probiotic dose mixture (5×10^8 CFU/day), and 20 subjects to a placebo group. The three groups were perfectly comparable at baseline for their demographic and nutritional characteristics and for values of all routine laboratory parameters. Per protocol analyses was performed to assess the effect of supplementation on systemic inflammation after 12 weeks of administration and after 24 weeks (12 weeks of administration and 12 weeks follow up). The plasma concentrations of IL-1 and IL-10 were undetectable at every time point, but in this study, the authors found that the values of TGF-β1 concentrations were significantly affected and reduced after the administration of probiotics in both the low-dose and high-dose probiotic groups compared to placebo ($p < 0.05$ after 12 weeks, $p < 0.01$ after 24 weeks).

In 2013, Moro-Garcia et al. analyzed the effect of supplementation with *Lactobacillus delbrueckii* supsp. *bulgaricus* 8481 on the innate and acquired immune response of older subjects tested in 2013 in [33]. Within a multi-centric, double-blind, placebo-controlled study, twenty-eight subjects who were assigned to the intervention group consumed three capsules/day containing 3×10^7 *L. delbruecki supsp. bulgaricus* 8481 for 6 months, twenty-four subjects consumed a placebo. Subjects from the two groups were perfectly comparable at baseline relatively to demographic data and hematological, biochemical, and immunological values. The authors tested numerous cytokines with pro and anti-inflammatory activities, both at 3 and at 6 months - IFN-γ, IL-1β, IL-2, IL-4, IL-5, IL-6, IL-10, IL-12p70, TNF-α, and TNF-β - and found that the 6 month consumption of *L. delbruecki supsp. bulgaricus* 8481 affected only IL-8 levels, which were significantly reduced in the probiotic group. In the same year, Dong et al. performed a randomized placebo-controlled, single-blind crossover study in a small sample of 30 healthy older volunteers (55–74 years old) to investigate the effect of *Lactobacillus casei Shirota* (LcS) contained in a commercial fermented probiotic drink on their immune function [34]. Subjects were randomized to enter two intervention arms—probiotic (16 subjects) and placebo (14 subjects)—and during the 4 weeks of the intervention period consumed two bottles of the product or placebo daily. After a 4 week post-administration washout period, subjects were crossed over to the other treatment. The effect of product on inflammation was assessed by measuring CRP and C5a markers, IL-10 and Il-12. The only statistical significance was registered relatively to the marginal increase in the ratio of IL-10/Il-12 during the period of treatment with probiotics compared to placebo treatment. In 2015, Valentini et al. compared the changes in high-sensitivity C-reactive protein (hsCRP) levels in 31 subjects who were consuming the personalized diet (Arm A) and 31 subjects who were consuming personalized diet and a probiotic supplement (Arm B) within a multicenter open label, randomized, controlled trial: the RISTOMED project [35]. The probiotic used contained 112×10^9 of lyophilized bacteria *Bifidobacterium infantis* DSM 24737, *B. longum* DSM 24736, *B. breve* DSM 24732, *Lactobacillus acidophilus* DSM 24735, *L. delbrückii* ssp. *Bulgaricus* DSM 24734, *L. paracasei* DSM 24733, *L. plantarum* DSM 24730, and *Streptococcus thermophilus* DSM 24731. The authors enrolled subjects whose baseline values of hsCRP were slightly above the normal range ($\geq$3 mg/L), suggesting some level of low-grade inflammation (68% of subjects from Arm A and 71% of subjects from Arm B, without significant differences between the two groups), and found that the eight-week consumption of probiotics was not efficient in modulating the values of inflammatory parameters. In the same year, Nyangale et al. performed a randomized, double-blind, placebo-controlled crossover study to test the efficacy of a commercially available spore-forming probiotic capsule containing 10^9 CFUs of *Bacillus coagulans* GBI-36, 6086 (BC30) in improving immune and gut function in healthy older subjects [36]. Forty-two volunteers aged 65–80 years, free from chronic diseases, were randomly allocated into group A (intervention) or B (placebo). The study contained two treatment periods consisting of 4 weeks separated by a 3 week washout period. For the first 4 weeks, subjects from group A consumed BC30 and subjects from group B consumed the placebo (microcrystalline cellulose). After the washout period, the products were inverted. Samples of feces and blood were analyzed at the beginning of each treatment (probiotic and/or placebo) and after the 4 week treatment to assess the comparative effects. Parameters tested were IL-10, TNF-α, and CRP but neither Nyangale et al. found any significant difference in the values between the two groups after the administration of *Bacillus coagulans* GBI-36, 6086 (BC30). Spaiser et al. also performed in the same year a 13 week randomized, double-blind, placebo-controlled crossover study in a small sample of healthy older adults (mean age 70 + 1 years) to assess the effect of a specific probiotic mixture of *Lactobacillus gasseri* KS-13, *Bifidobacterium bifidum* G9-1, and *Bifidobacterium longum* MM2 on circulating CD4+ lymphocytes, cytokine production, and intestinal microbiota [37]. Thirty-four participants were randomly assigned to one of two intervention sequences. All participants completed a one-week pre-intervention phase followed by a 3 week intervention and a one-week post-intervention for each period of the crossover, with 5 weeks of washout between the intervention periods. To evaluate the effect of probiotics on inflammation, cytokine concentrations were assessed at baseline and after the first and second intervention. Spaiser et al. identified some important changes in the values of parameters tested. IFN-γ increased after probiotic intervention versus placebo in period 1 and that difference was maintained during the washout period. During period 2, IFN-γ production increased significantly with both interventions ($p < 0.0001$) without differences between them. IL-2 increased with both interventions in the period 2, IL-5 and Il-10 also increased, but only with probiotic interventions during both periods. Finally, the most recent study assessing the efficacy of supplementation with probiotics on modulating the inflammatory parameters in healthy older subjects dates back to the year 2017. In that year, Lee et al. conducted an open-label, placebo-controlled study to investigate the impact of the consumption of yogurt containing *Lactobacillus paracasei* ssp. *paracasei* (*L. paracasei*), *Bifidobacterium animalis* ssp. *lactis* (*B. lactis*) and heat-treated *Lactobacillus plantarum* (*L. plantarum*), on immune function in a large sample of healthy volunteers older than 60 years [38]. Volunteers were randomly assigned to the intervention group (100 subjects) which consumed one bottle (120 mL) of dairy yogurt a day, containing probiotics, or to the placebo group (100 subjects) which consumed the same volume of milk (placebo), once a day. TNF-α, IL-12, IFN-γ, and high sensitivity C-reactive protein (hsCRP) were perfectly comparable at baseline between the two groups. After 12 weeks of treatment, the intervention group registered an increase in IFN-γ concentrations compared to placebo ($p < 0.041$) and in IL-12 ($p < 0.01$). HsCRP values registered a statistically significant increase in the placebo group (from 0.80 mg/L ± 0.007 at t0 to 2.01 mg/L ± 0.71 after 12 weeks; $p < 0.05$) and did not change in the intervention group (1.24 ± 0.26 vs. 1.77 ± 0.50, $p > 0.05$).

4. Discussion

The results of some studies on healthy centenarians suggest that the formula of longevity lies in the balancing low-grade inflammation, which is the basis of a large number of age-related diseases, with anti-inflammatory factors. Evidence is also available on capability of microorganisms contained in probiotics in treating the causes of dysbiosis, which is one of the main causes that increases chronic low-grade inflammation [39]. In this study, we searched human RCTs investigating the impact of probiotics on inflammation by assessing the values of biomarkers of inflammation, i.e., cytokines and C-reactive protein. The results of our research show that, despite the high expectations for probiotics, the clinical trials carried out with the aim of analyzing their effect on inflammation were few, extremely heterogeneous, and provided conflicting results. Therefore, the available evidence is not sufficient to support the concept that probiotics might be a useful tool to counteract inflammaging in healthy older adults. The main reasons underlying this inconclusiveness of published research might be related, at least in part, to the methodological limitations and heterogeneity of the different studies. Concerning the first point, the majority of trials were performed in small samples, with the only exception of Guillemart et al. ($n = 125$ subjects) and Lee et al. ($n = 152$). The inclusion of older people in clinical trials may actually be challenging given that older subjects may have cognitive impairment, which prevents them from being able to consent to participate in the trial, a higher likelihood of becoming sick, or sensory or mobility limitations that reduce their ability to participate without the help of a family member or caregiver [40,41]. Still, the sample dimensions are of great importance for generalization of study results. Secondly, the studies were characterized by short follow-up periods. Given that there are no clear indications by the scientific community on what would be the right duration of administration of probiotics, it seems that the administration periods were defined almost arbitrarily within each study. They went from 4 up to 24 weeks. Moreover, a number of inaccuracies in study design and statistical analysis may be highlighted that also limit the generalizability and reproducibility of their results. In most studies the recruitment, randomization, and allocation concealment are poorly described. Protocols used to guarantee the adherence and compliance are also rarely specified while that would be extremely important, especially for those studies where products were consumed several times a day and/or for a very long time. For data analyses, the final, per protocol analyses was prevalently used, while the intention to treat is a gold standard for RCTs. RCTs analyzed are also heterogeneous relatively to outcome measures assessed, probiotic strains, and doses administered. Given that the authors assessed the effects of probiotics on variables which differed from study to study—different pro- and anti-inflammatory cytokines, tumor necrosis factor and transforming growth factor, CRP, or hsCRP—even the results of studies that found probiotics effective in modulating the LGI are incomparable. Mane et al. reported on the effect of probiotics on TGF-β, Moro-Garcia on IL-8, Dong et al. on the IL-10/IL-12 ratio, Spaiser et al. on IL-5 and IL-10, and Lee et al. on IL-12 and IFN-γ. In addition, it has to be considered that different laboratories use different reagents and measurement techniques, that have different levels of accuracy and are not always adequate to answer the study questions. This is the case, for instance for CRP which, if measured with methods other than high-sensitivity ones, cannot be used to demonstrate a decrease at a value lower than 0.5 g/L. Microorganisms administered in different studies were mostly from the *Lactobacillus* and *Bifidobacterium* genera, but species and strains were quite different just like the combinations of microorganisms for each product. Furthermore, in some studies, probiotics were administered added to dairy products—fermented and non-fermented, which naturally contain probiotics, and given that the health effect is carried by the entire product and not only by bacterial strains, the results of those studies may be affected by this consideration. Just like the duration of the administration period, the dosage of probiotic bacterium administered daily varied consistently among the studies (from 10^7 to 10^{10} CFU). The definition of a proper dosage is a problem of primary importance in this field given that it is not clearly defined by the scientific evidence and/or by the relevant institutions [42]. Very few countries have regulations on probiotics, which differ consistently among each other. The Italian Ministry of Health, for example, developed the guidelines on probiotics and prebiotics in 2018 and according to those guidelines, probiotics must contain no less than 10^9 live cells of at least one strain [43]. The evidence collected through in vitro studies and studies on rats and humans regarding the functioning of the microbiota and the ability of probiotics, in particular those containing Lactobacillus and Bifidobacterium species, to modulate its composition, is available and is very promising. The ability of probiotics to affect positively different pathologies in different age groups was also tested and partially proved, but the evidence collected so far on the efficacy of probiotics in modulating LGI in older subjects is poor and inconsistent. As already pointed out, performing studies in this population is particularly difficult and challenging but considering the importance of the topic and some positive results found in other age groups, research in this area should continue. Future studies should be performed in significantly larger samples, with study designs which will overcome the weaknesses evidenced in this review. Within those studies it would be particularly useful to collect additional evidence on how the modulation of biomarkers of inflammation following the intake of probiotics is associated with clinical outcomes. Finally, when interpreting the results of studies, it is very important to keep in mind that immunosenescence and inflammaging, which until recently were considered exclusively negative factors, in reality are a result of physiological remodeling during aging. It has been shown, indeed, that in centenarians the increased inflammatory state does not have negative effects on the organism, as it is balanced by the production of anti-inflammatory substances [44].

5. Conclusions

Based on this narrative review, probiotic supplementation showed a limited effect on inflammatory markers in healthy subjects older than 65 years. Besides being few, the studies analyzed have methodological limitations, were heterogeneous, and provided results that are incomparable.

Author Contributions: Conceptualization, A.C. and P.O.; methodology N.J.P., G.D. and B.C.; software, N.J.P. and G.D.; data search N.J.P., G.D., B.C. and M.M.; data curation, N.J.P. and G.D.; original draft preparation, N.J.P., G.D. and A.C.; writing N.J.P., G.D., M.M. and A.C.; supervision, A.C. and P.O.; project administration, P.O. and A.C. All authors have read and agreed to the published version of the manuscript.

Funding: This research received no external funding.

Institutional Review Board Statement: Not applicable.

Informed Consent Statement: Not applicable.

Data Availability Statement: The data presented in this study are available on request from the corresponding author.

Conflicts of Interest: The authors declare no conflict of interest.

References

1. Vollset, S.E.; Goren, E.; Yuan, C.-W.; Cao, J.; E Smith, A.; Hsiao, T.; Bisignano, C.; Azhar, G.S.; Castro, E.; Chalek, J.; et al. Fertility, mortality, migration, and population scenarios for 195 countries and territories from 2017 to 2100: A forecasting analysis for the Global Burden of Disease Study. *Lancet* **2020**, *396*, 1285–1306. [CrossRef]
2. Ferrucci, L.; Fabbri, E. Inflammageing: Chronic inflammation in ageing, cardiovascular disease, and frailty. *Nat. Rev. Cardiol.* **2018**, *15*, 505–522. [CrossRef]
3. Franceschi, C.; Garagnani, P.; Morsiani, C.; Conte, M.; Santoro, A.; Grignolio, A.; Monti, D.; Capri, M.; Salvioli, S. The Continuum of Aging and Age-Related Diseases: Common Mechanisms but Different Rates. *Front. Med.* **2018**, *5*, 61. [CrossRef] [PubMed]
4. Fulop, T.; Larbi, A.; Dupuis, G.; Le Page, A.; Frost, E.H.; Cohen, A.A.; Witkowski, J.M.; Franceschi, C. Immunosenescence and Inflamm-Aging As Two Sides of the Same Coin: Friends or Foes? *Front. Immunol.* **2018**, *8*, 1960. [CrossRef]
5. Franceschi, C.; Bonafè, M. Centenarians as a model for healthy aging. *Biochem. Soc. Trans.* **2003**, *31*, 457–461. [CrossRef] [PubMed]
6. Franceschi, C.; Capri, M.; Monti, D.; Giunta, S.; Olivieri, F.; Sevini, F.; Panourgia, M.P.; Invidia, L.; Celani, L.; Scurti, M.; et al. Inflammaging and anti-inflammaging: A systemic perspective on aging and longevity emerged from studies in humans. *Mech. Ageing Dev.* **2007**, *128*, 92–105. [CrossRef] [PubMed]
7. Minciullo, P.L.; Catalano, A.; Mandraffino, G.; Casciaro, M.; Crucitti, A.; Maltese, G.; Morabito, N.; Lasco, A.; Gangemi, S.; Basile, G. Inflammaging and Anti-Inflammaging: The Role of Cytokines in Extreme Longevity. *Arch. Immunol. Ther. Exp.* **2016**, *64*, 111–126. [CrossRef] [PubMed]
8. Calabrese, V.; Santoro, A.; Monti, D.; Crupi, R.; di Paola, R.; Latteri, S.; Cuzzocrea, S.; Zappia, M.; Giordano, J.; Calabrese, E.J.; et al. Aging and Parkinson's Disease: Inflammaging, neuroinflammation and biological remodeling as key factors in pathogenesis. *Free Radic. Biol. Med.* **2018**, *115*, 80–91. [CrossRef]
9. Franceschi, C.; Garagnani, P.; Parini, P.; Giuliani, C.; Santoro, A. Inflammaging: A new immune–metabolic viewpoint for age-related diseases. *Nat. Rev. Endocrinol.* **2018**, *14*, 576–590. [CrossRef]
10. Furman, D.; Campisi, J.; Verdin, E.; Carrera-Bastos, P.; Targ, S.; Franceschi, C.; Ferrucci, L.; Gilroy, D.W.; Fasano, A.; Miller, G.W.; et al. Chronic inflammation in the etiology of disease across the life span. *Nat. Med.* **2019**, *25*, 1822–1832. [CrossRef]
11. Franceschi, C.; Campisi, J. Chronic Inflammation (Inflammaging) and Its Potential Contribution to Age-Associated Diseases. *J. Gerontol. Ser. A Biol. Sci. Med. Sci.* **2014**, *69* (Suppl. S1), S4–S9. [CrossRef]
12. Arboleya, S.; Watkins, C.; Stanton, C.; Ross, R.P. Gut Bifidobacteria Populations in Human Health and Aging. *Front. Microbiol.* **2016**, *7*, 1204. [CrossRef] [PubMed]
13. Minihane, A.M.; Vinoy, S.; Russell, W.R.; Baka, A.; Roche, H.M.; Tuohy, K.M.; Teeling, J.L.; Blaak, E.E.; Fenech, M.; Vauzour, D.; et al. Low-grade inflammation, diet composition and health: Current research evidence and its translation. *Br. J. Nutr.* **2015**, *114*, 999–1012. [CrossRef]
14. Biagi, E.; Nylund, L.; Candela, M.; Ostan, R.; Bucci, L.; Pini, E.; Nikkïla, J.; Monti, D.; Satokari, R.; Franceschi, C.; et al. Through Ageing, and Beyond: Gut Microbiota and Inflammatory Status in Seniors and Centenarians. *PLoS ONE* **2010**, *5*, e10667. [CrossRef]
15. O'Toole, P.W.; Jeffery, I. Gut microbiota and aging. *Science* **2015**, *350*, 1214–1215. [CrossRef] [PubMed]
16. Bernardi, S.; Del Bo', C.; Marino, M.; Gargari, G.; Cherubini, A.; Andrés-Lacueva, C.; Liberona, N.H.; Peron, G.; González-Domínguez, R.; Kroon, P.A.; et al. Polyphenols and Intestinal Permeability: Rationale and Future Perspectives. *J. Agric. Food Chem.* **2019**, *68*, 1816–1829. [CrossRef] [PubMed]
17. Del Bo', C.; Bernardi, S.; Cherubini, A.; Porrini, M.; Gargari, G.; Hidalgo-Liberona, N.; González-Domínguez, R.; Zamora-Ros, R.; Peron, G.; Marino, M.; et al. A polyphenol-rich dietary pattern improves intestinal permeability, evaluated as serum zonulin levels, in older subjects: The MaPLE randomised controlled trial. *Clin. Nutr.* **2021**, *40*, 3006–3018. [CrossRef] [PubMed]
18. Carding, S.; Verbeke, K.; Vipond, D.T.; Corfe, B.M.; Owen, L.J. Dysbiosis of the gut microbiota in disease. *Microb. Ecol. Health Dis.* **2015**, *26*, 26191. [CrossRef]
19. Binda, S.; Hill, C.; Johansen, E.; Obis, D.; Pot, B.; Sanders, M.E.; Tremblay, A.; Ouwehand, A.C. Criteria to Qualify Microorganisms as "Probiotic" in Foods and Dietary Supplements. *Front. Microbiol.* **2020**, *11*, 1662. [CrossRef]

20. Kim, S.-K.; Guevarra, R.B.; Kim, Y.-T.; Kwon, J.; Kim, H.; Cho, J.H.; Kim, H.B.; Lee, J.-H. Role of Probiotics in Human Gut Microbiome-Associated Diseases. *J. Microbiol. Biotechnol.* **2019**, *29*, 1335–1340. [CrossRef]
21. Sonnenburg, J.L.; Fischbach, M.A. Community Health Care: Therapeutic Opportunities in the Human Microbiome. *Sci. Transl. Med.* **2011**, *3*, 78ps12. [CrossRef]
22. Hemarajata, P.; Versalovic, J. Effects of probiotics on gut microbiota: Mechanisms of intestinal immunomodulation and neuromodulation. *Ther. Adv. Gastroenterol.* **2013**, *6*, 39–51. [CrossRef] [PubMed]
23. Madsen, K.L. Enhancement of Epithelial Barrier Function by Probiotics. *J. Epithel. Biol. Pharmacol.* **2012**, *5*, 55–59. [CrossRef]
24. Preidis, G.; Versalovic, J. Targeting the Human Microbiome With Antibiotics, Probiotics, and Prebiotics: Gastroenterology Enters the Metagenomics Era. *Gastroenterology* **2009**, *136*, 2015–2031. [CrossRef] [PubMed]
25. Mohr, A.E.; Basile, A.; Crawford, M.S.; Sweazea, K.L.; Carpenter, K.C. Probiotic Supplementation Has a Limited Effect on Circulating Immune and Inflammatory Markers in Healthy Adults: A Systematic Review of Randomized Controlled Trials. *J. Acad. Nutr. Diet.* **2019**, *120*, 548–564. [CrossRef]
26. Calder, P.; Bosco, N.; Bourdet-Sicard, R.; Capuron, L.; Delzenne, N.; Doré, J.; Franceschi, C.; Lehtinen, M.J.; Recker, T.; Salvioli, S.; et al. Health relevance of the modification of low grade inflammation in ageing (inflammageing) and the role of nutrition. *Ageing Res. Rev.* **2017**, *40*, 95–119. [CrossRef]
27. Hutchinson, A.; Tingö, L.; Brummer, R. The Potential Effects of Probiotics and ω-3 Fatty Acids on Chronic Low-Grade Inflammation. *Nutrients* **2020**, *12*, 2402. [CrossRef]
28. Gui, Q.; Wang, A.; Zhao, X.; Huang, S.; Tan, Z.; Xiao, C.; Yang, Y. Effects of probiotic supplementation on natural killer cell function in healthy elderly individuals: A meta-analysis of randomized controlled trials. *Eur. J. Clin. Nutr.* **2020**, *74*, 1630–1637. [CrossRef]
29. Page, M.J.; McKenzie, J.E.; Bossuyt, P.M.; Boutron, I.; Hoffmann, T.C.; Mulrow, C.D.; Shamseer, L.; Tetzlaff, J.M.; A Akl, E.; Brennan, S.E.; et al. The PRISMA 2020 statement: An updated guideline for reporting systematic reviews. *BMJ* **2021**, *372*, n71. [CrossRef]
30. De Simone, C.; Ciardi, A.; Grassi, A.; Gardini, S.L.; Tzantzoglou, S.; Trinchieri, V.; Moretti, S.; Jirillo, E. Effect of Bifido bacterium bifidum and Lactobacillus acidophilus on gut mucosa and peripheral blood B lymphocytes. *Immunopharmacol. Immunotoxicol.* **1992**, *14*, 331–340. [CrossRef]
31. Guillemard, E.; Tondu, F.; Lacoin, F.; Schrezenmeir, J. Consumption of a fermented dairy product containing the probiotic Lactobacillus casei DN-114001 reduces the duration of respiratory infections in the elderly in a randomised controlled trial. *Br. J. Nutr.* **2009**, *103*, 58–68. [CrossRef] [PubMed]
32. Mañé, J.; Pedrosa, E.; Lorén, V.; A Gassull, M.; Espadaler, J.; Cuñé, J.; Audivert, S.; A Bonachera, M.; Cabré, E. A mixture of Lactobacillus plantarum CECT 7315 and CECT 7316 enhances systemic immunity in elderly subjects. A dose-response, double-blind, placebo-controlled, randomized pilot trial. *Nutr. Hosp.* **2011**, *26*, 228–235. [PubMed]
33. Moro-García, M.A.; Alonso-Arias, R.; Baltadjieva, M.; Benítez, C.F.; Barrial, M.A.F.; Ruisánchez, E.D.; Santos, R.A.; Sánchez, M.Á.; Miján, J.S.; López-Larrea, C. Oral supplementation with Lactobacillus delbrueckii subsp. bulgaricus 8481 enhances systemic immunity in elderly subjects. *AGE* **2013**, *35*, 1311–1326. [CrossRef] [PubMed]
34. Dong, H.; Rowland, I.; Thomas, L.; Yaqoob, P. Immunomodulatory effects of a probiotic drink containing Lactobacillus casei Shirota in healthy older volunteers. *Eur. J. Nutr.* **2013**, *52*, 1853–1863. [CrossRef]
35. Valentini, L.; Pinto, A.; Bourdel-Marchasson, I.; Ostan, R.; Brigidi, P.; Turroni, S.; Hrelia, S.; Hrelia, P.; Bereswill, S.; Fischer, A.; et al. Impact of personalized diet and probiotic supplementation on inflammation, nutritional parameters and intestinal microbiota—The "RISTOMED project": Randomized controlled trial in healthy older people. *Clin. Nutr.* **2015**, *34*, 593–602. [CrossRef]
36. Nyangale, E.P.; Farmer, S.; Cash, H.A.; Keller, D.; Chernoff, D.; Gibson, G.R. Bacillus coagulans GBI-30, 6086 Modulates Faecalibacterium prausnitzii in Older Men and Women. *J. Nutr.* **2015**, *145*, 1446–1452. [CrossRef]
37. Spaiser, S.J.; Culpepper, T.; Nieves, C.; Ukhanova, M.; Mai, V.; Percival, S.S.; Christman, M.C.; Langkamp-Henken, B. Lactobacillus gasseri KS-13, Bifidobacterium bifidum G9-1, and Bifidobacterium longum MM-2 Ingestion Induces a Less Inflammatory Cytokine Profile and a Potentially Beneficial Shift in Gut Microbiota in Older Adults: A Randomized, Double-Blind, Placebo-Controlled, Crossover Study. *J. Am. Coll. Nutr.* **2015**, *34*, 459–469. [CrossRef]
38. Lee, A.; Lee, Y.J.; Yoo, H.J.; Kim, M.; Chang, Y.; Lee, D.S.; Lee, J.H. Consumption of Dairy Yogurt Containing *Lactobacillus paracasei* ssp. paracasei, *Bifidobacterium animalis* ssp. lactis and Heat-Treated Lactobacillus plantarum Improves Immune Function Including Natural Killer Cell Activity. *Nutrients* **2017**, *9*, 558. [CrossRef]
39. Tilg, H.; Zmora, N.; Adolph, T.E.; Elinav, E. The intestinal microbiota fuelling metabolic inflammation. *Nat. Rev. Immunol.* **2020**, *20*, 40–54. [CrossRef]
40. Pérez-Zepeda, M.U.; Cherubini, A.; García-Peña, C.; Zengarini, E.; Gutiérrez-Robledo, L.M. Clinical Trials on Aging Research. In *Aging Research—Methodological Issues*; Springer Science and Business Media LLC: Berlin/Heidelberg, Germany, 2018; pp. 115–127.
41. Cherubini, A.; Gasperini, B. How to increase the participation of older subjects in research: Good practices and more evidence are needed! *Age Ageing* **2017**, *46*, 878–881. [CrossRef]
42. Ouwehand, A.C. A review of dose-responses of probiotics in human studies. *Benef. Microbes* **2017**, *8*, 143–151. [CrossRef] [PubMed]

43. Ministero Della Salute. Direzione Generale per L'igiene e la Sicurezza Degli Alimenti e la Nutrizione-Ufficio 4. In *Linee Guida su Probiotici e Prebiotici, Roma, Revisione Marzo*; 2018. Available online: https://www.salute.gov.it/imgs/C_17_pubblicazioni_1016_allegato.pdf (accessed on 23 August 2021).
44. Foligne, B.; Zoumpopoulou, G.; Dewulf, J.; Ben Younes, A.; Chareyre, F.; Sirard, J.-C.; Pot, B.; Grangette, C. A Key Role of Dendritic Cells in Probiotic Functionality. *PLoS ONE* **2007**, *2*, e313. [CrossRef] [PubMed]

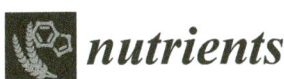

Article

Dietary Pattern Accompanied with a High Food Variety Score Is Negatively Associated with Frailty in Older Adults

Won Jang [1], Yoonjin Shin [1] and Yangha Kim [1,2,*]

[1] Department of Nutritional Science and Food Management, Ewha Womans University, Seoul 03760, Korea; jangwon1011@naver.com (W.J.); yjin19@hotmail.com (Y.S.)
[2] Graduate Program in System Health Science and Engineering, Ewha Womans Universty, Seoul 03760, Korea
* Correspondence: yhmoon@ewha.ac.kr; Tel.: +82-2-3277-3101

Abstract: Proper nutrition is a modifiable factor in preventing frailty. This study was conducted to identify the association between dietary patterns and frailty in the older adult population. The cross-sectional analysis was performed on 4632 subjects aged ≥65 years enrolled in the Korea National Health and Nutrition Examination Survey from 2014–2018. Food variety score (FVS) was defined as the number of foods items consumed over a day. Three dietary patterns were identified using factor analysis: "white rice and salted vegetables," "vegetables, oils, and fish," and "noodles and meat." The higher "white rice and salted vegetables" pattern score was related to significantly lower FVS, whereas higher "vegetables, oils, and fish" and "noodles and meat" pattern scores were associated with a higher FVS. Participants with higher FVS showed a low risk of frailty (odds ratio (OR) (95% confidence interval, CI) = 0.44 (0.31–0.61), p-trend = 0.0001) than those with lower FVS. Moreover, the "vegetables, oils, and fish" pattern score was significantly associated with a low risk of frailty (OR (95% CI) = 0.55 (0.40–0.75), p-trend = 0.0002). These results suggested that consuming a dietary pattern based on vegetables, oils, and fish with high FVS might ameliorate frailty in older adults.

Keywords: frailty; dietary pattern; food variety score

Citation: Jang, W.; Shin, Y.; Kim, Y. Dietary Pattern Accompanied with a High Food Variety Score Is Negatively Associated with Frailty in Older Adults. *Nutrients* 2021, *13*, 3164. https://doi.org/10.3390/nu13093164

Academic Editors: Emiliana Giacomello and Luana Toniolo

Received: 13 August 2021
Accepted: 7 September 2021
Published: 10 September 2021

Publisher's Note: MDPI stays neutral with regard to jurisdictional claims in published maps and institutional affiliations.

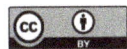

Copyright: © 2021 by the authors. Licensee MDPI, Basel, Switzerland. This article is an open access article distributed under the terms and conditions of the Creative Commons Attribution (CC BY) license (https://creativecommons.org/licenses/by/4.0/).

1. Introduction

Given the rapid aging of the world's population, the prevention of frailty is becoming more important than ever. Frailty is a geriatric syndrome characterized by a reduced physical and psychological function and a decline in the ability to maintain homeostasis [1]. Frailty in older adults is a risk factor for falls, morbidity, disability, and even mortality [2] and is often viewed as a major challenge for medical and health care services [3]. Thus, preventing frailty can help reduce medical and related costs and address the challenges of successful aging.

Nutritional status is considered one of the modifiable risk factors for frailty. It is well known that inadequate protein and micronutrients can contribute to frailty [4]. However, understanding the nutrition–health interface requires shifting the focus from individual nutrients toward food-based approaches. In this regard, investigating the impact of dietary patterns on frailty may be more useful than analyzing the effects of a single nutrient in establishing a frailty prevention strategy. In Western countries, adherence to a Mediterranean diet has been associated with a reduced incidence of frailty among older people [4–6], but whether there is an association between frailty and dietary patterns other than the Mediterranean diet is still unknown [7]. It is difficult to compare the results of dietary patterns between populations because dietary patterns are strongly related to the study population's diet.

Therefore, it would be interesting to understand the relationship between dietary patterns and frailty and the impact of dietary quality to identify the most appropriate diets for decreasing frailty prevalence. The food variety score (FVS) is a simple count of food items and has been proven to be a useful indicator of the nutritional adequacy of the diet [8]. Consuming a wide variety of food groups increases the chances of providing the various nutrients and phytochemicals needed for optimal health, which could reduce the risk of frailty [9]. In contrast, inadequate nutrient intake that accompanies poor dietary variety causes oxidative stress [10] and inflammatory reactions [11], contributing to the risk of frailty. In some studies, frailty decreased as a result of high overall diet quality [12], characterized by increased consumption of fruits and vegetables [13] and optimal intakes of antioxidant nutrients [14].

Dietary variation is important for health maintenance and disease prevention in older adults. Many prior studies have reported the association between healthy dietary patterns and frailty, but most of them have been focused on Western populations [5–7]. Very few studies have been conducted with Asian population [8,10,15], and the results are not consistent. Thus, in-depth research on the association between dietary factors and frailty is highly needed. Therefore, this study aimed to identify dietary patterns related to frailty in a larger sample of older Korean adults. Moreover, we investigate not only dietary patterns but also dietary variety that is comprehensively available in various food culture as an indicator of dietary factors related to frailty.

2. Materials and Methods

2.1. Data Collection

This study used the data from the 2014–2018 Korea National Health and Nutrition Examination Survey (KNHANES), which included KNHANES VI (2013–2015) and KNHANES VII (2016–2018), conducted by the Korea Centers for Disease Control and Prevention (KCDC). The KNHANES is an ongoing cross-sectional survey designed to use complex, multistage, stratified, and probability cluster sampling to obtain nationally representative estimates [16]. The investigation included a health questionnaire, health examination, and nutrition surveys. The Institutional Review Board (IRB) of the KCDC approved this study (2013-07CON-03-4C, 2013-12EXP-03-5C, 2018-01-03-P-A). Detailed information about the data and survey is available on the KNHANES website (http://knhanes.cdc.go.kr accessed on 9 September 2021).

2.2. Subjects

The participants in the 2014–2018 survey totaled 39,199. The present analysis was limited to adults aged 65 or older who completed the survey (n = 7166). Participants with incomplete data on frailty classification were excluded (n = 1229). Those with missing dietary intake data, having energy intakes below 500 kcal and over 5000 kcal, and unusual intake on the previous day were also excluded (n = 1232). In addition, we excluded subjects with missing data on other covariates, such as sociodemographic information, smoking, and alcohol consumption (n = 73). Thus, 4632 subjects were included in the study.

2.3. Frailty Classification

Frailty was measured using a slight modification of the five criteria for the frailty phenotype developed by Fried et al. [17]: (1) unintentional weight loss (self-reported unintentional weight loss in the last year of >3 kg) [18], (2) exhaustion (if self-perception of stress is extremely high, it is considered to be emotional/physical exhaustion) [19], (3) weakness (handgrip strength <26 kg for men and <18 kg for women based on the Asian Working Group criteria for sarcopenia) [20], (4) walking difficulties (if the subjects responded to the mobility question of the European Quality of Life 5-Dimensions (EuroQoL-5D) questionnaire that walking was difficult, it was classified as walking difficulties) [21], and (5) low physical activity (physical activity was measured using the Global Physical Activity Questionnaire (GPAQ) developed by the World Health Organization (WHO) and was classified as low physical activity when recreational activity was <2 h per week) [22]. Participants were classified as robust if they fulfilled none of the criteria, pre-frail if they fulfilled one or two criteria, and frail if they fulfilled three or more criteria.

2.4. Dietary Assessment

Dietary intake information was obtained from a nutrition survey of the KNHANES using the 24 h recall method [16]. Skilled and well-trained dietary interviewers conducted the 24 h recall by face-to-face interview. The participants reported all the food and beverage that was consumed the previous day, including food name, types of ingredients, and amount of food intake per meal. For the analysis of dietary patterns, food items from the 24 h recall data were integrated into 18 food groups based on similarities. The grains and grain products group accounted for nearly half of the daily energy intake, so this food group was further divided into white rice, grains, noodles and dumplings, flour, bread and rice cakes, and pizza and hamburgers. Salted vegetables, including kimchi, were separated from other raw vegetables because, as a traditional fermented food in Korea, it has a high frequency of consumption and contains high sodium. Beverages were divided into alcohol, coffee and tea, and sugar-sweetened beverages. Our final analysis included a total of 24 food groups. The difference in weight between solid and liquid foods was corrected by representing the food groups as a percentage of energy.

To assess diet quality, the overall FVS was adopted. FVS was calculated by the simple count of the number of food items consumed by each subject during the last 24 h [23]. If the main ingredients were the same, they were classified as the same food items even if prepared by different cooking methods. The amount of food consumed and the frequency of consumption were not taken into account.

2.5. Assessment of Other Variables

Information on demographic and socioeconomic characteristics, including age, body mass index (BMI; kg/m^2), living status (living alone, living with others), residential area (urban, rural), education level ($\leq$elementary school, $\geq$middle school), household income level ($\leq$the lowest quartile, $\geq$middle–low), smoking status (current smoker or non-current smoker), high-risk alcohol consumption (yes or no), and comorbidity (whether subjects suffered from three or more simultaneous diseases diagnosed by a doctor), was obtained using a general questionnaire and health interview questionnaire.

2.6. Statistical Analysis

All statistical analyses were performed using SAS software version 9.4 (SAS Institute, Inc., Cary, NC, USA). Due to the complex sampling design of the KNHANES study, sample weights, stratifying variables (*k* strata), and primary sampling units were included in our analysis. The dietary pattern was derived using factor analysis with the FACTOR procedure and VARIMAX rotation function that maintains uncorrelated factors and increases interpretability. Eigenvalues, scree plot, and interpretability ability were considered in deciding the number of factors. Significance was given to the food group whose factor load value exceeded 0.25 or −0.25. Scores of the individual dietary patterns of the whole population were categorized into tertiles and used for comparison of FVS, nutrient intake, and other general characteristics. Differences in the distribution of characteristics between tertiles of dietary pattern scores were analyzed using the SURVEY FREQ procedure for categorical variables or the SURVEY MEAN procedure for continuous variables. Significant differences between tertiles of dietary patterns were determined using the χ^2 test or a general linear model (Scheffe's test of multiple comparisons). Multinomial SURVEYLOGISTIC analysis was performed to estimate the odds ratios (ORs) and 95% confidence intervals (CIs) for frailty (robust vs. pre-frail vs. frail, with robust as the reference) across tertiles of dietary pattern scores and FVS. Adjustments were performed for potential confounding variables, selected based on the prior knowledge from the scientific literature and whether they are related to the independent and dependent variables. Confounders included age, gender, BMI, residential area, family income, education level, smoking status, high-risk alcohol consumption, total energy intake, and comorbidity and there was no significant multicollinearity among these variables. All reported probability tests were two-sided, with a *p*-value < 0.05 considered statistically significant.

3. Results

3.1. General Characteristics of Study Subjects

The general characteristics of the study population are presented in Table 1. Of the 2184 males (48.8%) and 2448 females (51.2%) included in the study, 17.5% lived alone, 21.6% were rural residents, and 78.4% were urban residents. The average age of the study subjects was 72.5 ± 0.1 years. More than half of the subjects had education levels below elementary school (56.2%), and 44.9% had income levels below the lowest quartile. Comorbidity, defined as having more than three diseases simultaneously, was seen in 19.7% of the subjects.

Table 1. General characteristics of the study subjects.

Variables	Total (n = 4632)
Age (years, mean ± SE)	72.5 ± 0.1
Age range	
65–69	1538 (33.6)
70–79	2411 (51.9)
≥80	683 (14.5)
Gender	
Male	2184 (48.8)
Female	2448 (51.2)
Living status	
Living alone	990 (17.5)
Living with others	3642 (82.5)
Residence	
Rural	1300 (21.6)
Urban	3332 (78.4)
Education	
≤Elementary school	2708 (56.2)
≥Middle school	1924 (43.8)
Family income	
≤The lowest quartile	2164 (44.9)
≥Middle–low	2468 (55.1)
Current smoking status	
Current smoker	439 (9.6)
Non-current smoker	4193 (90.4)
High-risk alcohol consumption	
Yes	187 (4.1)
No	4444 (95.9)
Body mass index (kg/m^2, mean ± SE)	24.0 ± 0.1
Body mass index range	
<18.5	120 (2.6)
18.5–24.9	2833 (61.7)
≥25.0	1679 (35.7)
Comorbidity	
Yes	925 (19.7)
No	3707 (80.3)

Values are presented as mean ± standard error (SE) or n (%).

3.2. Dietary Patterns in the Study Population

Table 2 gives the three dietary patterns identified by factor analysis. Pattern 1 showed the highest factor loadings for white rice and kimchi and salted vegetables and negative loadings for flour, pizza, snacks, and fruits. We named Pattern 1 "white rice and salted vegetables." Pattern 2 had the highest factor loadings for non-salted vegetables, seasonings, oils, and fish and shellfish, so we described Pattern 2 as "vegetables, oils, and fish." Pattern 3 had high factor loadings for noodles and dumplings, meat, alcohol, and coffee and tea, and negative loadings for fruits and non-salted vegetables. We named Pattern 3 "noodles and meat." These three patterns accounted for 19.5% of the total variance in food intakes.

Table 2. Factor loading matrix for the three dietary patterns of older Korean adults.

Food Group	Pattern 1	Pattern 2	Pattern 3
	White Rice and Kimchi	Vegetables, Oils, and Fish	Noodles and Meat
White rice	0.83902		−0.27383
Grains			
Noodles and dumplings	−0.2601		0.54391
Flour, bread, and rice cakes	−0.41547		
Hamburgers, pizza, and snacks			
Potatoes	−0.30472		
Sweets			
Beans			
Nuts	−0.3071		−0.33496
Non-salted vegetables		0.61885	
Kimchi and salted vegetables	0.32283		
Mushrooms			
Fruits	−0.40244		−0.34568
Meats			0.42253
Processed meats			
Eggs	−0.32273		
Fish and shellfish		0.47125	
Seaweed			
Milk and dairy products	−0.38096		
Oils		0.51915	
Alcohol		0.27234	0.38311
Coffee and tea			0.37365
Sugar-sweetened beverages			
Seasonings		0.53593	
Variance explained (%)	8.15%	5.85%	5.53%

Factor loading values < |0.25| were excluded for simplicity. The patterns were derived based on the energy contribution ratio of food groups by factor analysis.

3.3. Comparison of General Characteristics by Tertiles of Dietary Pattern Scores

The subjects' general characteristics across the tertiles of the dietary pattern scores are summarized in Table 3. Subjects in the highest tertile of the "white rice and salted vegetables" dietary pattern tended to be male, older, rural residents of high-risk alcohol consumption with a lower education level and lower family income level than those in the lowest tertile. Meanwhile, subjects in the highest tertile of the "vegetables, oils, and fish" pattern tended to be younger, living alone, urban residents, and highly educated, with higher family income and lower comorbidity than their lowest tertile counterparts. Lastly, the highest tertile of the "noodles and meat" pattern was associated with subjects with high-risk alcohol consumption that were less educated and more likely to smoke than those in the lowest tertile of this dietary pattern (Table 3).

Table 3. General characteristics across tertiles of dietary pattern scores.

Variables	Pattern 1 White Rice and Salted Vegetables				Pattern 2 Vegetables, Oils, and Fish				Pattern 3 Noodles and Meat			
	Tertile 1 (Lowest) (n = 1544)	Tertile 2 (Middle) (n = 1544)	Tertile 3 (Highest) (n = 1544)	p-Value	Tertile 1 (Lowest) (n = 1544)	Tertile 2 (Middle) (n = 1544)	Tertile 3 (Highest) (n = 1544)	p-Value	Tertile 1 (Lowest) (n = 1544)	Tertile 2 (Middle) (n = 1544)	Tertile 3 (Highest) (n = 1544)	p-Value
Age (years, mean ± SE)	71.6 ± 0.2	72.5 ± 0.2	73.6 ± 0.1	<0.0001	73.1 ± 0.1	72.7 ± 0.2	71.8 ± 0.2	<0.0001	72.2 ± 0.2	72.9 ± 0.1	72.5 ± 0.2	0.0037
Age range (years)				<0.0001				<0.0001				0.0448
65–69	622 (41.3)	518 (33.6)	398 (25.6)		415 (27.9)	516 (32.7)	607 (39.9)		548 (36.3)	487 (30.8)	503 (33.7)	
70–79	745 (47.1)	811 (53.1)	855 (55.7)		850 (55.4)	807 (52.3)	754 (48.2)		796 (51.0)	809 (53.8)	806 (50.9)	
80≤	177 (11.5)	215 (13.3)	291 (18.7)		279 (16.7)	221 (15.0)	183 (11.9)		200 (12.7)	248 (15.4)	235 (15.4)	
Gender (male, %)	612 (41.2)	782 (52.5)	790 (52.8)	<0.0001	630 (41.0)	736 (50.4)	818 (54.7)	<0.0001	581 (39.6)	710 (47.5)	893 (59.2)	<0.0001
Living status (living alone, %)	317 (17.3)	314 (16.7)	359 (18.5)	0.4475	414 (21.9)	276 (14.8)	300 (16.1)	<0.0001	343 (18.0)	326 (17.3)	321 (17.3)	0.8580
Residence (rural, %)	302 (15.0)	442 (21.4)	556 (28.7)	<0.0001	495 (24.2)	419 (21.7)	386 (19.2)	0.0147	393 (19.8)	453 (22.4)	454 (22.7)	0.1996
Education (≤elementary school, %)	707 (43.5)	910 (56.5)	1091 (68.9)	<0.0001	1042 (64.9)	896 (57.1)	770 (46.8)	<0.0001	895 (54.4)	951 (60.3)	862 (53.7)	0.0031
Family income level (≤low, %)	549 (34.9)	715 (44.9)	900 (55.3)	<0.0001	851 (52.0)	695 (43.1)	618 (39.9)	<0.0001	721 (44.0)	750 (47.5)	693 (43.2)	0.0974
Current smoker (%)	102 (2.3)	145 (9.8)	192 (12.3)	<0.0001	135 (9.0)	138 (8.8)	166 (11.0)	0.1539	94 (6.0)	127 (8.8)	218 (14.0)	<0.0001
High-risk alcohol consumption (%)	42 (2.6)	61 (3.8)	84 (5.7)	0.0002	38 (2.4)	47 (3.1)	102 (6.6)	<0.0001	38 (2.3)	43 (2.8)	106 (7.0)	<0.0001
Body mass index (kg/m², mean ± SE)	24.2 ± 0.1	24.1 ± 0.1	23.9 ± 0.1	0.1164	24.0 ± 0.1	24.0 ± 0.1	24.1 ± 0.1	0.5946	24.0 ± 0.1	24.0 ± 0.1	24.1 ± 0.1	0.6819
Body mass index range (kg/m²)				0.0157				0.0222				0.5585
<18.5	28 (1.8)	35 (2.2)	57 (3.9)		53 (3.8)	37 (2.4)	30 (1.7)		35 (2.1)	43 (3.1)	42 (2.7)	
18.5–24.9	934 (60.9)	949 (61.9)	950 (62.2)		923 (59.7)	963 (63.2)	947 (62.1)		963 (63.1)	930 (60.7)	940 (61.3)	
≥25.0	582 (37.3)	560 (35.8)	537 (33.9)		568 (36.5)	544 (34.4)	567 (36.2)		546 (34.8)	571 (36.2)	562 (36.0)	
Comorbidity (%)	334 (21.2)	307 (20.1)	284 (17.6)	0.0692	324 (20.6)	328 (21.4)	273 (17.1)	0.0192	340 (21.2)	296 (18.9)	289 (19.0)	0.2871

Values are presented as mean ± standard error (SE) or n (%). All p-values were determined by the chi-square test and general linear model.

3.4. FVS and Nutrient Intakes across Tertiles of Dietary Pattern Scores

Table 4 lists the age- and sex-adjusted mean values for FVS and nutrient intakes across the tertiles of the dietary pattern scores. Both the "vegetables, oils, and fish" and the "noodles and meat" patterns showed a significant positive trend of FVS. On the contrary, the "white rice and salted vegetables" pattern showed a significant negative tendency for FVS. The "white rice and salted vegetables" pattern showed a significant negative association with energy, energy from protein, energy from fat, and intake of nutrients, such as fiber, calcium, phosphorus, potassium, thiamin, riboflavin, vitamin C, ω-3/-6 polyunsaturated fatty acids (PUFA), flavonoids, and carotenoids. Conformability to the "vegetables, oils, and fish" pattern was significantly positively related to energy, energy from protein, energy from fat, and intake of nutrients, such as fiber, calcium, iron, sodium, potassium, thiamin, riboflavin, niacin, vitamin C, ω-3/-6 PUFA, flavonoids, and carotenoids. In the "noodles and meat" pattern, there was a significantly positive tendency to consume energy and iron but a negative tendency for other nutrients.

3.5. Association of Frailty with Dietary Pattern Scores Considering FVS

The prevalence of frail and pre-frail in this study was 11.9% ($n = 572$) and 62.5% ($n = 2945$), respectively. From the results of the multinomial logistic analysis for the association of frailty with the tertile of FVS (Figure 1), frailty was inversely associated with each tertile of FVS. The OR of pre-frail and frail was significantly lower in the highest tertile of FVS (OR (95% CI) = 0.44 (0.31–0.61), p-trend < 0.0001) compared to the lowest tertile.

The results of the multinomial logistic analysis for the association between frailty and dietary pattern score are presented in Figure 2. The highest tertile of the "vegetables, oils, and fish" pattern was significantly inversely associated with frailty (OR (95% CI) = 0.55 (0.40–0.75), p-trend = 0.0002). The ORs (95% CI) of frailty for those in the highest tertile compared to the lowest tertile of pattern scores were 1.39 (1.02–1.91) for the "white rice and salted vegetables" pattern (p-trend = 0.0376) and 1.55 (1.13–2.13) for the "noodles and meat" pattern (p-trend = 0.0066).

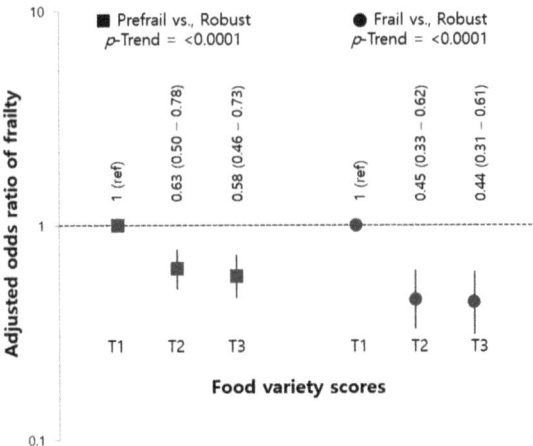

Figure 1. Adjusted ORs (95% CI) for pre-frailty and frailty according to the tertile of food variety scores. Ref.: reference category; OR: odds ratio; CI: confidence interval. Data were calculated using the multinomial SURVEYLOGISTIC model. ORs (95% CIs) were adjusted for gender, age, BMI, living status, residential area, family income, education level, smoking status, high-risk alcohol consumption, comorbidity, and energy intake.

Table 4. Age- and sex-adjusted mean daily energy and nutrient intake across tertiles of food variety scores and dietary pattern scores.

	Pattern 1 White Rice and Salted Vegetables				Pattern 2 Vegetables, Oils, and Fish				Pattern 3 Noodles and Meat			
	Tertile 1	Tertile 2	Tertile 3	p-Trend	Tertile 1	Tertile 2	Tertile 3	p-Trend	Tertile 1	Tertile 2	Tertile 3	p-Trend
Food variety score	34.7 ± 0.4	32.9 ± 0.4	25.5 ± 0.4	<0.0001	24.4 ± 0.4	32.7 ± 0.4	36.0 ± 0.5	<0.0001	29.9 ± 0.4	31.4 ± 0.4	32.0 ± 0.4	0.0077
Total energy (kcal)	1803.4 ± 21.0	1722.2 ± 18.4	1548.4 ± 19.3	<0.0001	1655.0 ± 19.7	1701.7 ± 19.2	1719.9 ± 20.1	<0.0001	1659.0 ± 21.5	1648.4 ± 17.8	1771.2 ± 20.9	<0.0001
percentage from energy												
Carbohydrates (%)	68.7 ± 0.3	71.1 ± 0.3	74.8 ± 0.3	<0.0001	76.3 ± 0.3	72.2 ± 0.3	66.1 ± 0.3	<0.0001	74.5 ± 0.3	73.4 ± 0.3	66.6 ± 0.3	<0.0001
Protein (%)	13.4 ± 0.1	13.2 ± 0.1	12.1 ± 0.1	<0.0001	11.2 ± 0.1	13.1 ± 0.1	14.4 ± 0.1	<0.0001	13.1 ± 0.1	12.7 ± 0.1	13.0 ± 0.1	0.7579
Fat (%)	17.3 ± 0.2	13.4 ± 0.2	8.8 ± 0.2	<0.0001	10.6 ± 0.2	12.9 ± 0.2	16.0 ± 0.3	<0.0001	12.2 ± 0.2	11.8 ± 0.2	15.6 ± 0.2	<0.0001
Fiber (g)	29.7 ± 0.5	25.8 ± 0.4	21.0 ± 0.4	<0.0001	22.3 ± 0.5	26.2 ± 0.5	28.1 ± 0.5	<0.0001	31.2 ± 0.5	23.6 ± 0.4	21.9 ± 0.4	<0.0001
Calcium (mg)	507.7 ± 9.7	444.7 ± 9.3	365.4 ± 8.9	<0.0001	364.0 ± 6.8	433.1 ± 8.1	520.8 ± 11.7	<0.0001	515.4 ± 12.3	416.8 ± 7.7	387.6 ± 6.7	<0.0001
Phosphorus (mg)	1003.6 ± 13.1	934.9 ± 11.7	779.2 ± 11.8	<0.0001	780.2 ± 10.7	916.9 ± 11.7	1020.6 ± 14.1	<0.0001	985.4 ± 14.8	877.7 ± 10.9	857.9 ± 11.6	<0.0001
Iron (mg)	13.3 ± 0.3	13.7 ± 0.3	11.9 ± 0.2	0.2458	11.4 ± 0.2	13.0 ± 0.3	14.6 ± 0.3	<0.0001	14.6 ± 0.3	12.7 ± 0.2	11.7 ± 0.2	<0.0001
Sodium (mg)	3179.9 ± 61.9	3097.1 ± 60.8	2725.9 ± 59.1	0.4835	2465.6 ± 51.9	2913.5 ± 55.1	3615.2 ± 71.7	<0.0001	2782.3 ± 62.9	2818.5 ± 51.9	3413.0 ± 64.5	<0.0001
Potassium	3069.1 ± 47.7	2715.1 ± 34.8	2197.7 ± 34.8	<0.0001	2302.9 ± 37.6	2680.9 ± 38.5	3001.7 ± 46.8	<0.0001	3028.9 ± 49.3	2555.7 ± 36.4	2409.7 ± 37.2	<0.0001
Vitamin A (μg RAE)	341.0 ± 9.9	318.3 ± 10.8	293.2 ± 22.8	0.9197	204.6 ± 11.1	294.7 ± 8.7	450.8 ± 20.6	<0.0001	391.5 ± 21.7	292.6 ± 9.4	269.0 ± 10.6	<0.0001
Thiamin (mg)	1.3 ± 0.0	1.5 ± 0.0	1.3 ± 0.0	<0.0001	1.2 ± 0.0	1.4 ± 0.0	1.5 ± 0.0	<0.0001	1.4 ± 0.0	1.4 ± 0.0	1.3 ± 0.0	<0.0001
Riboflavin (mg)	1.4 ± 0.0	1.1 ± 0.0	0.8 ± 0.0	<0.0001	0.9 ± 0.0	1.1 ± 0.0	1.3 ± 0.0	<0.0001	1.2 ± 0.0	1.0 ± 0.0	1.1 ± 0.0	<0.0001
Niacin (mg)	11.9 ± 0.1	11.8 ± 0.2	10.1 ± 0.2	0.6320	9.6 ± 0.2	11.8 ± 0.2	13.0 ± 0.2	<0.0001	11.9 ± 0.2	10.8 ± 0.2	11.2 ± 0.2	<0.0001
Vitamin C (mg)	91.4 ± 3.4	75.9 ± 3.6	48.7 ± 1.8	<0.0001	63.2 ± 3.9	68.9 ± 2.3	84.3 ± 2.7	<0.0001	97.0 ± 4.1	64.0 ± 2.0	55.6 ± 2.3	<0.0001
ω-3 PUFA (g)	1.8 ± 0.1	1.5 ± 0.0	1.1 ± 0.1	<0.0001	0.8 ± 0.0	1.4 ± 0.0	2.2 ± 0.1	<0.0001	1.8 ± 0.1	1.4 ± 0.1	1.3 ± 0.0	<0.0001
ω-6 PUFA (g)	8.6 ± 0.2	6.2 ± 0.1	3.9 ± 0.1	<0.0001	4.4 ± 0.1	6.0 ± 0.1	8.3 ± 0.2	<0.0001	6.5 ± 0.2	5.4 ± 0.1	6.9 ± 0.2	0.8982
Flavonoids (mg)	102.3 ± 2.6	91.2 ± 2.3	75.9 ± 2.3	<0.0001	79.6 ± 2.6	91.6 ± 2.4	98.4 ± 2.7	<0.0001	114.9 ± 3.0	82.0 ± 2.0	73.0 ± 2.1	<0.0001
Carotenoids (mg)	11.6 ± 0.4	9.4 ± 0.2	6.8 ± 0.2	<0.0001	7.3 ± 0.3	98.4 ± 2.7	11.5 ± 0.4	<0.0001	11.8 ± 0.4	6.9 ± 0.2	7.0 ± 0.2	<0.0001

Values are presented as means (least-square means) ± standard error adjusted for gender and age. PUFA, polyunsaturated fatty acid.

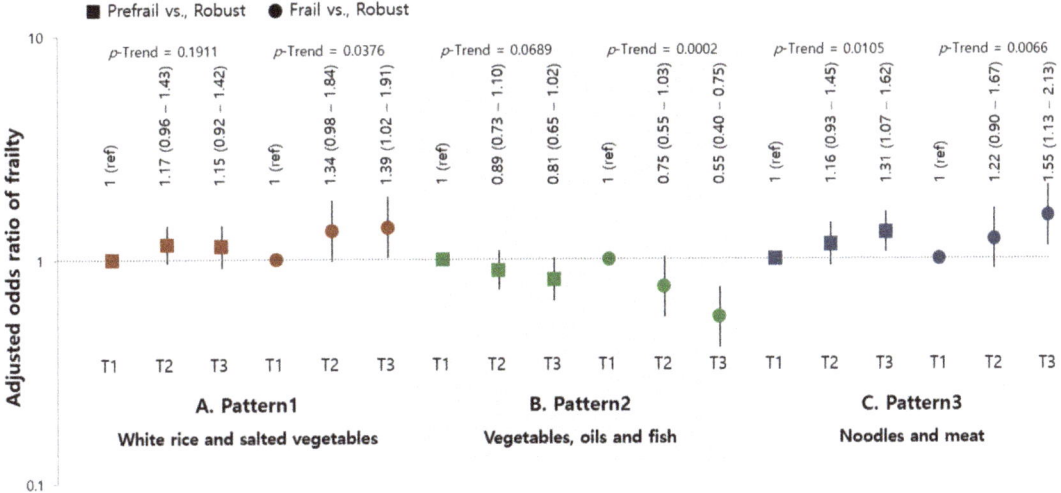

Figure 2. Adjusted ORs (95% CI) for pre-frailty and frailty according to the tertile of dietary pattern scores. (**A**) "White rice and salted vegetables"; (**B**) "Vegetables, oils, and fish"; (**C**) "Noodles and meat." Ref.: reference category; OR: odds ratio; CI: confidence interval. Data were calculated using the multinomial SURVEYLOGISTIC model. ORs (95% CIs) were adjusted for gender, age, BMI, living status, residential area, family income, education level, smoking status, high-risk alcohol consumption, comorbidity, and energy intake.

4. Discussion

This study was conducted to identify the relationship of dietary patterns with frailty considering food variety. A greater food variety was significantly associated with lower odds of frailty. Three major dietary patterns were identified in this study of older Korean adults: "white rice and salted vegetables," "vegetables, oils, and fish," and "noodles and meat." Among these patterns, "vegetables, oils, and fish" was associated positively with FVS and showed an inverse relationship with the risk of frailty.

Assessing the relationship between individual nutrients and frailty may not take into consideration the interactions between nutrients. An increasing number of investigations in recent years has evaluated the association between dietary patterns and frailty. As mentioned above, some studies in Western countries have reported that adherence to Mediterranean dietary patterns protects against frailty [4,5]. In this current study of the specific dietary pattern of Koreans, we found that the highest tertile of the "vegetables, oils, and fish" pattern was associated with a low prevalence of frailty. A prospective study of older Spanish adults [6] found that a "prudent" dietary pattern (characterized by a high intake of olive oil and vegetables) was inversely associated with frailty incidence. Furthermore, in a study of Taiwanese older adults, a reduced prevalence of frailty was observed in those with a dietary pattern high in ω-3-rich deep-sea fish, phytonutrient-rich plant foods, and other protein-rich foods, such as shellfish and milk [24]. In another study involving a large cohort of older European subjects, high consumption of fruits and vegetables was associated with a reduced frailty risk [5]. A sufficient intake of fish or oils rich in ω-3 and vegetables rich in antioxidants and phytonutrients could have the effect of preventing frailty through various mechanisms, including anti-oxidative, anti-inflammatory, and muscle decomposition prevention. Similar to our research, one study of the Korean population reported that dietary patterns with high consumption of meat, fish, and vegetables lower the risk of pre-frailty. It suggests a potentially protective effect against frailty of a protein-rich and vegetable-rich food pattern [15]. Dietary patterns are analyzed based on the diet of the study reference population, so the dietary patterns extracted from each study may be different. In the present study, a dietary pattern of "white rice and salted vegetables" or "noodles and meat" was associated with an increased risk of frailty. This outcome might also be linked to oxidative stress and inflammation because high intakes of carbohydrates, sodium, red meat, and N-nitroso compounds found in processed meat products are related to oxidative stress and inflammation [25,26].

In a prospective investigation of older Chinese people there was no association between a dietary pattern including a "vegetable–fruit" pattern and the incidence of frailty [7]. The FVS refers to the total number of different food items consumed individually over a particular time. It is the main measure used to assess the overall diet and has been associated with the nutrient adequacy ratio of the nutrients and diet quality [8]. A previous study reported that the FVS could reflect the overall dietary quality and is related to the health status of Korean adults [27]. In this current study, considering both dietary pattern and food diversity, the higher the compliance with the "vegetable, oils, and fish" pattern, the higher the FVS and the lower the prevalence of frailty. On the contrary, the "white rice and salted vegetables" pattern was inversely associated with FVS and an increased risk of frailty. Furthermore, we found that a lower diet diversity, indicated by a significantly low FVS, was also associated with frailty. This finding is consistent with another study that found frailty was intimately related to low dietary diversity in older adults [9]. Low food variety and a narrow range of food choices may result in an inadequate intake of micronutrients and phytochemicals [28]. Antioxidant nutrients could reduce the risk of frailty through different biological pathways, such as oxidative stress [10] and inflammation [11]. Antioxidant nutrients have been shown to protect against oxidative stresses that may cause muscle atrophy and loss of muscle fibers [10]. Inflammation is an inevitable reaction to the aging process and plays an important role in frailty pathogenesis by influencing key components of the frailty syndrome. Moreover, increased pro-inflammatory cytokines and interleukin-6 have been associated with slow walking speed and reduced muscle strength [29]. High levels of C-reactive protein have also been associated with frailty [30].

In our study, we found no detail confirming whether frailty was related to individual macronutrients, such as carbohydrates, proteins, and fats. Protein intake has been a major focus of literature studies evaluating specific nutrients related to frailty because of the progressive loss of muscle mass and strength with aging. Amino acids stimulate muscle protein synthesis. However, previous studies on protein intake and frailty showed somewhat contradictory results [31–34]. Bartali et al. [31] reported an association of low protein intake and frailty after adjusting for energy intake. Kobayashi et al. [32] showed that increased total protein intake was associated with a decreased prevalence of frailty among older Japanese women. However, our research did not follow these results. As with our findings, Schoufour et al. [33] and Shikany et al. [34] did not observe an association between frailty and energy-adjusted protein intake. Although the overall quality of meals and dietary patterns are more important than single nutrients, the importance of protein intake in older adults should not be overlooked in relation to muscle strength, the main cause of aging. In our study, the positive association of the "vegetables, oils, and fish" pattern, which was inversely related to frailty, and the protein-energy intake, might provide some evidence to support the relationship between frailty and protein. Detailed research on frailty and proteins is needed, considering not only amount of protein intake but also the source of protein.

The present study has some limitations. First, because of the cross-sectional nature of KNHANES, we could not define the causality of frailty and dietary factors. Further investigation is warranted to identify the causal relationship. Second, as a retrospective study, we developed a modified frailty index using the variables investigated in KNHANES to analyze the association between frailty with nutritional factors. In addition to the phenotype of frailty, there may be several other operations and definitions of frailty. Third, our dietary data were derived from a single 24 h dietary recall, which may not be sufficient to estimate usual dietary intake. However, only minor variations were observed between a single-day (24 h) dietary recall and data obtained over 2–10 days (3.9% for energy, within

10% for macronutrients and micronutrients) in the 2009 KNHANES [35]. Nevertheless, to the best of our knowledge, this current study is the first to report that a dietary pattern of "vegetables, oils, and fish" that includes diverse food items might be a therapeutic approach to decreasing frailty among older adults, based on a nationally representative population.

5. Conclusions

Our findings revealed that dietary pattern characterized by a high intake of vegetables, oils, and fish with a wide variety of foods might decrease frailty among older adults. To prevent frailty in older adults, encouraging the consumption of various kinds of food based on an increased intake of vegetables, oils, and fish may be one of the most straightforward and effective public nutrition strategies for the aging population. Future longitudinal study may be promising to confirm the causal association between dietary pattern and the risk of frailty.

Author Contributions: Y.K. and W.J. conceived and designed the study; W.J. performed the statistical analysis; W.J. and Y.S. wrote the paper; Y.K. contributed to the critical review of the manuscript. All authors have read and agreed to the published version of the manuscript.

Funding: This research was supported by the academic-research cooperation program in the Korea Maritime Institute (KMI) (No.2021-0010-1002).

Institutional Review Board Statement: The study was conducted according to the guidelines of the Declaration of Helsinki. The Institutional Review Board (IRB) of the KCDC approved this study (2013-07CON-03-4C, 2013-12EXP-03-5C, 2018-01-03-P-A).

Informed Consent Statement: Informed consent was obtained from all subjects involved in the study.

Data Availability Statement: Data are available from the Korea National Health and Nutrition Examination Survey (KNHANES VI and VII), conducted by the Korea Centers for Disease Control and Prevention (KCDCP), and are freely available from KCDCP (https://knhanes.cdc.go.kr, accessed on 9 September 2021).

Conflicts of Interest: The authors declare no conflict of interest.

References

1. Morley, J.E.; Haren, M.T.; Rolland, Y.; Kim, M.J. Frailty. *Med. Clin.* **2006**, *90*, 837–847. [CrossRef]
2. Sieber, C.C. Frailty–from concept to clinical practice. *Exp. Gerontol.* **2017**, *87*, 160–167. [CrossRef]
3. Lacas, A.; Rockwood, K. Frailty in primary care: A review of its conceptualization and implications for practice. *BMC Med.* **2012**, *10*, 4. [CrossRef]
4. Veronese, N.; Stubbs, B.; Noale, M.; Solmi, M.; Rizzoli, R.; Vaona, A.; Demurtas, J.; Crepaldi, G.; Maggi, S. Adherence to a Mediterranean diet is associated with lower incidence of frailty: A longitudinal cohort study. *Clin. Nutr.* **2018**, *37*, 1492–1497. [CrossRef] [PubMed]
5. Rahi, B.; Ajana, S.; Tabue-Teguo, M.; Dartigues, J.-F.; Peres, K.; Feart, C. High adherence to a Mediterranean diet and lower risk of frailty among French older adults community-dwellers: Results from the Three-City-Bordeaux Study. *Clin. Nutr.* **2018**, *37*, 1293–1298. [CrossRef]
6. León-Muñoz, L.M.; García-Esquinas, E.; López-García, E.; Banegas, J.R.; Rodríguez-Artalejo, F. Major dietary patterns and risk of frailty in older adults: A prospective cohort study. *BMC Med.* **2015**, *13*, 11. [CrossRef]
7. Chan, R.; Leung, J.; Woo, J. Dietary Patterns and Risk of Frailty in Chinese Community-Dwelling Older People in Hong Kong: A Prospective Cohort Study. *Nutrients* **2015**, *7*, 7070–7084. [CrossRef] [PubMed]
8. Foote, J.A.; Murphy, S.P.; Wilkens, L.R.; Basiotis, P.P.; Carlson, A. Dietary Variety Increases the Probability of Nutrient Adequacy among Adults. *J. Nutr.* **2004**, *134*, 1779–1785. [CrossRef] [PubMed]
9. Motokawa, K.; Watanabe, Y.; Edahiro, A.; Shirobe, M.; Murakami, M.; Kera, T.; Kawai, H.; Obuchi, S.; Fujiwara, Y.; Ihara, K. Frailty severity and dietary variety in Japanese older persons: A Cross-sectional study. *J. Nutr. Health Aging* **2018**, *22*, 451–456. [CrossRef]
10. Soysal, P.; Isik, A.T.; Carvalho, A.F.; Fernandes, B.S.; Solmi, M.; Schofield, P.; Veronese, N.; Stubbs, B. Oxidative stress and frailty: A systematic review and synthesis of the best evidence. *Maturitas* **2017**, *99*, 66–72. [CrossRef] [PubMed]
11. De Martinis, M.; Franceschi, C.; Monti, D.; Ginaldi, L. Inflammation markers predicting frailty and mortality in the elderly. *Exp. Mol. Pathol.* **2006**, *80*, 219–227. [CrossRef]
12. Bollwein, J.; Diekmann, R.; Kaiser, M.J.; Bauer, J.M.; Uter, W.; Sieber, C.C.; Volkert, D. Dietary quality is related to frailty in community-dwelling older adults. *J. Gerontol. Ser. A Biomed. Sci. Med. Sci.* **2012**, *68*, 483–489. [CrossRef] [PubMed]

13. García-Esquinas, E.; Rahi, B.; Peres, K.; Colpo, M.; Dartigues, J.-F.; Bandinelli, S.; Feart, C.; Rodríguez-Artalejo, F. Consumption of fruit and vegetables and risk of frailty: A dose-response analysis of 3 prospective cohorts of community-dwelling older adults. *Am. J. Clin. Nutr.* **2016**, *104*, 132–142. [CrossRef]
14. Balboa-Castillo, T.; Struijk, E.A.; Lopez-Garcia, E.; Banegas, J.R.; Rodríguez-Artalejo, F.; Guallar-Castillon, P. Low vitamin intake is associated with risk of frailty in older adults. *Age Ageing* **2018**, *47*, 872–879. [CrossRef]
15. Kim, J.; Lee, Y.; Won, C.; Kim, M.; Kye, S.; Shim, J.-S.; Ki, S.; Yun, J.-H. Dietary Patterns and Frailty in Older Korean Adults: Results from the Korean Frailty and Aging Cohort Study. *Nutrients* **2021**, *13*, 601. [CrossRef] [PubMed]
16. Kweon, S.; Kim, Y.; Jang, M.-J.; Kim, Y.; Kim, K.; Choi, S.; Chun, C.; Khang, Y.-H.; Oh, K. Data Resource Profile: The Korea National Health and Nutrition Examination Survey (KNHANES). *Int. J. Epidemiol.* **2014**, *43*, 69–77. [CrossRef]
17. Fried, L.P.; Tangen, C.M.; Walston, J.; Newman, A.B.; Hirsch, C.; Gottdiener, J.; Seeman, T.; Tracy, R.; Kop, W.J.; Burke, G.; et al. Frailty in Older Adults: Evidence for a Phenotype. *J. Gerontol. Ser. A Biol. Sci. Med. Sci.* **2001**, *56*, M146–M157. [CrossRef]
18. Jönsson, A.; Lindgren, I.; Norrving, B.; Lindgren, A. Weight loss after stroke: A population-based study from the Lund Stroke Register. *Stroke* **2008**, *39*, 918–923. [CrossRef] [PubMed]
19. Grossi, G.; Perski, A.; Osika, W.; Savic, I. Stress-related exhaustion disorder–clinical manifestation of burnout? A review of as-sessment methods, sleep impairments, cognitive disturbances, and neuro-biological and physiological changes in clinical burnout. *Scand. J. Psychol.* **2015**, *56*, 626–636. [CrossRef]
20. Chen, L.-K.; Liu, L.-K.; Woo, J.; Assantachai, P.; Auyeung, T.-W.; Bahyah, K.S.; Chou, M.-Y.; Chen, L.-Y.; Hsu, P.-S.; Krairit, O.; et al. Sarcopenia in Asia: Consensus Report of the Asian Working Group for Sarcopenia. *J. Am. Med. Dir. Assoc.* **2014**, *15*, 95–101. [CrossRef]
21. Kim, S.-H.; Ahn, J.; Ock, M.; Shin, S.; Park, J.; Luo, N.; Jo, M.-W. The EQ-5D-5L valuation study in Korea. *Qual. Life Res.* **2016**, *25*, 1845–1852. [CrossRef] [PubMed]
22. Savela, S.L.; Koistinen, P.; Stenholm, S.; Tilvis, R.S.; Strandberg, A.Y.; Pitkälä, K.H.; Salomaa, V.V.; Strandberg, T.E. Leisure-time physical activity in midlife is related to old age frailty. *J. Gerontol. Ser. A Biomed. Sci. Med. Sci.* **2013**, *68*, 1433–1438. [CrossRef] [PubMed]
23. Krebs-Smith, S.M.; Smiciklas-Wright, H.; Guthrie, H.A.; Krebs-Smith, J. The effects of variety in food choices on dietary quality. *J. Am. Diet. Assoc.* **1987**, *87*, 897–903. [CrossRef]
24. Lo, Y.; Hsieh, Y.; Hsu, L.; Chuang, S.; Chang, H.; Hsu, C.; Chen, C.; Pan, W. Dietary pattern associated with frailty: Results from nutrition and health survey in Taiwan. *J. Am. Geriatr. Soc.* **2017**, *65*, 2009–2015. [CrossRef]
25. Chai, W.; Morimoto, Y.; Cooney, R.V.; Franke, A.A.; Shvetsov, Y.B.; Le Marchand, L.; Haiman, C.A.; Kolonel, L.N.; Goodman, M.T.; Maskarinec, G. Dietary Red and Processed Meat Intake and Markers of Adiposity and Inflammation: The Multiethnic Cohort Study. *J. Am. Coll. Nutr.* **2017**, *36*, 378–385. [CrossRef] [PubMed]
26. Tan, B.L.; Norhaizan, M.E.; Liew, W.-P.-P. Nutrients and Oxidative Stress: Friend or Foe? *Oxidative Med. Cell. Longev.* **2018**, *2018*, 9719584. [CrossRef]
27. Kim, S.H.; Kim, J.Y.; Ryu, K.A.; Sohn, C.M. Evaluation of the dietary diversity and nutrient intakes in obese adults. *Korean J. Community Nutr.* **2007**, *12*, 583.
28. Bernstein, M.A.; Tucker, K.L.; Ryan, N.D.; O'Neill, E.F.; Clements, K.M.; Nelson, M.E.; Evans, W.J.; Singh, M.A.F. Higher dietary variety is associated with better nutritional status in frail elderly people. *J. Am. Diet. Assoc.* **2002**, *102*, 1096–1104. [CrossRef]
29. Ferrucci, L.; Penninx, B.W.; Volpato, S.; Harris, T.B.; Bandeen-Roche, K.; Balfour, J.; Leveille, S.G.; Fried, L.P.; Md, J.M.G. Change in muscle strength explains accelerated decline of physical function in older women with high interleukin-6 serum levels. *J. Am. Geriatr. Soc.* **2002**, *50*, 1947–1954. [CrossRef]
30. Walston, J.; McBurnie, M.A.; Newman, A.; Tracy, R.P.; Kop, W.J.; Hirsch, C.H.; Gottdiener, J.; Fried, L.P. Frailty and activation of the in-flammation and coagulation systems with and without clinical comorbidities: Results from the Cardiovascular Health Study. *Arch. Intern. Med.* **2002**, *162*, 2333–2341. [CrossRef]
31. Bartali, B.; Frongillo, E.A.; Bandinelli, S.; Lauretani, F.; Semba, R.D.; Fried, L.P.; Ferrucci, L. Low nutrient intake is an essential compo-nent of frailty in older persons. *J. Gerontol. Ser. A Biol. Sci. Med. Sci.* **2006**, *61*, 589–593. [CrossRef] [PubMed]
32. Kobayashi, S.; Asakura, K.; Suga, H.; Sasaki, S. High protein intake is associated with low prevalence of frailty among old Japa-nese women: A multicenter cross-sectional study. *Nutr. J.* **2013**, *12*, 164. [CrossRef] [PubMed]
33. Schoufour, J.D.; Franco, O.H.; Kiefte-de Jong, J.C.; Trajanoska, K.; Stricker, B.; Brusselle, G.; Rivadeneira, F.; LaHousse, L.; Voortman, T. The association between dietary protein intake, energy intake and physical frailty: Results from the Rotterdam Study. *Br. J. Nutr.* **2019**, *121*, 393–401. [CrossRef] [PubMed]
34. Shikany, J.M.; Barrett-Connor, E.; Ensrud, K.E.; Cawthon, P.M.; Lewis, C.E.; Dam, T.L.; Shannon, J.; Redden, D.T.; Osteoporotic Fractures in Men (MrOS) Research Group. Macronutrients, diet quality, and frailty in older men. *J. Gerontol. Ser. A Biomed. Sci. Med. Sci.* **2013**, *69*, 695–701. [CrossRef]
35. Korea Health Industry Development Institute. *National Food & Nutrition Statistics: Based on 2009 Korea National Health and Nutrition Examination Survey*; Korea Health Industry Development Institute: Osong, Korea, 2011.

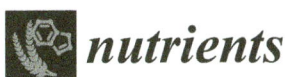

Review

Using Nature to Nurture: Breast Milk Analysis and Fortification to Improve Growth and Neurodevelopmental Outcomes in Preterm Infants

Katherine Marie Ottolini [1], Elizabeth Vinson Schulz [1], Catherine Limperopoulos [2,3,4] and Nickie Andescavage [4,5,*]

1. Department of Pediatrics, Division of Neonatal-Perinatal Medicine, Uniformed Services University of the Health Sciences, Bethesda, MD 20814, USA; katherine.ottolini@usuhs.edu (K.M.O.); elizabeth.schulz@usuhs.edu (E.V.S.)
2. Department of Pediatrics, George Washington University School of Medicine, Washington, DC 20037, USA; climpero@childrensnational.org
3. Department of Radiology, George Washington University School of Medicine, Washington, DC 20037, USA
4. Developing Brain Research Laboratory, Children's National Hospital, Washington, DC 20010, USA
5. Department of Neonatology, Children's National Hospital, Washington, DC 20010, USA
* Correspondence: NNiforat@childrensnational.org; Tel.: +1-202-476-3920

Abstract: Premature infants are born prior to a critical window of rapid placental nutrient transfer and fetal growth—particularly brain development—that occurs during the third trimester of pregnancy. Subsequently, a large proportion of preterm neonates experience extrauterine growth failure and associated neurodevelopmental impairments. Human milk (maternal or donor breast milk) is the recommended source of enteral nutrition for preterm infants, but requires additional fortification of macronutrient, micronutrient, and energy content to meet the nutritional demands of the preterm infant in attempts at replicating in utero nutrient accretion and growth rates. Traditional standardized fortification practices that add a fixed amount of multicomponent fortifier based on assumed breast milk composition do not take into account the considerable variations in breast milk content or individual neonatal metabolism. Emerging methods of individualized fortification—including targeted and adjusted fortification—show promise in improving postnatal growth and neurodevelopmental outcomes in preterm infants.

Keywords: preterm; breast milk; fortification; neurodevelopment

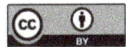

1. Introduction

The third trimester of pregnancy represents a period of rapid fetal growth resulting from increased placental nutrient and energy transfer. The rate of fetal protein accretion during the second half of pregnancy is estimated to be approximately 2 g/kg/day [1,2]. Fat accretion occurs almost entirely after 25 weeks' gestation, increasing exponentially thereafter and peaking at 7 g/day by term [3]. Adequate nutrient transfer during this timeframe is particularly essential for the developing human brain, with cerebral and cerebellar volumes increasing by 230% and 384%, respectively, between 25- and 37-weeks' gestation in healthy fetuses [4].

In comparison to the developing fetus, preterm infants born during this critical developmental window are exposed to unique environmental stressors and systemic illness within the extrauterine environment that pose additional nutritional demands to achieve growth rates that parallel in utero nutrient accretion [2]. Despite advances in neonatal nutrition, half of all very low birth weight (VLBW, <1500 g) infants continue to experience extrauterine growth restriction, which has been closely tied to poor neurodevelopmental outcomes [5–7]. Postnatal growth has major implications for preterm brain development, as greater increases in weight, linear growth, and head circumference have all been associated with improved long-term neurodevelopment outcomes [8,9].

Substrates for enteral nutrition in these high-risk infants include bovine or human-milk-derived products. Human milk administration has several well-established benefits in this population, conferring protection against common morbidities associated with impaired growth and neurodevelopment—including sepsis, necrotizing enterocolitis, and bronchopulmonary dysplasia [10,11]. Breast milk intake has also been associated with superior brain growth and microstructural development, as well as short and long-term neurodevelopmental outcomes compared to preterm formula, likely as a result of its unique bioactive and nutritional components [11,12]. Exclusive human milk feeding is therefore recommended as the standard of care for preterm infants, with the provision of donor breast milk when the mother's own milk is not available [10,13]. However, unfortified human milk does not adequately meet the nutritional demands of the growing preterm infant, warranting fortification with additional macro- and micronutrients [10,14]. In this review, we aim to discuss current and evolving methods of breast milk fortification with the aim of optimizing postnatal growth rates and neurodevelopment, including the use of individualized fortification and human milk analysis.

2. Human Milk Analysis

2.1. Crematocrit

Human milk analysis began in the late 1970s based on a microcentrifugation technique originally used for estimating the fat content in goats' milk [15]. This method for estimation of human milk's energy and fat content advertised a "rapid and cheap" analysis of the percentage of cream within the milk, thus named the "*crematocrit*" [15]. In this process, a homogenized sample of human milk is drawn into a standard capillary tube. The sample is centrifuged and then immediately removed and placed upright, and the layer of fat at the top of the tube is then measured with calipers [15,16]. This value represents a percentage of the total volume of milk in the tube, and an estimation of fat and energy content (kcal/30 mL) may subsequently be derived using the following calculations [14,15,17].

$$\text{fat (g/L)} = \frac{(creamatocrit\ [\%] - 0.59)}{0.146} \quad (1)$$

$$\text{kcal/L} = (290 + 66.8) \times creamatocrit\ (\%) \quad (2)$$

Unfortunately, despite the simplicity of obtaining a *crematocrit*, this tool only provides data for the fat content of the milk. Lucas et al. additionally reported the potential for overestimation of the *crematocrit*, dependent upon what location along the meniscus (superior versus inferior border) the calipers measured [15]. This concern was confirmed by O'Neill et al., who demonstrated an overestimation of the fat and energy content of human milk using the *crematocrit* microanalysis method in comparison to a human milk analyzer (mid-infrared spectroscopy method) [16]. With newer technologies, the *crematocrit* has become a historical means of fat content analysis in human milk but may have utility for late preterm and term infants in low-resource settings when alternate technologies are unavailable. Nevertheless, this practice is cautioned for use in VLBW and extremely low birth weight (ELBW, <1000 g) infants due to their increased nutritional demands and the vast changes in breast milk content that take place over the initial weeks of lactation for their mothers.

2.2. Biochemical Methods

Originating from the bovine dairy industry in Europe, several standardized laboratory biochemical approaches to assess macronutrient content in human milk exist, including the Gerber method for fat concentration, the biuret method for protein content, and Marier and Boulet's phenol-sulphuric acid colorimetric method for lactose content [18–23]. In the Gerber method, homogenized milk is combined with sulfuric acid and amyl alcohol with centrifugation to produce separation of the fat [24]. This reaction utilizes a butyrometer, a specialized scaled container that measures the percentage of fat following separation, with each percentage representing a specific volume. For total protein analysis, the biuret assay aims to induce formation of a complex between peptide molecules and copper salts under alkaline conditions [23]. If the biuret reaction occurs, the complex will become violet in appearance and a spectrophotometer is then utilized to measure the absorbance at ~540 nm in order to calculate the concentration of protein within the sample [23]. Lastly, colorimetry may be utilized for determining the lactose content in human milk in which a homogenized milk sample is mixed with phenol-sulphuric acid or a combination of zinc sulfate and barium hydroxide and then centrifuged. The resultant clear supernatant is further processed, and absorbance read at ~520 nm to calculate lactose concentration [25]. It should be noted that alternative biochemical methods are available for the measurement of each of these macronutrients.

2.3. Spectroscopy

As with the previous methods of human milk analysis, spectroscopy use originated in the bovine milk industry. Although human milk analyzers, which use either near-infrared or mid-infrared spectroscopy (NIRS/MIRS, respectively), are reported in the literature for targeted nutrition for premature infants since the 1980s, approval by the United States Food and Drug Administration (FDA) for the use of a breast milk analyzer did not occur until 2018 [26,27]. Current human milk analyzers primarily use spectrophotometry to assess the fat, carbohydrate (lactose), protein, and energy content [28]. The principle behind the use of infrared analysis in human milk is the identification of chemical groups (fat, lactose, and protein) through their absorbance of infrared energy [29]. The output from the various analyzers represents each of these components (i.e., macronutrients) based on their wavelength. Near-infrared spectroscopy differs from mid-infrared spectroscopy in the portion of the wavelength spectrum the spectrophotometry is taking place; NIRS utilizes a wavelength spectrum of 1200 to 2400 nm, while MIRS utilizes 1300 to 3000 nm [29].

There is considerable variation in the accuracy of spectroscopy as it compares to traditional biochemical techniques in the dairy industry [16,21]. Much of this variability arises from the multiple types of milk analyzers (e.g., different brands, near-infrared versus mid-infrared) and the variety of biochemical techniques that are utilized globally for the estimation of macronutrients. As such, the comparisons between different types and brands of analyzers differ depending on the various biochemical techniques used. However, when standardization and rigorous calibration are maintained, human milk analyzers provide accurate, reliable, and rapid measurements of macronutrient and energy content [30–32].

2.4. Breast Milk Content

Numerous studies have revealed nutrient variability in human milk from lactating mothers of preterm infants [33–35]. Although the estimated energy average of breast milk for the purposes of standardizing fortification is 19–20 kcal/30 mL, human milk is a dynamic fluid that yields varying macronutrient and energy densities depending on time of day, degree of premature delivery, and stage of lactation. Because of these variations, standardization of the fortification process may not meet the individual nutritional needs for optimal growth and neurodevelopment in VLBW and ELBW infants. Maternal colostrum, which is the early, small volume supply of human milk, constitutes the maximum density of protein (reported as g/100 mL) during lactation [36]. As lactation continues, in addition to diurnal variations, the content of protein continues to drop, such that premature human milk resembles that of term milk within weeks of delivery (Figure 1) [33].

When an adequate supply of mother's own milk is not available, supplementation with pasteurized donor breast milk from an established human milk bank is recommended [10]. In an effort to protect infants of mothers who donate their expressed milk, most milk banks and donor human milk companies will not accept human milk donations until several weeks postpartum and, in many cases, require demonstration of appropriate growth in the mother's own infant. Therefore, donated human milk products and their macronutrients more often resemble term milk and/or later stages of postpartum lactation—including decreased protein, fat, and energy content as compared to preterm milk [37]. One strategy utilized by international milk banking associations is to pool milk from multiple donors for the collective benefits of variable macronutrient content and a uniform batch of donor milk [38]. Nevertheless, the energy content of even pooled donor milk remains, before and after pasteurization, less than mother's own milk (Figure 1) [39,40]. Fortification of either mother's own milk or donor human milk with a bovine milk-derived or human-milk-derived fortifier aims to increase the macro- and micronutrient content to promote optimal growth of the high-risk preterm neonate [13].

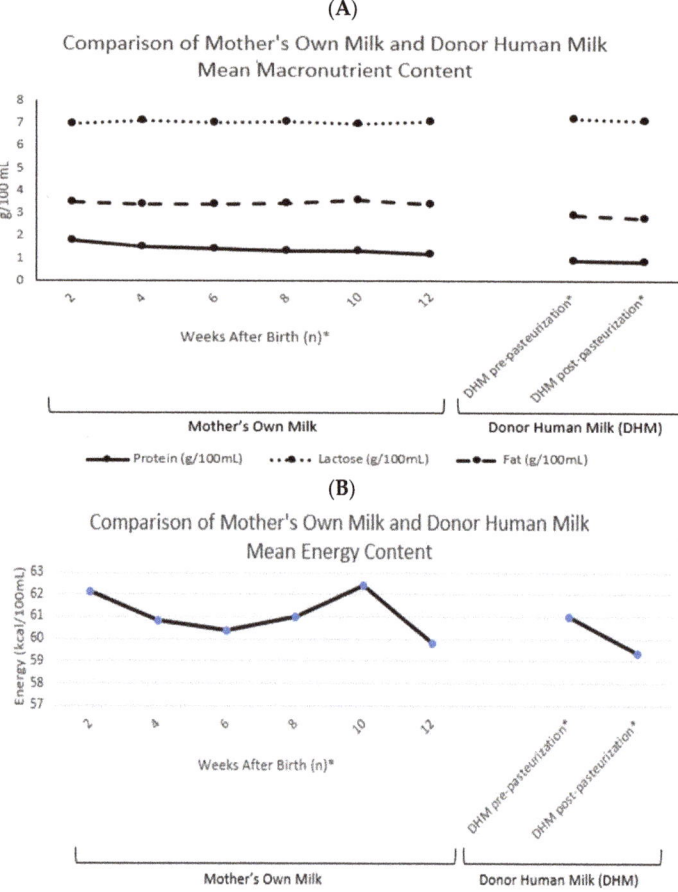

Figure 1. (**A**) Comparison of mother's own milk and donor human milk mean macronutrient content (protein, lactose and fat; g/100 mL). (**B**) Comparison of mother's own milk and donor human milk mean energy content. Means extracted from Piemontese et al. and Zachariassen et al. The values presented represent native (unfortified) human milk [37,41]. * Values representing the weeks after delivery are indicative of the mother's own milk averages, whereas the donor human milk (DHM) averages represent over 90% of donor milk mothers who delivered after 37 weeks' gestation. Donation began 2.9 ± 2.3 months after delivery [37].

3. Breast Milk Fortification

3.1. Standardized Fortification

Standardized (also known as "fixed-dose" and "blind") fortification is based on assumed breast milk macronutrient (protein, fat, carbohydrate), micronutrient, and energy content from reference values, wherein mother's own milk and donor human milk are both estimated at ~20 kcal/30 mL [13]. Typically, a multicomponent fortifier is added to the human milk substrate to achieve a desired energy content between 22–26 kcal/30 mL. As mentioned previously, variations in diurnal and week-to-week maternal milk content throughout lactation bring caution to the assumptions of a standard milk composition. The variable composition of donor human milk, due to inter-donor variations in lactation phase and the impact of pasteurization on nutritional content, raises added concerns (Figure 1). Additionally, the differences between bovine and human-milk-derived fortifiers may affect the ability to tailor the human milk substrate to optimal macronutrient content [13]. A variety of concentrated bovine milk-derived fortifiers exist on the market to not only enhance caloric density, but also improve delivery of higher protein content. Similarly, commercially available human-milk-derived fortifiers incorporate a selection of macronutrient additives with the aim to provide an exclusive human milk or human-milk-derived diet comparable to the bovine milk-derived products (Figure 1) [41].

3.2. Individualized Fortification

With the variable content human milk over time, as well as the unique nutritional requirements of individual infants, it is not surprising that standardized fortification may not provide optimal macronutrient content in half of very low birth weight infants [5,42,43]. Nutritional and technological advances, including the development of modular macronutrient fortifiers and the increased availability of breast milk analysis within the neonatal intensive care unit (NICU), have led to a growing wave of 'lacto-engineering' and customized nutrition for the high-risk neonate. Strategies for individualized breast milk fortification include adjusted and targeted fortification, as well as combinations of both methods. Results from a recent national survey of U.S. NICUs demonstrated that only 12% of respondents currently utilize human milk analysis, whereas 41% employ adjusted fortification methods and 98% use modular macronutrient products [44].

In targeted fortification, a sample of human milk (via NIRS/MIRS) is analyzed to determine its specific macronutrient and energy content, and then additional macronutrient supplementation is provided to achieve goal values. Targeted values for the macronutrient and energy content of enteral feeds are typically based on consensus recommendations for preterm infants, including 3.5–4.5 g/kg/day protein, 4.8–6.6 g/kg/day lipids, 11.6–13.2 g/kg/day carbohydrates, 110–135 kcal/kg/day, and protein/energy ratios of 3.2–4.1 g/100 kcal [2]. Fortification may be achieved through a combination of multicomponent fortifiers, as well as specific modular macronutrient products such as medium-chain triglycerides, safflower oil, whey protein, casein-based liquid protein, maltrodextrin, and glucose polymers [43,45–49]. A human-milk-derived cream fortifier is also commercially available to provide additional fat, protein, and carbohydrate content [45]. The frequency of human milk analysis in studies of targeted fortification has ranged from twice daily to weekly [43,45,46,48–50]. In a study evaluating the effects of differing sampling intervals ranging from daily to weekly, Rochow et al. found that twice weekly milk analysis achieved macronutrient intake within 5% of targeted goals [50]. Although targeted fortification is an appealing method of providing customized nutrition to preterm neonates, the process can be time- and labor-intensive as well as cost-prohibitive. It requires the purchase of a human milk analyzer, of which there is currently only one U.S. FDA-approved device. In addition to equipment expenses, specialized training is also required to properly analyze milk and provide tailored fortification. Coordination with lactating mothers is also necessary to obtain accurate milk samples that are reflective of average macronutrient content. This process may involve large, multidisciplinary care teams including pharmacy or milk laboratory technicians, registered dieticians, lactation consultants, and physicians [44].

Adjustable fortification poses a less labor-intensive approach to individualized fortification, in which neonatal growth velocity along with laboratory markers of protein metabolism are utilized to estimate protein requirements [13]. Blood urea nitrogen (BUN) level is the most commonly utilized laboratory value in this tailored approach, although additional markers that have been cited in the literature include the BUN-to-creatine ratio and corrected serum urea nitrogen (adjusted for the serum creatinine level) [51–56]. The majority of published protocols aim for BUN levels ranging from 9–16 mg/dL, although targets as low as >3–5 mg/dL have been utilized [10,51–56]. Laboratory values are monitored once or twice weekly and protein fortification is adjusted accordingly utilizing either multi-component fortifiers or modular protein additives. Recently, the urinary urea-to-creatinine ratio has been explored as a potential non-invasive marker of protein metabolism, demonstrating a high correlation between the urinary urea-to-creatinine ratio, serum BUN levels, and actual protein intake in preterm neonates [57]. In contrast to targeted fortification, adjustable fortification only allows for estimation of an infant's protein requirements, but it is more easily implemented and titrates protein administration based on an individual neonate's metabolic response [13].

Some individualized fortification protocols have utilized a combination of targeted and adjustable fortification. In one such approach, the mother's milk is first analyzed and fortified to achieve preset targeted goals for macronutrient and energy content. Protein supplementation is then further tailored based on laboratory monitoring [58].

4. Growth Outcomes

4.1. Standardized Fortification

Before the fortification of breast milk in preterm neonates became the standard of care, several small studies were conducted beginning in the 1980s comparing growth rates between infants receiving standardized fortification and unfortified breast milk. In a 2016 Cochrane review of randomized-controlled trials, Brown et al. found evidence supporting increased in-hospital weight gain, length, and head circumference in infants receiving standardized fortification compared to unfortified breast milk, although included studies were characterized as being small with weak methodology [59]. For infants born small-for-gestational-age (SGA), one study suggested a greater positive effect of fortification on growth rates compared to those born appropriate-for-gestational age (AGA) [60]. A recent large umbrella review of breast milk fortification in VLBW infants found evidence that the multicomponent fortification—with the addition of protein and energy (as fat or carbohydrate)—led to significant increases in weight, length, and head circumference [61].

Human-milk-derived fortifiers are an appealing option to provide an exclusive human milk diet to preterm infants [62]. In a recent systematic review of randomized-controlled trials, Ananathan et al. noted significantly lower weight gain infants receiving human-milk-derived fortifiers in comparison to bovine-derived, without any difference in length or head growth between groups [63]. O'Connor et al. also noted slower weight gain in infants receiving human versus bovine-derived fortification, although this difference was no longer significant when weights were converted into z-scores [64]. In a large study of SGA infants, those receiving human-milk-derived fortification exhibited greater length z-scores by hospital discharge than those receiving bovine milk-derived fortification [62].

In evaluating the timing of fortification, one large cohort study found a significant association between earlier fortification and improved in-hospital length and weight gain in neonates receiving both human-milk-derived and bovine-based fortification [65]. However, these results were not replicated in three randomized controlled trials that showed no difference in growth velocities between infants receiving early versus delayed fortification with either human or cow's milk-derived products [66–68].

There is no consensus on the optimal post-discharge feeding regimen for breast milk-fed preterm infants, and few studies have evaluated the use of multicomponent breast milk fortifiers in the outpatient setting. When fortification was provided in 50% of daily feeds for 12 weeks, infants demonstrated significantly greater weight and length at 12 months of age compared to those receiving unfortified milk, with additional benefits in head growth seen in those born <1250 g [64,69]. Similar growth benefits at one year of age were seen in a study that provided fortifier via breast milk 'shots' given prior to direct breastfeeding through 2 months corrected age [70]. In contrast, no benefits from fortification were noted when a considerably lower volume of fortifier was administered once a day through 4 months corrected age [71].

4.2. Individualized Fortification

Targeted fortification utilizing human milk analysis has been associated with improved growth rates compared to standardized methods [43,45,46]. Studies using a combination of multicomponent fortifier and modular macronutrient supplements have demonstrated superior weight, length, and head circumference in infants receiving targeted fortification [43,46]. One study that achieved targeted fortification utilizing the addition of a human milk-based cream also found superior growth velocities for weight and length compared to standardized fortification [45]. In two studies that did not find any growth benefits from targeted fortification, the macronutrient content of analyzed milk was actually greater than assumed reference values, such that infants in the targeted fortification group received less supplementation compared to controls receiving standardized fortification [48,49].

Recent studies of adjustable fortification strategies utilizing goal BUN values of >3 mg/dL, >5 mg/dL, 9–14 mg/dL, and 10–16 mg/dL have all demonstrated superior growth rates compared to standardized fortification [51–56]. Studies of in-hospital growth have revealed improved weight, length, and head circumference in infants receiving adjustable fortification [51,52,56]. Picauld et al. similarly demonstrated improved weight, length, and head circumference z-scores following the implementation of adjustable fortification [53]. Biasini et al. did not observe an overall effect of adjustable fortification on in-hospital growth rates, but infants who received adjustable fortification experienced greater post-discharge length at 9 months corrected age compared to standardized fortification [54]. ELBW infants managed with adjustable versus standardized fortification have demonstrated superior in-hospital growth velocities for weight, length, and head circumference, as well as greater post-discharge head circumference through 24 months corrected age [54,55].

A recent systematic review evaluating growth outcomes following individualized fortification revealed stronger evidence for the growth benefits of adjustable versus targeted fortification based on available studies [72]. One study comparing targeted versus adjustable fortification strategies noted a greater daily increase in weight and head circumference in the targeted group, although a low BUN threshold (>5 mg/dL) was utilized in the adjustable fortification group [73]. A study by Simsek et al. found that both targeted and adjustable fortification methods achieved greater weight and head circumference compared to standardized fortification [74].

5. Neurodevelopment

5.1. Standardized Fortification

Few studies have specifically evaluated the effects of breast milk fortification on neurodevelopmental outcomes. Lucas et al. did not find any significant differences in Bayley Scale of Infant Development (BSID) scores at 9 and 18 months between infants receiving bovine-derived standardized fortification versus unfortified breast milk. However, these results should be interpreted with caution, as this study was performed more than two decades ago and breast milk comprised less than 50% of milk intake in both groups [75]. Kashaki et al. followed preterm neonates through 3 years of age to evaluate the long-term neurodevelopmental impact of high protein administration versus lower protein administration utilizing a bovine-based multicomponent fortifier. The high-protein group demonstrated greater communication and gross motor scores based on the Ages and Stages Questionnaire, as well as improved development in auditory, verbal language and perception, and cognitive domains using the Newsha Developmental Scale [76].

A comparison of BSID-III scores at 18 months corrected age between human and bovine-milk derived fortification found no significant differences between groups, although investigators acknowledged that the study may not have been powered to detect all clinically-significant differences [77]. Similarly, a study of ELBW infants who received human versus bovine-derived fortification failed to demonstrate any significant differences in BSID III cognitive scores through 18 months corrected age [78]. A potential neuroprotective effect of human versus bovine-derived fortification was noted in a study of ELBW infants, which found that fortification with a human-milk-derived fortifier was associated with a decreased incidence of severe intraventricular hemorrhage or periventricular leukomolacia [79].

Studies of post-discharge fortification have demonstrated modest, if any, neurodevelopmental benefits [69,80,81]. Twice daily supplementation of breast milk with a bovine-based fortifier through 4–6 months corrected age was not associated with any improvements in 12-month BSID-III scores [81]. Fortification of 50% of breast milk feeds with a bovine-based fortifier for 12 weeks was associated with improved visual acuity at 4 and 6 months corrected age, although no significant impact on BSID-III scores was seen at 18 months corrected age [69,80].

5.2. Individualized Fortification

Adjustable fortification has been associated with improved neurodevelopmental outcomes through 2 years of age [52,54,55]. Ergenekon et al. found significantly higher BSID-III scores at 18 months corrected age in preterm neonates who had received adjustable versus standardized fortification for both the mental and psychomotor developmental index [52]. Using the Griffiths Mean Developmental Score (GMDS), Biasini et al. demonstrated significantly higher hearing and language scores at 12 and 18 months corrected age in infants receiving adjustable fortification. The greatest developmental benefits of adjustable fortification were seen in the subset of SGA infants, who exhibited superior GDMS scores in nearly all domains at 18 and 24 months corrected age [54]. Those ELBW infants who received adjustable fortification demonstrated higher GDMS performance scores at 3 months and hearing and language scores at 12 months corrected age. In a study comparing ELBW infants managed with the same adjustable fortification protocol to controls receiving standardized fortification, Mariani et al. noted a drop in GMDS scores between 12 and 24 months corrected age in the standardized but not the adjustable fortification group [55].

5.3. Future Directions

It is difficult to elucidate the precise impact of early breast milk feeding on long-term neurodevelopment, especially when the decision to breastfeed is highly correlated with a multitude of genetic and environmental factors that may also influence brain development including maternal race/ethnicity, socio-economic status, intelligence quotient, and educational level [82]. Novel quantitative magnetic resonance imaging (MRI) techniques—including volumetric segmentation and diffusion tensor imaging—are emerging as non-invasive methods for evaluating the impact of early nutritional interventions on preterm brain development at the microstructural level [12]. Quantitative MRI has already been utilized to demonstrate the effects of early breast milk, macronutrient, and energy intake on preterm brain development by term-equivalent age, and could potentially be utilized as a future tool in determining ideal breast milk fortification practices [12,82–84].

6. Conclusions

The evolving practices of individualized human milk fortification through targeted and adjustable methods show promise in improving postnatal growth and neurodevelopmental outcomes in preterm neonates. Additional research is needed to elucidate the ideal fortification method to support adequate postnatal growth and long-term neurodevelopment in this vulnerable population.

Author Contributions: K.M.O. and E.V.S. conceptualized, prepared the original draft, and edited the manuscript. C.L. and N.A. conceptualized, reviewed, and edited the manuscript. All authors have read and agreed to the published version of the manuscript.

Funding: This research received no external funding.

Institutional Review Board Statement: Not applicable.

Informed Consent Statement: Not applicable.

Data Availability Statement: Not applicable.

Conflicts of Interest: The authors declare no conflict of interest. The contents of this article are solely the responsibility of the authors and do not necessarily represent the official views of the Department of Defense or the United States Air Force.

References

1. Poindexter, B.B.; Denne, S.C. Protein Needs of the Preterm Infant. *NeoReviews* **2003**, *4*, e52–e59. [CrossRef]
2. Agostoni, C.; Buonocore, G.; Carnielli, V.P.; Darmaun, D.; Decsi, T.; Domellof, M.; Ebleton, N.D.; Fusch, C.; Genzel-Boroviczeny, O.; Goulet, O.; et al. Enteral nutrient supply for preterm infants: Commentary from the European society of paediatric gastroenterology, hepatology and nutrition committee on nutrition. *J. Pediatr. Gastroenterol. Nutr.* **2010**, *50*, 85–91. [CrossRef]
3. Haggarty, P. Fatty acid supply to the human fetus. *Annu. Rev. Nutr.* **2010**, *30*, 237–255. [CrossRef] [PubMed]
4. Clouchoux, C.; Guizard, N.; Evans, A.C.; du Plessis, A.J.; Limperopoulos, C. Normative fetal brain growth by quantitative in vivo magnetic resonance imaging. *Am. J. Obstet. Gynecol.* **2012**, *206*, 173.e1–173.e8. [CrossRef] [PubMed]
5. Horbar, J.D.; Ehrenkranz, R.A.; Badger, G.J.; Edwards, E.M.; Morrow, K.A.; Soll, R.F.; Buzas, J.S.; Bertino, E.; Gagliardi, L.; Bellù, R. Weight growth velocity and postnatal growth failure in infants 501 to 1500 grams: 2000–2013. *Pediatrics* **2015**, *136*, e84–92. [CrossRef] [PubMed]
6. Ramel, S.E.; Demerath, E.W.; Gray, H.L.; Younge, N.; Boys, C.; Georgieff, M.K. The relationship of poor linear growth velocity with neonatal illness and two-year neurodevelopment in preterm infants. *Neonatology* **2012**, *102*, 19–24. [CrossRef] [PubMed]
7. Latal-Hajnal, B.; von Siebenthal, K.; Kovari, H.; Bucher, H.U.; Largo, R.H. Postnatal growth in VLBW infants: Significant association with neurodevelopmental outcome. *J. Pediatr.* **2003**, *143*, 63–170. [CrossRef]
8. Ehrenkranz, R.A.; Dusick, A.M.; Vohr, B.R.; Wright, L.L.; Wrage, L.A.; Poole, W.K. Growth in the neonatal intensive care unit influences neurodevelopmental and growth outcomes of extremely low birth weight infants. *Pediatrics* **2006**, *117*, 1253–1261. [CrossRef]
9. Sammallahti, S.; Kajantie, E.; Matinolli, H.-M.; Pyhälä, R.; Lahti, J.; Heinonen, K.; Lahti, M.; Pesonen, A.-K.; Eriksson, J.G.; Hovi, P.; et al. Nutrition after preterm birth and adult neurocognitive outcomes. *PLoS ONE* **2017**, *12*, e0185632. [CrossRef]
10. Moro, G.E.; Minoli, I.; Ostrom, M.; Jacobs, J.R.; Picone, T.A.; Räihä, N.C.; Ziegler, E.E. Fortification of human milk: Evaluation of a novel fortification scheme and of a new fortifier. *J. Pediatr. Gastroenterol. Nutr.* **1995**, *20*, 162–172. [CrossRef]
11. Chetta, K.E.; Schulz, E.V.; Wagner, C.L. Outcomes improved with human milk intake in preterm and full-term infants. *Semin. Perinatol.* **2021**, *45*, 151384. [CrossRef]
12. Ottolini, K.M.; Andescavage, N.; Keller, S.; Limperopoulos, C. Nutrition and the developing brain: The road to optimizing early neurodevelopment: A systematic review. *Pediatr. Res.* **2020**, *87*, 194–201. [CrossRef] [PubMed]
13. Arslanoglu, S.; Boquien, C.-Y.; King, C.; Lamireau, D.; Tonetto, P.; Barnett, D.; Bertino, E.; Gaya, A.; Gebauer, C.; Grovslien, A.; et al. Fortification of human milk for preterm infants: Update and recommendations of the European Milk Bank Association (EMBA) working group on human milk fortification. *Front. Pediatr.* **2019**, *7*, 76. [CrossRef] [PubMed]
14. De Curtis, M.; Rigo, J. The nutrition of preterm infants. *Early Hum. Dev.* **2012**, *88*, S5–S7. [CrossRef]
15. Lucas, A.; Gibbs, J.A.; Lyster, R.L.; Baum, J.D. Creamatocrit: Simple clinical technique for estimating fat concentration and energy value of human milk. *Br. Med. J.* **1978**, *1*, 1018–1020. [CrossRef]
16. O'Neill, E.F.; Radmacher, P.G.; Sparks, B.; Adamkin, D.H. Creamatocrit analysis of human milk overestimates fat and energy content when compared to a human milk analyzer using mid-infrared spectroscopy. *J. Pediatr. Gastroenterol. Nutr.* **2013**, *56*, 569–572. [CrossRef] [PubMed]
17. Lemons, J.A.; Schreiner, R.L.; Gresham, E.L. Simple method for determining the caloric and fat content of human milk. *Pediatrics* **1980**, *66*, 626–628.

18. Fusch, G.; Rochow, N.; Choi, A.; Fusch, S.; Poeschl, S.; Ubah, A.O.; Lee, S.-Y.; Raja, P.; Fusch, C. Rapid measurement of macronutrients in breast milk: How reliable are infrared milk analyzers? *Clin. Nutr.* **2015**, *34*, 465–476. [CrossRef]
19. Casadio, Y.S.; Williams, T.M.; Lai, C.T.; Olsson, S.E.; Hepworth, A.R.; Hartmann, P.E. Evaluation of a mid-infrared analyzer for the determination of the macronutrient composition of human milk. *J. Hum. Lact.* **2010**, *26*, 376–383. [CrossRef]
20. Menjo, A.; Mizuno, K.; Murase, M.; Nishida, Y.; Taki, M.; Itabashi, K.; Shimono, T.; Namba, K. Bedside analysis of human milk for adjustable nutrition strategy. *Acta Paediatr.* **2009**, *98*, 380–384. [CrossRef] [PubMed]
21. Silvestre, D.; Fraga, M.; Gormaz, M.; Torres, E.; Vento, M. Comparison of mid-infrared transmission spectroscopy with biochemical methods for the determination of macronutrients in human milk. *Matern. Child Nutr.* **2014**, *10*, 373–382. [CrossRef]
22. Bosset, J.; Blanc, B.; Plattner, E. New method of automatic photometric determination of proteins in whole milk. I. theoretical basis and improvements in the principle parameters of the test. *Anal. Chim. Acta* **1974**, *70*, 327–329. [CrossRef]
23. Gornall, A.G.; Bardawill, C.J.; David, M.M. Determination of serum proteins by means of the biuret reaction. *J. Biol. Chem.* **1949**, *177*, 751–766. [CrossRef]
24. Mlcek, J.; Dvorak, L.; Sustova, K.; Szwedziak, K. Accuracy of the FT-NIR method in evaluating the fat content of milk using calibration models developed for the reference methods according to röse-gottlieb and gerber. *J. AOAC Int.* **2016**, *99*, 1305–1309. [CrossRef] [PubMed]
25. Feitosa Teles, F.F.; Young, C.K.; Still, J.W. A method for rapid determination of lactose. *J. Dairy Sci.* **1978**, *61*, 506–508. [CrossRef]
26. Michaelsen, K.F.; Pedersen, S.B.; Skafte, L.; Jaeger, P.; Peitersen, B. Infrared analysis for determining macronutrients in human milk. *J. Pediatr. Gastroenterol. Nutr.* **1988**, *7*, 229–235. [CrossRef]
27. Food and drug administration. FDA Permits Marketing of a Diagnostic Test to Aid in Measuring Nutrients in Breast Milk. 21 December 2018. Available online: https://www.fda.gov/news-events/press-announcements/fda-permits-marketing-diagnostic-test-aid-measuring-nutrients-breast-milk (accessed on 15 October 2021).
28. Sauer, C.W.; Kim, J.H. Human milk macronutrient analysis using point-of-care near-infrared spectrophotometry. *J. Perinatol.* **2011**, *31*, 339–343. [CrossRef]
29. Lynch, J.M.; Barbano, D.M.; Schweisthal, M.; Fleming, J.R. Precalibration evaluation procedures for mid-infrared milk analyzers. *J. Dairy Sci.* **2006**, *89*, 2761–2774. [CrossRef]
30. Perrin, M.T.; Festival, J.; Starks, S.; Mondeaux, L.; Brownell, E.A.; Vickers, A. Accuracy and reliability of infrared analyzers for measuring human milk macronutrients in a milk bank setting. *Curr. Dev. Nutr.* **2019**, *3*, nzz116. [CrossRef]
31. Zhu, M.; Yang, Z.; Ren, Y.; Duan, Y.; Gao, H.; Liu, B.; Ye, W.; Wang, J.; Yin, S. Comparison of macronutrient contents in human milk measured using mid-infrared human milk analyser in a field study vs. chemical reference methods. *Matern. Child Nutr.* **2017**, *13*. [CrossRef]
32. Giuffrida, F.; Austin, S.; Cuany, D.; Sanchez-Bridge, B.; Longet, K.; Bertschy, E.; Sauser, J.; Thakkar, S.K.; Lee, L.Y.; Affolter, M. Comparison of macronutrient content in human milk measured by mid-infrared human milk analyzer and reference methods. *J. Perinatol.* **2019**, *39*, 497–503. [CrossRef]
33. Gidrewicz, D.A.; Fenton, T.R. A systematic review and meta-analysis of the nutrient content of preterm and term breast milk. *BMC Pediatr.* **2014**, *14*, 216. [CrossRef]
34. Fischer Fumeaux, C.J.; Garcia-Rodenas, C.L.; De Castro, C.A.; Courtet-Compondu, M.C.; Thakkar, S.K.; Beauport, L.; Tolsa, J.F.; Affolter, M. Longitudinal analysis of macronutrient composition in preterm and term human milk: A prospective cohort study. *Nutrients* **2019**, *11*, 1525. [CrossRef] [PubMed]
35. Sahin, S.; Ozdemir, T.; Katipoglu, N.; Akcan, A.B.; Kaynak Turkmen, M. Comparison of changes in breast milk macronutrient content during the first month in preterm and term infants. *Breastfeed. Med.* **2020**, *15*, 56–62. [CrossRef] [PubMed]
36. Adamkin, D.H.; Radmacher, P.G. Fortification of human milk in very low birth weight infants (VLBW <1500 g birth weight). *Clin. Perinatol.* **2014**, *41*, 405–421. [CrossRef] [PubMed]
37. Piemontese, P.; Mallardi, D.; Liotto, N.; Tabasso, C.; Menis, C.; Perrone, M.; Roggero, P.; Mosca, F. Macronutrient content of pooled donor human milk before and after holder pasteurization. *BMC Pediatr.* **2019**, *19*, 58. [CrossRef]
38. Updegrove, K.; Festival, J.; Hackney, R. HMBANA Standards for Donor Human Milk Banking: An Overview, Public Version 1.0. September 2020. Available online: https://www.hmbana.org/our-work/publications.html (accessed on 15 October 2021).
39. García-Lara, N.R.; Vieco, D.E.; De la Cruz-Bértolo, J.; Lora-Pablos, D.; Velasco, N.U.; Pallás-Alonso, C.R. Effect of holder pasteurization and frozen storage on macronutrients and energy content of breast milk. *J. Pediatr. Gastroenterol. Nutr.* **2013**, *57*, 77–382. [CrossRef] [PubMed]
40. Vieira, A.A.; Soares, F.V.; Pimenta, H.P.; Abranches, A.D.; Moreira, M.E. Analysis of the influence of pasteurization, freezing/thawing, and offer processes on human milk's macronutrient concentrations. *Early Hum. Dev.* **2011**, *87*, 577–580. [CrossRef] [PubMed]
41. Zachariassen, G.; Fenger-Gron, J.; Hviid, M.V.; Halken, S. The content of macronutrients in milk from mothers of very preterm infants is highly variable. *Dan. Med. J.* **2013**, *60*, A4631.
42. Henriksen, C.; Westerberg, A.C.; Rønnestad, A.; Nakstad, B.; Veierød, M.B.; Drevon, C.A.; Iversen, P.O. Growth and nutrient intake among very-low-birth-weight infants fed fortified human milk during hospitalisation. *Br. J. Nutr.* **2009**, *102*, 1179–1186. [CrossRef]

43. Rochow, N.; Fusch, G.; Ali, A.; Bhatia, A.; So, H.Y.; Iskander, R.; Chessell, L.; El Helou, S.; Fusch, C. Individualized target fortification of breast milk with protein, carbohydrates, and fat for preterm infants: A double-blind randomized controlled trial. *Clin. Nutr.* **2021**, *40*, 54–63. [CrossRef]
44. Ramey, S.R.; Merlino Barr, S.; Moore, K.A.; Groh-Wargo, S. Exploring innovations in human milk analysis in the neonatal intensive care unit: A survey of the United States. *Front. Nutr.* **2021**, *8*, 692600. [CrossRef] [PubMed]
45. Hair, A.B.; Blanco, C.L.; Moreira, A.G.; Hawthorne, K.M.; Lee, M.L.; Rechtman, D.J.; Abrams, S.A. Randomized trial of human milk cream as a supplement to standard fortification of an exclusive human milk-based diet in infants 750–1250 g birth weight. *J. Pediatr.* **2014**, *165*, 915–920. [CrossRef] [PubMed]
46. Morlacchi, L.; Mallardi, D.; Giannì, M.L.; Roggero, P.; Amato, O.; Piemontese, P.; Consonni, D.; Mosca, F. Is targeted fortification of human breast milk an optimal nutrition strategy for preterm infants? an interventional study. *J. Transl. Med.* **2016**, *14*, 195. [CrossRef]
47. Salas, A.A.; Jerome, M.; Finck, A.; Razzaghy, J.; Chandler-Laney, P.; Carlo, W.A. Body composition of extremely preterm infants fed protein-enriched, fortified milk: A randomized trial. *Pediatr. Res.* **2021**, 1–7. [CrossRef]
48. Agakidou, E.; Karagiozoglou-Lampoudi, T.; Parlapani, E.; Fletouris, D.J.; Sarafidis, K.; Tzimouli, V.; Diamanti, E.; Agakidis, C. Modifications of own mothers' milk fortification protocol affect early plasma IGF-I and ghrelin levels in preterm infants. A randomized clinical trial. *Nutrients* **2019**, *11*, 3056. [CrossRef]
49. McLeod, G.; Sherriff, J.; Hartmann, P.E.; Nathan, E.; Geddes, D.; Simmer, K. Comparing different methods of human breast milk fortification using measured v. assumed macronutrient composition to target reference growth: A randomised controlled trial. *Br. J. Nutr.* **2016**, *115*, 431–439. [CrossRef]
50. Rochow, N.; Fusch, G.; Zapanta, B.; Ali, A.; Barui, S.; Fusch, C. Target fortification of breast milk: How often should milk analysis be done? *Nutrients* **2015**, *7*, 2297–2310. [CrossRef]
51. Alan, S.; Atasay, B.; Cakir, U.; Yildiz, D.; Kilic, A.; Kahvecioglu, D.; Erdeve, O.; Arsan, S. An intention to achieve better postnatal in-hospital-growth for preterm infants: Adjustable protein fortification of human milk. *Early Hum. Dev.* **2013**, *89*, 1017–1023. [CrossRef] [PubMed]
52. Ergenekon, E.; Soysal, Ş.; Hirfanoğlu, İ.; Baş, V.; Gücüyener, K.; Turan, Ö.; Beken, S.; Kazancı, E.; Türkyılmaz, C.; Önal, E.; et al. Short- and long-term effects of individualized enteral protein supplementation in preterm newborns. *Turk. J. Pediatr.* **2013**, *55*, 365–370. [PubMed]
53. Picaud, J.C.; Houeto, N.; Buffin, R.; Loys, C.M.; Godbert, I.; Haÿs, S. Additional protein fortification is necessary in extremely low-birth-weight infants fed human milk. *J. Pediatr. Gastroenterol. Nutr.* **2016**, *63*, 103–105. [CrossRef]
54. Biasini, A.; Monti, F.; Laguardia, M.C.; Stella, M.; Marvulli, L.; Neri, E. High protein intake in human/maternal milk fortification for ≤1250 gr infants: Intrahospital growth and neurodevelopmental outcome at two years. *Acta Biomed.* **2018**, *88*, 470–476. [CrossRef]
55. Mariani, E.; Biasini, A.; Marvulli, L.; Martini, S.; Aceti, A.; Faldella, G.; Corvaglia, L.; Sansavini, A.; Savini, S.; Agostini, F.; et al. Strategies of increased protein intake in ELBW infants fed by human milk lead to long term benefits. *Front. Public Health* **2018**, *6*, 272. [CrossRef] [PubMed]
56. Arslanoglu, S.; Moro, G.E.; Ziegler, E.E. Adjustable fortification of human milk fed to preterm infants: Does it make a difference? *J. Perinatol.* **2006**, *26*, 614–621. [CrossRef]
57. Mathes, M.; Maas, C.; Bleeker, C.; Vek, J.; Bernhard, W.; Peter, A.; Poets, C.F.; Franz, A.R. Effect of increased enteral protein intake on plasma and urinary urea concentrations in preterm infants born at <32 weeks gestation and <1500 g birth weight enrolled in a randomized controlled trial—A secondary analysis. *BMC Pediatr.* **2018**, *18*, 154. [CrossRef] [PubMed]
58. Quan, M.; Wang, D.; Gou, L.; Sun, Z.; Ma, J.; Zhang, L.; Wang, C.; Schibler, K.; Li, Z. Individualized human milk fortification to improve the growth of hospitalized preterm infants. *Nutr. Clin. Pract.* **2020**, *35*, 680–688. [CrossRef]
59. Brown, J.V.; Embleton, N.D.; Harding, J.E.; McGuire, W. Multi-nutrient fortification of human milk for preterm infants. *Cochrane Database Syst. Rev.* **2016**. [CrossRef]
60. Mukhopadhyay, K.; Narnag, A.; Mahajan, R. Effect of human milk fortification in appropriate for gestation and small for gestation preterm babies: A randomized controlled trial. *Indian Pediatr.* **2007**, *44*, 286–290.
61. North, K.; Marx Delaney, M.; Bose, C.; Lee, A.C.C.; Vesel, L.; Adair, L.; Semrau, K. The effect of milk type and fortification on the growth of low-birthweight infants: An umbrella review of systematic reviews and meta-analyses. *Matern. Child. Nutr.* **2021**, *17*, e13176. [CrossRef]
62. Fleig, L.; Hagan, J.; Lee, M.L.; Abrams, S.A.; Hawthorne, K.M.; Hair, A.B. Growth outcomes of small for gestational age preterm infants before and after implementation of an exclusive human milk-based diet. *J. Perinatol.* **2021**, *41*, 1859–1864. [CrossRef]
63. Ananthan, A.; Balasubramanian, H.; Rao, S.; Patole, S. Human milk-derived fortifiers compared with bovine milk-derived fortifiers in preterm infants: A systematic review and meta-analysis. *Adv. Nutr.* **2020**, *11*, 1325–1333. [CrossRef]
64. O'Connor, D.L.; Kiss, A.; Tomlinson, C.; Bando, N.; Bayliss, A.; Campbell, D.M.; Daneman, A.; Francis, J.; Kotsopoulos, K.; Shah, P.S.; et al. Nutrient enrichment of human milk with human and bovine milk-based fortifiers for infants born weighing <1250 g: A randomized clinical trial. *Am. J. Clin. Nutr.* **2018**, *108*, 108–116. [CrossRef]
65. Huston, R.K.; Markell, A.M.; McCulley, E.A.; Gardiner, S.K.; Sweeney, S.L. Improving growth for infants ≤1250 grams receiving an exclusive human milk diet. *Nutr. Clin. Pract.* **2018**, *33*, 671–678. [CrossRef]

66. Sullivan, S.; Schanler, R.J.; Kim, J.H.; Patel, A.L.; Trawöger, R.; Kiechl-Kohlendorfer, U.; Chan, G.M.; Blanco, C.L.; Abrams, S.; Cotton, C.M.; et al. An exclusively human milk-based diet is associated with a lower rate of necrotizing enterocolitis than a diet of human milk and bovine milk-based products. *J. Pediatr.* **2010**, *156*, 562–567.e1. [CrossRef]
67. Shah, S.D.; Dereddy, N.; Jones, T.L.; Dhanireddy, R.; Talati, A.J. Early versus delayed human milk fortification in very low birth weight infants-A randomized controlled trial. *J. Pediatr.* **2016**, *174*, 126–131. [CrossRef]
68. Alizadeh Taheri, P.; Sajjadian, N.; Asgharyan Fargi, M.; Shariat, M. Is early breast milk fortification more effective in preterm infants: A clinical trial. *J. Perinat. Med.* **2017**, *45*, 953–957. [CrossRef] [PubMed]
69. Aimone, A.; Rovet, J.; Ward, W.; Jefferies, A.; Campbell, D.M.; Asztalos, E.; Feldman, M.; Vaughan, J.; Westall, C.; Whyte, H.; et al. Growth and body composition of human milk-fed premature infants provided with extra energy and nutrients early after hospital discharge: 1-year follow-up. *J. Pediatr. Gastroenterol. Nutr.* **2009**, *49*, 456–466. [CrossRef] [PubMed]
70. Marino, L.V.; Fudge, C.; Pearson, F.; Johnson, M.J. Home use of breast milk fortifier to promote postdischarge growth and breast feeding in preterm infants: A quality improvement project. *Arch. Dis. Child* **2019**, *104*, 1007–1012. [CrossRef]
71. Zachariassen, G.; Faerk, J.; Grytter, C.; Esberg, B.H.; Hjelmborg, J.; Mortensen, S.; Thybo Christesen, H.; Halken, S. Nutrient enrichment of mother's milk and growth of very preterm infants after hospital discharge. *Pediatrics* **2011**, *127*, e995–e1003. [CrossRef] [PubMed]
72. Fabrizio, V.; Trzaski, J.M.; Brownell, E.A.; Esposito, P.; Lainwala, S.; Lussier, M.M.; Hagadorn, J.I. Individualized versus standard diet fortification for growth and development in preterm infants receiving human milk. *Cochrane Database Syst. Rev.* **2020**, *11*, CD013465. [CrossRef]
73. Bulut, Ö.; Çoban, A.; İnce, Z. Macronutrient analysis of preterm human milk using mid-infrared spectrophotometry. *J. Perinat. Med.* **2019**, *47*, 785–791. [CrossRef]
74. Kadıoğlu Şimşek, G.; Alyamaç Dizdar, E.; Arayıcı, S.; Canpolat, F.E.; Sarı, F.N.; Uraş, N.; Oguz, S.S. Comparison of the effect of three different fortification methods on growth of very low birth weight infants. *Breastfeed. Med.* **2019**, *14*, 63–68. [CrossRef]
75. Lucas, A.; Fewtrell, M.S.; Morley, R.; Lucas, P.J.; Baker, B.A.; Lister, G.; Bishop, N.J. Randomized outcome trial of human milk fortification and developmental outcome in preterm infants. *Am. J. Clin. Nutr.* **1996**, *64*, 142–151. [CrossRef] [PubMed]
76. Kashaki, M.; Samghabadi, F.M.; Bordbar, A. Effect of fortification of breast milk in conjugation with protein supplement on neurodevelopment of preterm low birth weight infants at 3 years. *Med. Arch.* **2019**, *73*, 344–350. [CrossRef]
77. Hopperton, K.E.; O'Connor, D.L.; Bando, N.; Conway, A.M.; Ng, D.V.; Kiss, A.; Jackson, J.; Ly, L.; OptiMoMFeeding Group Unger, S.L. Nutrient enrichment of human milk with human and bovine milk-based fortifiers for infants born <1250 g: 18-month neurodevelopmental follow-up of a randomized clinical trial. *Curr. Dev. Nutr.* **2019**, *3*, nzz129. [CrossRef] [PubMed]
78. Carome, K.; Rahman, A.; Parvez, B. Exclusive human milk diet reduces incidence of severe intraventricular hemorrhage in extremely low birth weight infants. *J. Perinatol.* **2021**, *41*, 535–543. [CrossRef] [PubMed]
79. Colacci, M.; Murthy, K.; DeRegnier, R.O.; Khan, J.Y.; Robinson, D.T. Growth and development in extremely low birth weight infants after the introduction of exclusive human milk feedings. *Am. J. Perinatol.* **2017**, *34*, 130–137. [CrossRef]
80. O'Connor, D.L.; Weishuhn, K.; Rovet, J.; Mirabella, G.; Jefferies, A.; Campbell, D.M.; Asztalos, E.; Feldman, M.; Whyte, H.; Westall, C. Visual development of human milk-fed preterm infants provided with extra energy and nutrients after hospital discharge. *JPEN J. Parenter. Enter. Nutr.* **2012**, *36*, 349–353. [CrossRef]
81. da Cunha, R.D.; Lamy Filho, F.; Rafael, E.V.; Lamy, Z.C.; de Queiroz, A.L. Breast milk supplementation and preterm infant development after hospital discharge: A randomized clinical trial. *J. Pediatr (Rio J).* **2016**, *92*, 136–142. [CrossRef]
82. Griffiths, L.J.; Tate, A.R.; Dezateux, C. Millennium Cohort Study Child Health Group. Do early infant feeding practices vary by maternal ethnic group? *Public Health Nutr.* **2007**, *10*, 957–964. [CrossRef]
83. Ottolini, K.M.; Andescavage, A.; Kapse, K.; Jacobs, M.; Limperopoulos, C. Improved brain growth and microstructural development in breast milk-fed very low birth weight premature infants. *Acta Paediatr.* **2020**, *109*, 580–1587. [CrossRef] [PubMed]
84. Ottolini, K.M.; Andescavage, N.; Kapse, K.; Jacobs, M.; Murnick, J.; VanderVeer, R.; Basu, S.; Said, M.; Limperopoulos, C. Early lipid intake improves cerebellar growth in very-low-birth-weight preterm infants. *J. Parenter. Enter. Nutr.* **2021**, *45*, 587–595. [CrossRef] [PubMed]

MDPI
St. Alban-Anlage 66
4052 Basel
Switzerland
Tel. +41 61 683 77 34
Fax +41 61 302 89 18
www.mdpi.com

Nutrients Editorial Office
E-mail: nutrients@mdpi.com
www.mdpi.com/journal/nutrients

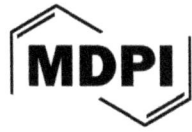